Plague and Empire in the Early Modern Mediterranean World
The Ottoman Experience, 1347–1600

This is the first systematic scholarly study of the Ottoman experience of plague during the Black Death pandemic and the centuries that followed. Using a wealth of archival and narrative sources, including medical treatises, hagiographies, and travelers' accounts, as well as recent scientific research, Nükhet Varlık demonstrates how plague interacted with the environmental, social, and political structures of the Ottoman Empire from the late medieval through the early modern era. The book argues that the empire's growth transformed the epidemiological patterns of plague by bringing diverse ecological zones into interaction and by intensifying the mobilities of exchange among both human and nonhuman agents. Varlık maintains that persistent plagues elicited new forms of cultural imagination and expression as well as a new body of knowledge about the disease. In turn, this new consciousness sharpened the Ottoman administrative response to the plague, while contributing to the makings of an early modern state.

Nükhet Varlık is Assistant Professor of History at Rutgers University–Newark. She is the author of several articles and is currently editing a collection of essays titled *Plague and Contagion in the Islamic Mediterranean*. She is the recipient of an NEH Fellowship by the American Research Institute in Turkey, a Senior Fellowship from Koç University's Research Center for Anatolian Civilizations, and a Turkish Cultural Foundation Post-Doctoral Fellowship.

Plague and Empire in the Early Modern Mediterranean World

The Ottoman Experience, 1347–1600

NÜKHET VARLIK

Rutgers University–Newark

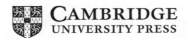

CAMBRIDGE
UNIVERSITY PRESS

University Printing House, Cambridge CB2 8BS, United Kingdom

One Liberty Plaza, 20th Floor, New York, NY 10006, USA

477 Williamstown Road, Port Melbourne, VIC 3207, Australia

4843/24, 2nd Floor, Ansari Road, Daryaganj, Delhi - 110002, India

79 Anson Road, #06-04/06, Singapore 079906

Cambridge University Press is part of the University of Cambridge.

It furthers the University's mission by disseminating knowledge in the pursuit of
education, learning and research at the highest international levels of excellence.

www.cambridge.org
Information on this title: www.cambridge.org/9781108412773

© Nükhet Varlık 2015

First published 2015
First paperback edition 2017

A catalogue record for this publication is available from the British Library

Library of Congress Cataloging in Publication data
Varlık, Nükhet.
Plague and empire in the early modern Mediterranean world : the Ottoman experience,
1347–1600 / Nükhet Varlık (Rutgers University–Newark).
pages cm
Includes bibliographical references and index.
ISBN 978-1-107-01338-4 (hardback)
1. Plague – Turkey – Epidemiology – History.   2. Black Death – Turkey – History.
3. Plague – Environmental aspects – Turkey – History.   4. Plague – Social
aspects – Turkey – History.   5. Plague – Political aspects – Turkey – History.
6. Imperialism – Social aspects – Turkey – History.   7. Turkey – History –
Ottoman Empire, 1288–1918.   8. Turkey – Environmental conditions –
History.   I. Title.
RC179.T9V37   2016
614.5′73209561–dc23   2015006206

ISBN 978-1-107-01338-4 Hardback
ISBN 978-1-108-41277-3 Paperback

To Ben, with love and gratitude

Contents

Figures, Maps, and Tables

Figures

Maps

Tables

Acknowledgments

This book is the result of my fascination with plague – a fascination that took me on a long and winding journey in life – but I first caught the "germs" at Boğaziçi University in Istanbul, and they gradually incubated and amplified at the University of Chicago; finally, the infection ran its course at Rutgers University. Along the twists and turns of the journey, I crossed paths with many people, who each in his or her special way left behind a mark on this project; their signatures are hidden in the pages of this book. I am deeply grateful to every one of those people with whom I exchanged ideas and shared long hours of discussion, frustration, and hope. This book would simply not have been brought to completion if it were not for the inspiration, support, and assistance I received from these individuals.

Going back in time to the first "seeds of disease" planted in my mind and the people who nurtured this curiosity, I would like to acknowledge the faculty in the Department of History at Boğaziçi University in Istanbul, in particular Nevra Necipoğlu, Edhem Eldem, Selim Deringil, Selçuk Esenbel, Tony Greenwood, Günay Kut, and Halil Berktay (now at Sabancı University). I would also like to acknowledge the support and encouragement I received from Nil Sarı, of Istanbul University, and Ekmeleddin İhsanoğlu, formerly of the Research Center of Islamic History, Art, and Culture (IRCICA) in Istanbul.

Chicago became a second home after Istanbul. Beyond all, I am deeply grateful to Cornell Fleischer of the University of Chicago, who first saw merit in my project, welcomed me as a graduate student, and offered thorough training in Ottoman history, culture, and language. He was the one who unlocked the doors to a new cultural landscape and made me believe that I could venture into writing the history of Ottoman plagues. I thank him for his unwavering support, encouragement, and guidance and, most importantly, for being a model to emulate. As a graduate student at the University of Chicago, I had the privilege of working with Robert Dankoff,

Fred Donner, Adrian Johns, Holly Shissler, and the late Farouk Mustafa. I remain grateful for everything I have learned from them.

In more recent years, I have been blessed with the support, guidance, and encouragement of scholars who transformed my perception and understanding of past plagues. Ann Carmichael of Indiana University has been an invaluable mentor, guide, and friend in this journey. I thank her from the bottom of my heart for guiding me through the difficulties of writing in moments of self-doubt and for ever-rejuvenating my passion for plague. It was thanks to her that I discovered a larger community of scholars who shared a similar passion for the subject. I am truly grateful to Monica Green, for she has transformed my thinking about plague by opening my horizons to the world of research in other disciplines, especially the new plague science. With her inexhaustible energy, dedication, and resourcefulness, she continues to be an inspiration. I would also like to acknowledge Michelle Ziegler and the other members of the plague working group, which has been an invaluable resource for keeping each of us informed and updated about new research in the field. I have benefited from these conversations in numerous ways.

I would like to acknowledge the support and encouragement I have received from my colleagues formerly in the Department of History at James Madison University and currently in the Federated Department of History at Rutgers University–Newark and NJIT. Rutgers has been a home away from home, and my colleagues have been enormously supportive in every possible way. I am honored and humbled to have such colleagues, and I thank every single one of them. At Rutgers, I would also like to thank Tuna Artun, Nahyan Fancy (of DePauw University), and the RCHA "Networks of Exchange" seminar colleagues, in particular Toby Jones and James Delbourgo. The friendship of Zeynep Çelik at Rutgers has been like a breath of fresh air. I thank her for being a relentless source of support and guidance every step of the way.

Several institutions have been instrumental in supporting me as I researched and wrote this book. I am grateful for the financial support provided by the American Research Institute in Turkey (ARIT)–National Endowment for the Humanities (NEH) Advanced Research Fellowship; Koç University's Research Center for Anatolian Civilizations (RCAC) Senior Fellowship; and a Turkish Cultural Foundation Post-Doctoral Fellowship during the academic year 2010–11, which I spent in Istanbul. I am also grateful for research support provided by Rutgers University–Newark FASN and the Rutgers Center for Historical Analysis Faculty Fellowship in 2012–13.

I conducted research for this book in several libraries and archives across two continents. I thank the librarians and archivists of Koç University's RCAC, IRCICA, İslam Araştırmaları Merkezi (İSAM), the Department of Medical Ethics and History of Medicine at Istanbul University Cerrahpaşa Medical School, Atatürk Library, Bayezid Library, Süleymaniye Library, the

Topkapı Palace Museum Archives, the Prime Ministry Ottoman Archives in Istanbul, the Joseph Regenstein Library in Chicago (especially Basima Bezirgan and Marlis Saleh of the Middle East Collection), and, last but not least, the John Cotton Dana Library and its interlibrary loan staff. I would like to thank Esra Müyesseroğlu and Sevgi Ağca from the Topkapı Palace Museum and Lauren Jones from the Orientalist Museum, Doha for their help with publication permits.

I have had the privilege of presenting earlier versions of this work and benefiting from the feedback of colleagues at various institutions. I thank them for commenting on my work in progress, offering suggestions, and sharing insights. Among these, I would like to mention in particular John Brooke, Snjezana Buzov, and Carter Findley of Ohio State University; Scott Redford of Koç University–RCAC, Stefan Leder of Orient-Institut Beirut, Asa Eger of the University of North Carolina–Greensboro; the faculty at the Department of Medical History and Ethics at Istanbul University Cerrahpaşa Medical School; and Tolga Esmer and Tijana Krstić of Central European University. Over the many years of research and writing, several colleagues helped with research, shared sources, and answered questions about various issues. I would like to mention Zahit Atcıl, Günhan Börekçi, Rainer Brömer, John Curry, Canan Çakırlar, Semavi Eyice, Christopher Markiewicz, Miri Shefer-Mossensohn, Uli Schamiloglu, Justin Stearns, Kahraman Şakul, and Tunç Şen. I am grateful for the assistance of Israa Alhassani of James Madison University, Burçak Özlüdil Altın of NJIT, William Kynan-Wilson, and Erkan Karakoyun at various stages of the preparation of this book. I would like to thank Marigold Acland, who oversaw the first stages of this project; my editor, William Hammell; Sarika Narula and Kate Gavino; and the anonymous reviewers from Cambridge University Press.

I have also enjoyed the friendship of many kindred spirits who shared ideas, offered every imaginable type of help, and, most importantly, made the journey meaningful and enjoyable. I thank Mehmetcan Akpınar, Betül İpşirli Argıt, Abdurrahman Atcıl, Buket Kitapçı Bayrı, Betül Başaran, Peter Bondarenko, Lale Can, Esin Eğit, Pınar Emiralioğlu, Side Emre, Mayte Green, Kelda Jamison, Aslı Niyazioğlu, Ertuğrul Ökten, Ayşe Polat, Kaya Şahin, Kabir Tambar, Ece Turnator, Gökben Uluderya, Patrick Wing, Bike Yazıcıoğlu, Sara Nur Yıldız, and Betül Yılmaz. My thanks also go to my students, especially those in my recent Black Death seminar at Rutgers, for sharing my fascination with plague and resisting, against all bids, to call me Dr. Morbid.

Last but not least, I would like to mention the members of my family across two continents: my mother-in-law, Karen Hutchens; my brother, Aşkın Varlık, and his family; my parents, Nermin and İmdat Varlık; and my beloved children, Alanur and Evan Arda. I cannot thank them enough for their love, unwavering support, and help in every possible way. Benjamin Hutchens, my husband, love, and friend, has been absolutely the greatest source of support through this journey. I thank him for listening to me tirelessly even when the conversation was mostly about rats, fleas, and bacteria; for reading countless drafts of this work; and for making suggestions and comments, thus saving me from many embarrassing mistakes, not only thanks to his sound reasoning skills as a philosopher but also as a fervent student of history. To dedicate this book to him is the least I can do in the way of thanking him.

Abbreviations

Albèri	Eugenio Albèri, ed., *Relazioni degli Ambasciatori Veneti al Senato*, Series III, 3 vols. (Florence: Società editrice fiorentina, 1840–55)
BOA	Başbakanlık Osmanlı Arşivi (Prime Ministry Ottoman Archives), Istanbul
*EI*²	*Encyclopaedia of Islam 2*, electronic edition
IJMES	*International Journal of Middle East Studies*
IRCICA	Research Centre for Islamic History, Art, and Culture, Istanbul
JESHO	*Journal of the Economic and Social History of the Orient*
JHMAS	*Journal of the History of Medicine and Allied Sciences*
KK	Kamil Kepeci
MD	Mühimme Defteri
OS	Coşkun Yılmaz and Necdet Yılmaz, ed., *Osmanlılarda Sağlık*, 2 vols. (Istanbul: Biofarma, 2006)
PLoS	*Public Library of Science*
PNAS	*Proceedings of the National Academy of Sciences*
Sanudo	Marino Sanudo, *I diarii di Marino Sanuto (MCCCCXCVI–MDXXXIII) dall' autografo Marciano ital. cl. VII codd. CDXIX–CDLXXVII*, 58 vols. (Venice: F. Visentini, 1879–1903)
TDVİA	*Türkiye Diyanet Vakfı İslam Ansiklopedisi*, electronic edition
TSMA	Topkapı Sarayı Müzesi Arşivi, Istanbul (Topkapı Palace Museum Archives)
TTK	Türk Tarih Kurumu
WHO	World Health Organization

Note on Transliteration and Dates

To make reading easier for the nonspecialist, I have followed an eclectic and practical approach to transliteration. I have simplified book titles and personal names in Ottoman Turkish by following modern Turkish orthography and omitting diacritical marks as much as possible. Place-names, if within the boundaries of modern Turkey, are given in modern Turkish forms. For example, I have used "Trabzon" but not "Trebizond," with the exception of place-names that are well known in Anglicized form, for example, "Gallipoli" but not "Gelibolu." If outside Turkey, then modern English place-names are adopted, followed by the Ottoman Turkish name in parentheses the first time a place is mentioned in the text. For example, I have used "Rhodes" instead of "Rodos." When using terms pertaining to the Islamicate culture that are already established in modern English, I have preferred Anglicized forms over Turkicized versions. For this reason, I have used "ulama" instead of "*ulema*," "hadith" instead of "*hadis*," "waqf" instead of "*vakıf*," and so on. For other such terms where an Anglicized form is not used commonly, the Turkicized version has been used, without transliteration, for example, "*taun*" or "*askeri*." Names and book titles in Arabic and Persian in the text follow a simplified version of the *IJMES* transliteration system. Full transliteration is given in the bibliography. Long vowel markers have been omitted as much as possible. Unless otherwise noted, all translations are mine.

For Turkish pronunciation, the readers are kindly referred to the following guidelines prepared by Erika H. Gilson: www.princeton.edu/~ehgilson/alpha.html.

Dates in the main text are given in the Common Era. In the notes, documents from the Ottoman archives are given in the original Hijri date followed by the Common Era date. Conversion of Hijri dates to the Gregorian calendar follows the conversion software of Tarih Çevirme Kılavuzu, offered online at http://193.255.138.2/takvim.asp.

I have used the Hijri months in the following forms:

Muharrem
Safer
Rebiülevvel
Rebiülahir
Cemaziyelevvel
Cemaziyelahir
Receb
Şaban
Ramazan
Şevval
Zilkade
Zilhicce

Introduction

This book could not have been written ten years ago – at least with the confidence we have today – without the recent spectacular new leap in plague scholarship that has transformed both humanistic and scientific research. Research in molecular archeology, and genetics in particular, has made remarkable achievements by extracting and analyzing ancient DNA (aDNA) and mapping out the phylogenetic (evolutionary) history of *Yersinia pestis* (the pathogen that causes the plague). In 2011, this research culminated in the reconstruction of the full genome of *Y. pestis* entirely from fourteenth-century human remains. The implications of this endeavor are truly revolutionary. For plague historians in particular, this heralds liberation from decades-long reticence that dominated their field of scholarship: students of past epidemics were methodologically restrained and cautioned against the pitfalls of retrospective diagnosis, using a disease category drawn from modern microbiological knowledge and applying it anachronistically to a past where that knowledge did not exist. Today, recognizing the significance of what science has to offer, the student of past plagues can integrate nonwritten evidence into historical analysis with great confidence.

Presently, there is international scholarly consensus that the three historical pandemics that were believed to have been *Y. pestis*–caused plague were indeed so: the First Pandemic, known as the Justinianic Plague (541 to circa 750); the Second Pandemic, known as the Black Death (1346–53), and its recurrent waves, which continued for centuries after the initial outbreak; and the Third Pandemic, which spread globally after its eruption in Hong Kong in 1894.[1] This book is concerned with perhaps the most controversial,

---

[1] For the conventionally accepted periodization of historical pandemics of plague, see Lester K. Little, "Plague Historians in Lab Coats," *Past and Present* 213, no. 1 (2011): 270–71. For the Eurocentrism of this periodization and why the Ottoman experience of plague complicates it, see Nükhet Varlık, "New Science and Old Sources: Why the Ottoman Experience of Plague Matters," *The Medieval Globe* 1 (2014): 193–227. For the scholarly consensus and

the Second Pandemic. Although the new scientific research will transform what is already a monumental scholarship devoted to the Second Pandemic, there are certain historiographical caveats that one must bear in mind.

First of all, Europe has been the primary benefactor of Black Death studies and thus continues to hold a privileged position in the scholarship compared to other parts of the world that may have been at least as badly affected by it, if not more gravely. For example, our current knowledge about how various parts of Asia, the Middle East, and Africa were affected by the pandemic is at best fragmentary and disconnected. Even though fine historical studies have examined the plague experience of these areas, these are difficult to bring together owing to their temporal and spatial breadth of coverage.

Second, a substantial portion of the available plague scholarship is devoted to the initial outbreak of the mid-fourteenth-century Black Death and its consequences, at the expense of the recurrent outbreaks of the Second Pandemic that continued for several centuries. Although some exemplary studies are exceptions to this general trend, the privileged position of the Black Death itself in the scholarship is undeniable. This emphasis may feed into a distorted historical perception of post–Black Death epidemics. Bearing in mind the many waves of plague that continued after the dreadful but brief episode of the Black Death, it becomes all the more evident that the recurrent waves of the Second Pandemic are underrepresented in the scholarship.

Third, and perhaps stemming from this underrepresentation in the scholarship, how and why plague persisted for such a long time during the Second Pandemic has hitherto gone largely unexplored.[2] Focusing on the European case, the scholarship has often considered the Great Plague of London in 1665 or the Plague of Marseille in 1720-21 as the end of the pandemic and produced discussions of the "disappearance" of plague. However, it is well known that outbreaks of plague continued in Russia in the 1770s and in the areas controlled by the Ottoman Empire well into the nineteenth century. These cases beg for a reconsideration of the Second Pandemic's chronological and geographical framing, the historical conditions that helped sustain it, and its effects in areas outside of Europe.

Fourth, as far as the broader Mediterranean world is concerned, the traditional scholarship seems to suffer from assumptions of differences between Christian and Muslim (or Oriental and Occidental) societies with respect to their experiences of plague. Even in studies that aim to offer a unified

---

its implications for the plague historiography, see Monica H. Green, "Editor's Introduction to *Pandemic Disease in the Medieval World: Rethinking the Black Death*," *The Medieval Globe* 1 (2014): 9–26.

[2] Ann G. Carmichael's recent work pioneers this change in the scholarship. See Carmichael, "Plague Persistence in Western Europe: A Hypothesis," *The Medieval Globe* 1 (2014): 157–91.

Mediterranean vision, these divisions play an important role in explaining the very differences in the spread of plague and the responses it stirred.[3] These dichotomies not only bind the scholarly analyses to reductionist perceptions of past societies but also produce a rather thin sense of the historicity of plague epidemics and the means through which they were experienced in the Mediterranean world. In fact, there is compelling evidence in support of the Mediterranean as a unified disease zone, with shared epidemiological experiences, as well as a common heritage of medical traditions.[4] To achieve a more connected understanding of the historical epidemiology of the Mediterranean world, it is imperative to study the plague experiences of those regions that are assumed to be essentially different from Europe. This book aims to contribute to a connected vision of the post–Black Death Mediterranean by integrating the Ottoman experience into the historical narrative. In these pages, we carefully position the Ottoman case on the dissection table, with a view to identifying the major nodes that were attacked by persistent outbreaks of plague, tracing the main arteries that enabled the circulation of infection and the overall responses of its people in the face of these epidemic invasions. The goal is to make it clear to the reader that the Ottoman experience of plague is not only eminently comparable to other such historical experiences but also indispensable for a better understanding of the post–Black Death Mediterranean plagues.

Fifth, and in conjunction with the previous points, the present state of the scholarship does not afford a proper understanding of the Ottoman experience of plague during the Second Pandemic. The only extensive scholarly monograph on the history of plague in the Ottoman Empire covers the years between 1700 and 1850.[5] As such, the emphasis on the later centuries of the empire's history may obscure the nature of the Ottoman experience of plague in the late medieval and early modern eras. This may especially be misleading because it seems to reproduce a historical narrative that heavily draws from a nineteenth-century Eurocentric vision of the Ottoman society and projects this vision to earlier eras. According to this narrative, the Ottoman Empire, as the "sick man of Europe," came to represent a plague exporter, the home of all plagues that assailed Europe's shores. With this in view, Europe strove to protect itself by implementing quarantine measures and establishing cordons sanitaires. But how is it that the Ottoman Empire is understood to be the primary plague exporter to Europe when the Ottomans' own experience of plague still remains unknown in the scholarship: when

---

3 See, e.g., Jean-Noël Biraben, *Les hommes et la peste en France et dans les pays européens et méditerranéens* (Paris: Mouton, 1975).

4 Emmanuel Le Roy Ladurie, "Un concept: l'unification microbienne du monde (XIVe-XVIIe siècles)," *Revue Suisse d'Histoire* 23, no. 4 (1973): 627–96.

5 See Daniel Panzac, *La peste dans l'empire ottoman, 1700–1850* (Leuven: Peeters, 1985). For a more detailed discussion of the scholarship on Ottoman plagues, see Chapter 2.

and how did it arrive in the Ottoman world, how did it circulate there, how did its people perceive it, and what, if anything, did the administration of the empire do about it? Curiously, whereas scholars interested in the European experience of plague are satisfied with the conclusion that plague came from the Ottoman Empire and have little or no interest in how it originated there, the historians of the Ottoman Empire rarely assign much importance to the role of plague in the empire's history. Scholars working outside the field of Ottoman studies cannot be expected to interest themselves in plague in the Empire if the Ottomanist scholarship does not produce the research that would assist them in doing so. And yet the plague in the Ottoman-ruled areas before the eighteenth century has remained largely unexplored. Was there no plague in the empire before 1700 worth being the subject of a scholarly monograph? Surely there was, as allegedly all European plagues originated there, but silence prevails.

The reasons for the silence in the Ottomanist scholarship can barely be accounted for by the depiction of the Ottoman Empire in this particular manner. Rather, there is a complex web of historical and historiographical reasons why this subject remains a bête noire in this field of scholarship, especially for the first centuries of Ottoman history, as is discussed at length in these pages. However, suffice it to say here that despite the recent flurry of interest in the subject, there exists no systematic study of the geographical and chronological scope of plague epidemics that affected the Ottoman lands before the eighteenth century, let alone an exploration of the nature of the specific diseases involved in them; their social, economic, demographic, and other such effects on Ottoman society; or the Ottoman perceptions of (and responses to) this phenomenon. Indeed, these have hitherto remained largely unexplored in the Ottomanist historiography.

In view of these limitations in the scholarship, this book takes upon itself the twofold task of demonstrating that Ottomanist literature should take plague more seriously and that studies of historical epidemiology should grant the Ottoman experience its due consideration. For doing so, on one hand, we seek to answer the question of why the Ottoman experience matters for an understanding of the post–Black Death Mediterranean plagues. On the other hand, we deal with the question of why plague matters for an understanding of Ottoman history. By addressing these questions, this book seeks to demonstrate that the histories of plague in the Mediterranean world and that of the Ottoman Empire should be considered in conjunction with each other.

Plague and Empire

In the following pages, I argue that the growth of the Ottoman Empire and the expansion of plague epidemics are intimately entwined. With a view to demonstrating this entwinement, this book reconstructs a historical narrative of plagues that affected Ottoman-controlled areas from the Black Death to the end of the sixteenth century (1347–1600), traces their trajectories and recurrence, and establishes their links to the patterns of growth and consolidation of the Ottoman power, with a special emphasis on conquest, urbanization, and networks of exchange.

Why this chronological frame? It should be noted at the outset that the selection of this time frame has been a conscious one. The study of this two-and-a-half-century-long period is critical for demonstrating the intimate relationship of plague and empire: not least because this era coincides with both the expansion of the Ottoman power and that of the plague, but more importantly because this is when the basic trajectories of dissemination of the epidemics took shape. This is especially true for what is referred to in this book as the long sixteenth century, that is, from the conquest of Constantinople to the end of the sixteenth century. Plague outbreaks gradually became more frequent and widespread in Ottoman cities during this era; hence, tracing the spatial distribution and periodicity of plagues of the long sixteenth century promises to afford a better understanding of plagues of the post-1600 period. Moreover, this is also when we see a critical change in the Ottoman perceptions of (and responses to) plagues, which may help explain the developments that followed in the seventeenth and eighteenth centuries.

At this point, it may be useful to remember the observation made by a great historian of medicine about two decades ago. In his colossal book *The Greatest Benefit to Mankind*, the late Roy Porter pointed out that empires, like trade and wars, triggered the spread of epidemic diseases.[6] Even though Porter had the early modern Spanish example in mind, his insightful comment still holds true for other empires in that era. As a matter of fact, empires and plagues have often been mentioned in conjunction with each other in historical scholarship. One does not fall short of finding examples of "great plagues" in the "great empires" of history. It is interesting to note, however, that plagues more readily conjure up associations with the "fall" of empires.[7] Regardless, the relationship between the two historical phenomena remains insufficiently explored. Instead, there seems to be a stronger inclination to associate pandemics with historical phenomena that had effects on a larger, hemispheric scale. Perhaps because empires conjure up notions of borders and boundaries, large-scale events such as pandemics seem to have called historians to adopt a world-historical perspective. It

---

[6] Roy Porter, *The Greatest Benefit to Mankind: A Medical History of Humanity from Antiquity to the Present* (London: HarperCollins, 1997), 26.

[7] E.g., see William Rosen, *Justinian's Flea: Plague, Empire, and the Birth of Europe* (New York: Penguin, 2007).

is no coincidence that historical studies of epidemics and pandemics have often emphasized the process of globalization as the fundamental modality for facilitating the spread of disease. However, historians of empires caution us against overexploiting the concept of "globalization," especially for the premodern era. For the sixteenth century, for example, Jane Burbank and Frederick Cooper remind us that *"thinking about a history of connections"* can afford a better understanding than that offered by "globalization."[8] It is thus critical not to project modern definitions of globalization onto the premodern world, where the precise nature of disease spread is blurred. Even though it is true that regional systems emerged in the premodern world and that their gradual integration contributed to the formation of a global system, this was not a linear process by which globalization was achieved in a smooth and uncontested manner. Despite the insights offered by such notions as "microbial unification" or the emergence of "disease zones," how exactly the assumed process of gradual globalization furthered the spread of disease remains far from clear.[9] Hence, with regard to disease spread, thinking about *a history of connections* might serve our purposes better.

In the example of the early modern Mediterranean, the driving force for these connections seems to have been assumed by (multi-)regional empires: the growth of territorial or tributary empires,[10] rather than a process of global unification, seems to constitute a better context for understanding the spread of epidemic disease. These empires, not only as political entities but also as configurations of networks of exchange, seem to have been the principal agents of epidemic expansion in the early modern era. Conceived in this manner, empires exercise myriad forms of power (such as military, administrative, or economic) along the connections they nurture and proliferate. Plague, like trade goods, people, animals, and ideas, circulated along these networks. As this book shows, the growth of the Ottoman domains produced an increased level of communication, interaction, and mobility between individual regions brought together by conquest. These newly conquered regions came to be bound within an administrative, military, and commercial system. Indeed, it did not take long for widespread plagues to follow. Consolidating the intersecting trade networks connecting the Balkans, Caucasus and Central Asia, Asia Minor, the Arabian Peninsula, Persia, North Africa, and the eastern Mediterranean provided a new set of connections over which plague could spread extensively both within the Ottoman domains and beyond. In this manner, the rise and expansion of the

---

[8] Jane Burbank and Frederick Cooper, *Empires in World History: Power and the Politics of Difference* (Princeton, NJ: Princeton University Press, 2011), 180.

[9] E.g., see Janet Abu-Lughod, *Before European Hegemony: The World System ad 1250–1350* (New York: Oxford University Press, 1989); Le Roy Ladurie, "Un concept"; William McNeill, *Plagues and Peoples* (Garden City, NY: Anchor Press, 1976).

[10] For the Ottoman empire as a tributary empire, see Peter F. Bang and C. A. Bayly, *Tributary Empires in Global History* (New York: Palgrave Macmillan, 2011).

Ottoman Empire constituted a constellation of connections for the spread of plague in the post–Black Death Mediterranean.

Plague Ecologies

Plague is an infectious disease caused by a bacterium, *Y. pestis*, that attacks the lymph nodes, usually causing inflammation that produces painful swellings in the groin, armpit, or neck, called *buboes* – a characteristic symptom of bubonic plague. Other symptoms, such as fever, chill, headache, and extreme exhaustion, may accompany buboes. If the bacteria infect the lungs, pneumonic plague develops, which then can be transferred from person to person via infected droplets spread in the air as a result of coughing or sneezing. When the bacteria multiply in the bloodstream, fatal septicemia may develop, causing shock, organ failure, and sudden death. In bubonic form, plague may be fatal (between 40 to 70 percent mortality). Today, bubonic plague can be treated successfully with antibiotics if diagnosed early. Pneumonic plague, however, still remains a fatal condition that can kill within twenty-four hours if not treated promptly. Even though some may believe that plague is a disease of the past that conjures up images of the Middle Ages, it is very much alive in some parts of the world (e.g., the southwestern United States, Central Asia, Madagascar), where it is enzootic among rodent populations and may "spill over" to human populations.[11]

Once plague is introduced to a new environment, if the infection finds a rodent population to sustain it, it tends to form enzootic foci, either in the wild or in human settlements. The enzootic foci in the wild normally are not a direct threat for human societies. Only those individuals who come into close contact with infected or dead plague carriers (rodents or other mammals) or their arthropod vectors would be exposed to risk. Hence, it is possible to imagine that the infection can be carried to human settlements near enzootic foci. In such places, this sort of sporadic isolated breakout probably occurred often enough, without being documented in the historical sources. Even when the infection is communicated to the commensal rodents living in close proximity to humans, there would be local and perhaps repeated outbreaks. Even if no communication existed among infected human settlements (no trade, no travel, etc.), enzootic plague could still continue and produce epizootics and epidemics at times. Such breakouts would allow us to identify their area of origin, spread, range, and periodicity, in some recognizable patterns. For example, when plague was introduced (or reintroduced) to Anatolia and the Balkans during the Black Death, it affected

---

[11] Nils Chr Stenseth et al., "Plague: Past, Present, and Future," *PLoS Medicine* 5, no. 1 (2008): e3; Elisabeth Carniel, "Plague Today," in *Pestilential Complexities: Understanding Medieval Plague*, ed. Vivian Nutton, 115–22 (London: Wellcome Trust for the History of Medicine at UCL, 2008).

certain locations, circulated along main routes, and eventually died down each time, to recur every ten to fifteen years. This being the typical behavior of the plague, it continued more or less in this manner until the mid-fifteenth century or so.

Starting in the second half of the fifteenth century, plagues occurring in Ottoman lands diverged from these patterns. From then on, the spread and frequency of the outbreaks become unrecognizably different, so much so that, for example, there is a recorded incidence of plague in Istanbul almost every year. This divergence certainly demands an explanation. I argue that this explanation needs to be sought in the formation of the Ottoman Empire. To build a centralized empire, the Ottoman polity regulated, mobilized, and organized its "natural" resources, including crops, livestock, people, and minerals. These items circulated in a manner imposed by the empire's administration – the effects of such ecological engineering have been shown convincingly in recent works.[12] As an unintended consequence, the very same constellation of connections helped circulate plague. This book is an attempt to demonstrate the effects of the empire's ecological management with respect to plague.

Plague Networks

Throughout the book, the reader will encounter terms, such as *plague networks*, *networks of exchange*, or *networks of disease exchange*, that will be used almost interchangeably. In addition, I also refer to *plague hubs* (major and minor) and *plague nodes* along these networks. What do I mean by these terms? I refer to a plague network as a dynamic set of relationships that not only enable the flow of the disease but also simultaneously circulate its meaning and effects as well as perceptions and knowledge about it along each node and segment of these connections. Thus, at its simplest level, one can conceive of a plague network as a set of circuits or pathways that connect a plague focus (a reservoir of plague, in which the infection is kept alive by animal hosts without causing large-scale mortality) to a human settlement, where the disease may assume an epidemic form. At a slightly more complex level of analysis, several urban and rural human settlements that are connected to one another with commercial, diplomatic, or economic relationships can be superimposed onto the simple set of trajectories that connected plague foci to them. In this picture, plague nodes and hubs are useful conceptual tools. Further expanding the scope spatially can help us identify larger zones of plague exchange. Each of these sets of relationships can be conceptualized as a plague network.

---

[12] See, e.g., Sam White, *The Climate of Rebellion in the Early Modern Ottoman Empire* (New York: Cambridge University Press, 2011); Alan Mikhail, *Nature and Empire in Ottoman Egypt: An Environmental History* (New York: Cambridge University Press, 2011).

Why plague networks? Looking at the experience and effects of plague in a given city or region can tell a lot. For example, it is possible to reconstruct the experience of a community with the disease at the local level. However, expanding the scope of the inquiry both temporally and geographically can offer new ways of understanding. Thus, tracing change through mobility and movement can add tremendous insight to the analysis. It may be possible, for instance, to detect patterns of spread, trajectories, and frequency.

More importantly, a conceptualization of disease along a set of relations in time and space can also expose social, political, and economic structures and inequalities. For example, the effects of plague were more visibly dramatic in Istanbul than elsewhere in the Ottoman realm. If not entirely an artifact of the sources, then plague, along with its opportunistic rodent hosts and parasitic vectors, was a free rider that moved toward centers of affluence. It may have moved toward the Ottoman capital in the same way that silk, wool, and fur did; just as sugar, spice, and rice did; and just as the same people, knowledge, and texts did. Istanbul was where multiple networks converged. Hence, most of our story is in or about Istanbul, and in this sense the picture that emerges in this book is heavily Istanbul-centric. To be sure, there were cases of plague in other cities and villages of the empire, but they do not receive equal attention in these pages. Yet, this should not be read as an apology owing to the emphasis given to Istanbul in the sources. Being fully aware of this methodological predicament, the historical analysis in this book aims to demonstrate an epidemiological phenomenon that may be called the *capital effect*. According to this, large urban areas, especially capitals of empires, tend to be visited by a greater number of epidemics than smaller towns or villages. Large cities like Istanbul worked like magnets; just as they attracted goods, people, capital, and knowledge, they also attracted disease. In the context of the political economy of an early modern empire, Istanbul's history can be reconstructed as the capital of plague.[13]

Furthermore, studying plague networks allows glimpses of how the imperial power was operationalized. Not only the circulation of plague along those networks but also the flow of reports and regulations about the disease may help in understanding this. As the case may be, the empire projected power from the center, but this power was not felt and exercised everywhere in the exact same manner. The imperial power was mediated within a given set of relationships at the local level. As a rule, the center sent agents to provinces in charge of carrying messages, documents, and papers on which imperial decrees were formulated. Provincial administrators

---

[13] A similar pattern can be observed during the city's Byzantine past. See Dionysios Stathakopoulos, *Famine and Pestilence in the Late Roman and Early Byzantine Empire: A Systematic Survey of Subsistence Crises and Epidemics* (Aldershot, UK: Ashgate, 2004), 30–32.

formulated responses and translated, mediated, and negotiated these decisions while drawing from firsthand knowledge of local circumstances. As far as cases of reporting plague are concerned, it may be possible to trace the processes, identify the agencies, and witness how local knowledge was used to define, refine, and modify the imperial vision of power. Taken as a whole, then, the empire itself consisted of a set of connections, operationalized at every step of the way through projections, mediations, and negotiations of power. Just like the plague, the empire operated on a porous, uneven, and patchy space, amid the nodes and trajectories that constantly strove to bring them together. Thus, this was as much an empire of paper, politics, and power as it was an empire of plague.

Last, we may need to address briefly the question of whether the recorded increase of plague reflects a real increase or a historical artifact. Both narrative and archival sources suggest an increase in recorded incidence of plagues in the sixteenth century and especially in its latter half. However, there is also an overall increase in record keeping in the very same period. Although this problem seems not an easily quantifiable one and may have had its share in shaping our historical perception, it may nevertheless prove itself to be framed, not in terms of an either-or dichotomy, but instead as concomitant manifestations of a larger force at work. In other words, instead of situating *more plague* in opposition to *better recording*, I propose apposing them as signs and symptoms of the formation of an imperial body and its vital networks facilitating collecting, recording, and distributing information, on one hand, and circulating disease, on the other. Hence, I suggest that the very same mechanisms sustained and enabled both plague and its mobilities of exchange.

Periodization, Sources, and Terminology

This book follows a system of periodization that draws from Ottoman political and military history, more specifically, from key Ottoman conquests, as well as from major plague outbreaks. For reasons elaborated at length in the following pages of this book, Ottoman conquests had a significant effect on plagues. Hence, the selection of dates such as 1453 or 1517 is owed to the lasting effects of those conquests for studying the Ottoman history of plagues. Such dates are used in conjunction with a periodization drawn from dates of outbreaks, such as the cases of 1347 and 1570. The obvious methodological complications of developing a system of periodization of plague notwithstanding, the approach adopted here offers some practical advantages. The secondary literature on the history of plague in the Mediterranean world (especially for the areas adjacent to the Ottomans and/or those conquered by them) has followed this system of periodization – for example, historians of the Byzantine Empire generally tend to study the history of plague until 1453.[14] Similarly, historians working on Syria and Egypt limit their history of plague chronologically to the end of the Mamluk era, that is, the Ottoman conquest of 1516–17.[15] Therefore adopting this system of periodization facilitates the production of comparable data with respect to epidemiological patterns, such as frequency and spread.

As concerning sources, this work utilizes a range and variety. Given the uncharted nature of the early Ottoman plagues, bringing a mixture of sources has been indispensable. As always, the usual suspects for the Ottoman historian, the archival and narrative sources, have been critical for establishing the basic structure of plague outbreaks and for tracing their movements, effects, and the like. However, those sources tend to run short when it comes to exploring the meaning and mentalities of plague, especially in the early part of this study's time frame. Hence, it is worthwhile to complement them with hagiographies, legal and medical discussions of plague, and, when possible, works of poetry. In addition, works of travel literature penned by visitors to Ottoman lands, as well as a rather limited pool of Byzantine, Mamluk, Armenian, and Venetian sources, were also exploited. In due course, an unusually helpful body of knowledge came from the latest scientific literature on plague, including in the areas of bioarcheology, zoology, entomology, and microbiology.

The problems concerning the Ottoman terminology of plague may benefit from some clarification here. *Ṭā ʿūn* and *vebā*' were the most commonly used terms by the Ottomans in reference to plague. These terms had their origins in classical Arabic, *ṭā ʿūn* and *wabā*', respectively. In theory, while *ṭā ʿūn* was used in reference to bubonic plague specifically, *wabā*' referred to pestilence or epidemic disease in general. Yet, much confusion accompanied their use, leading scholars to formulate a clarification. Thus, the scholars writing in Arabic after the Black Death of the mid-fourteenth century suggested that "every *ṭā ʿūn* is a *wabā*', but not every *wabā*' is a *ṭā ʿūn*."[16] Ottoman sources seem to have taken on this distinction, at least in theory. In practice, however, *ṭā ʿūn* and *vebā*' could be used almost interchangeably for emphasis or stylistic purposes, especially in nonmedical sources. In addition to these terms of Arabic origin, there were other terms used in reference to epidemic diseases in the vernacular Turkish, in both medical and nonmedical Ottoman sources. For example, *yumurcak* (or *yumrucuk*, "plague bubo") and *hıyarcık*

[14] There are of course exceptions, such as Kōstas Kōstēs, *Ston kairo tēs panōlēs: eikones apo tis koinōnies tēs Hellēnikēs chersonēsou, 140s-190s aiōnas* (Hērakleio: Panepistēmiakes Ekdoseis Krētēs, 1995); Marie-Hélène Congourdeau, "La peste noire à Constantinople de 1348 à 1466," *Medicina nei secoli* 11, no. 2 (1999): 377–89.
[15] E.g., see Michael Dols, *The Black Death in the Middle East* (Princeton, NJ: Princeton University Press, 1977).
[16] Lawrence Conrad, "*Ṭā ʿūn* and *Wabā*': Conceptions of Plague and Pestilence in Early Islam," *JESHO* 25, no. 3 (1982): 268–307; Dols, *Black Death in the Middle East*, 315–19.

were often used to refer to bubonic plague, particularly before the sixteenth century. In addition, *ölet*, which was used mainly in nonmedical works, can perhaps best be translated as "pestilence" or "mortality."[17]

While the Ottoman medical sources have from the outset maintained a clear identification of plague (*ṭāʿūn*) as distinct from other epidemic diseases, nonmedical sources could use *ṭāʿūn* and *vebāʾ* indiscriminately. Nevertheless, members of the Ottoman society had come to possess at least a basic working knowledge of the plague to identify and distinguish it from other diseases. After all, as is shown here, from 1347 onward, plague was an integral part of life for members of Ottoman society – a disease any adult would have witnessed at least a few times in a lifetime, if he was fortunate enough to survive it.

As Ottoman society became more and more familiar with plague – I situate this process somewhere in the late sixteenth century – the use of the term *ṭāʿūn* (as well as *yumurcak* and *ölet*) started to diminish. As the plague (*ṭāʿūn*) came to establish itself as *the* epidemic disease in Ottoman life, it gradually lost its original name as plague (*ṭāʿūn*) and came to be referred to as *the* epidemic (*vebāʾ*) or *the* disease (*hastalık* or *maraz*). The terminology used in reference to plague is discussed later in the book, but suffice it to give here an example for such use. A late-sixteenth-century letter sent to the Topkapı Palace in the midst of a plague outbreak reads, "Hiç ol mübarek hastalıksuz yer yokdur" (There is no place free from that blessed disease).[18] To its contemporaries, the reference was clear: the plague! Perhaps the living testimony of the persistence of plague and the growing familiarity of Ottoman society with it left behind its legacy in the late Ottoman and modern Turkish usage of the term, whereupon the term *veba* came to mean "plague."

Structure of the Chapters

The book has three parts. Part I is mainly conceived as a background, which seeks to situate the Ottoman plague experience in the larger context of history and historiography. In three chapters, it tackles the double problem of explaining why plague matters for Ottoman history to the Ottomanists and why the Ottoman experience of plague matters to the non-Ottomanist plague historians. To this end, it gives a critical account of the plague scholarship of the Second Pandemic, highlights some of the issues relevant to the Ottoman experience, and focuses on how the Ottoman experience enables us to explain those issues. Chapter 1 is a natural history of plague as experienced in the Ottoman areas. It largely relies on scientific evidence but, whenever possible, draws from historical sources to flesh out the natural

---

[17] Ünver, "Taun Nedir? Veba Nedir?," *Dirim* 3–4 (1978): 363–66.
[18] TSMA, E.4214. See Figure 2.

history of plague. It can be read as a synthesis of the latest scientific research on plague in the particular climatic, environmental, and social context of early modern Ottoman life. Chapter 2 addresses problems of the historiography of plague, both in the Ottomanist and non-Ottomanist scholarship. It tells the story of why the history of early Ottoman plagues has not been explored until now. In doing so, it offers a corrective to misconceptions about the Ottoman experience of plague, such as in the example of the trope of the fatalistic Turk, whose genealogy is sketched. Chapter 3 presents a brief account of the Black Death and the century that followed it (1347–1453), as experienced by the Ottomans and in the areas adjacent to them. It includes a first attempt to trace the trajectory of the spread of the Black Death in the interior of the Anatolian peninsula, as opposed to the current emphasis on coastal spread. The chapter also addresses the historical links between the Black Death and early Ottoman expansion.

Part II of the book aims to demonstrate the influence of the Ottoman territorial expansion on the spread, periodicity, and effects of plague outbreaks. In three chapters, it reconstructs the narrative history of Ottoman plagues in the long sixteenth century (1453–1600). As a first attempt to create a systematic compilation of Ottoman plagues in this era, it traces the movement of the disease both spatially and temporally. For doing so, it presents the material in three distinct phases, each presented in one chapter. Chapter 4 is devoted to the first phase of epidemiological activity (1453–1517), which is mainly characterized by plagues moving eastward, from the European ports of the Mediterranean toward Ottoman cities. The chapter aims to shed light on the relationship between Ottoman urban growth and plagues in this era. Chapter 5 focuses on the second phase (1517–70), which is underscored by the multiplication of trajectories of plague spread in the growing Ottoman domains. Following the movement of plagues, the chapter seeks to explore the changing patterns of epidemiological activity in the entangled histories of Ottoman conquests, trade, and urbanization. Chapter 6 surveys the third phase (1570–1600), which epitomizes the consolidation of Ottoman plague networks. It focuses on the emergence of Istanbul as the plague hub of the empire and examines the modalities of epidemiological exchange between the capital and the provinces.

Part III of the book explores how this plague experience affected Ottoman society. In two chapters, it seeks to examine how this experience shaped the beliefs and ideas of the Ottomans about plague and their responses to it. Chapter 7 aims to reconstruct how the Ottomans understood plague, what they knew about it, and how they conducted themselves in the face of it. It seeks to demonstrate that the Ottomans' perceptions and knowledge of plague as well as their attitudes toward it changed considerably over the course of the sixteenth century, as they watched plague persist in their lands. The chapter examines these changes in the context of the political, economic, social, and cultural changes of early modern Ottoman history.

In the light of the findings, Chapter 8 reconstructs the Ottoman administrative response to plagues by surveying the efforts at healthscaping in early modern Istanbul and, to a lesser extent, in other Ottoman cities. It seeks to demonstrate that the persisting plague outbreaks forced the hand of the Ottoman administration in developing measures to deal with the consequences of high mortality. By keeping records of plague mortality, regulating burial space, and cleansing cities of perceived sources of filth (both physical and moral), the Ottoman administration started to experiment with new technologies of governance and surveillance of bodies. Taken as a whole, the combined efforts of the politics of bodies not only laid the foundations of a system of public health but also contributed to the making of the early modern Ottoman state.

These three parts in eight chapters are followed by a brief epilogue, which makes some general remarks about the implications of this research. It highlights the areas of research that await scholarly interest and calls for comparison of the Ottoman experience of plague to other contemporary or near-contemporary historical examples.

PART I

PLAGUE

History and Historiography

I

A Natural History of Plague

Ne pire her biri bir zerk idici div-i hücum
Ne pire bilmez aman, vermez aman cana kıyar
Pire bir heybet ile halka hücum eyledi kim
Div bu yerde eğer bağlasalar ide firar

O'what a flea! Each one is an injecting attack-demon
O'what a flea! Has no mercy, shows no mercy, takes life
Fleas attacked people with such majesty that
Demon would flee this place even tied down[1]

The opportunity to write a natural history of plague in the Ottoman lands is a mixed blessing. On one hand, there is an embarrassment of riches in both the scientific and historical literature on plague, which is generally helpful for understanding plague's emergence, transmission, and effects. On the other, this literature has little bearing on the Ottoman experience of plague in the late medieval and early modern eras. My task in this chapter is to reconstruct a natural history of plague in the areas where the Ottomans came to rule, drawing from the scientific literature and from Ottoman sources. This effort will involve highlighting plague's main protagonists (its host and vector organisms and its causative agent or pathogen) and their interactions in the context of the physical, climatic, and environmental conditions of Ottoman history.

Plague is a zoonosis (animal-to-human disease) that primarily affects rodents; humans are only accidental hosts to it. It has a complex etiology that involves a system of entanglements between rodent hosts, arthropod vectors, the pathogen, human populations, and the environment. These agents interact with one another, while they themselves change in response to their

---

[1] Evliya Çelebi, *Evliyâ Çelebi Seyahatnâmesi* (Istanbul: Yapı Kredi Yayınları, 1999), 4:214–15. Evliya Çelebi claims to quote these couplets by Baba Abdi-i Horasani, composed during the latter's visit to Balıkesir, complaining of the fleas there.

interactions with other organisms and the broader environment. To get a holistic sense of this dynamic, it may be useful to consider the actors one by one. However, before introducing plague's protagonists, it may be useful to comment briefly about the phases of epidemiological activity, especially as they manifested in the Ottoman case. When historical sources mention outbreaks of plague, they are referring to the epidemic phase of the disease, that is, when it affects human populations, causing a certain degree of mortality. Even without any attempt to control, contain, or cure the disease, the epidemic phase of plague does not last very long. In the Ottoman areas with moderate climate, plague epidemics typically started slowly, gradually peaked, and then receded. The climatic and environmental conditions of a city could shape plague's *seasonal signature* (the temporal patterns of epidemic activity) – an unambiguous marker of plague. As far as the early modern Ottoman cities are concerned, we know fairly well how this took place, as did the Ottomans themselves. For example, in Istanbul, plague would typically start in April or May, peak in August and September, and recede in November and December. In the warmer temperatures and (higher) humidity of Thessaloniki, the right conditions for sustaining such outbreaks were between April and July; plague would normally break out in March, peak in June and July, and lose intensity by late summer to recede in September or October. In yet warmer cities, the timing could be slightly earlier. For example, in Alexandria, plague would usually break out in January, peak in April, and finish in June or July.[2]

Decreasing mortality signaled that the plague was on the wane and the end of the *plague season*, but not necessarily the end of the epidemic. The disease could return the following spring and follow a similar seasonal pattern. Hence, the epidemics came and went in waves, sometimes lasting several

[2] Panzac, *La peste*, 223–25, 628–29. Panzac noted that plague started in Istanbul when temperatures reached 11–12 degrees Celsius with an average humidity between 67 and 79 percent throughout the year; peaked in August when temperatures reached their maximum average (23.9 degrees); and continued in the fall with milder temperatures (20.2 degrees) and a high level of humidity (70 percent). As for Thessaloniki, plague started when temperatures were around 11 degrees Celsius and humidity between 60 and 70 percent. It peaked in June when temperatures were 23.9 degrees and humidity was around 50–55 percent. Increasing temperatures in July (27 degrees Celsius) and a fall in humidity (57 percent) impeded further activity of plagues. For the seasonality of plague epidemics in Thessaloniki, see Eleni Xoplaki et al., "Variability of Climate in Meridional Balkans during the Periods 1675–1715 and 1780–1830 and Its Impact on Human Life," *Climatic Change* 48, no. 4 (2001): 581–615, esp. 584–87. As for Alexandria, Panzac indicated that it broke out in January when both the temperature (14.4 degrees Celsius) and humidity (66 percent) were high enough, continued into a mild spring, and ended when higher temperatures were reached in June and July. Compare with the discussion "the season of plague" in Egypt in Alan Mikhail, "Plague and Environment in Late Ottoman Egypt," in *Water on Sand: Environmental Histories of the Middle East and North Africa*, ed. Alan Mikhail (Oxford: Oxford University Press, 2012), 120–23. For the most part, these figures for temperature and humidity represent the eighteenth and nineteenth centuries and may need to be compared with those of earlier eras of Ottoman history.

years in a row, at other times skipping a year or two but returning again later. Epidemic waves were separated by interepidemic phases of nonactivity (or low-level activity) among the human populations, depending on a variety of factors, including climate, the availability of a replenished pool of human and rodent hosts that lacked immunity, and flea-to-host ratios.

The epidemic phase of the disease, however, is not its only manifestation. In a plague focus or reservoir, the disease is sustained by ground-burrowing rodents that are resistant to the infection (*enzootic* phase), until it breaks out and starts affecting the rodents that are susceptible to it (*epizootic* phase). Typically, epizootics last for a period of one to two years, sometimes longer. Similar to epidemics affecting human populations, epizootics display a bell-shaped curve of activity with a slow onset, gradual increase, and decrease after peaking. Like epidemics, they come and go in waves, with interepizootic phases that depend on a complex web of factors, such as climate and the fluctuations in the host and vector populations.

The Hosts

Many species of mammals, such as cats, rabbits, goats, deer, and camels, can become infected with plague and thus serve as incidental hosts to the disease.[3] However, rodents are known to be particularly important in maintaining the disease in naturally occurring enzootic cycles, between hosts (some burrow-dwelling wild rodent species, such as marmots, voles, prairie dogs, ground squirrels, and gerbils) and their fleas. Today, several of these rodent species maintain the infection in the plague foci of the tropical and subtropical belt.[4]

Unless the disease becomes epizootic among susceptible rodents, it is normally not a direct threat to human populations. This being the case, the

---

[3] Handling Y. *pestis*–infected dead or live animals and eating their meat can transmit the disease to humans. Didier Raoult et al., "Plague: History and Contemporary Analysis," *Journal of Infection* 66, no. 1 (2013): 18–26; Abdulaziz A. Bin Saeed et al., "Plague from Eating Raw Camel Liver," *Emerging Infectious Diseases* 11, no. 9 (2005): 1456–57; A. B. Christie et al., "Plague in Camels and Goats: Their Role in Human Epidemics," *Journal of Infectious Diseases* 141, no. 6 (1980): 724–26; V. N. Fedorov, "Plague in Camels and Its Prevention in the USSR," *Bulletin of the World Health Organization* 23, nos. 2–3 (1960): 275–81. For the involvement of mammals, such as pigs, dogs, and cats, in the transmission process during the Black Death in Europe, see Stephen R. Ell, "Some Evidence for Interhuman Transmission of Medieval Plague," *Reviews of Infectious Diseases* 1, no. 3 (1979): 563–66; Ell, "Immunity as a Factor in the Epidemiology of Medieval Plague," *Reviews of Infectious Diseases* 6, no. 6 (1984): 866–79.

[4] Kenneth L. Gage and Michael Y. Kosoy, "Natural History of Plague: Perspectives from More Than a Century of Research," *Annual Review of Entomology* 50, no. 1 (2005): 505–28. More than two hundred species of wild rodents that inhabit all continents except Australia can host plague. See Andrey P. Anisimov, Luther E. Lindler, and Gerald B. Pier, "Intraspecific Diversity of *Yersinia pestis*," *Clinical Microbiology Reviews* 17, no. 2 (2004): 434–64.

presence of plague among ground-burrowing rodents could easily go unnoticed in the historical sources. Even though the sources would record plague epidemics that affected human populations, the epizootic and enzootic forms of the disease remain largely invisible. Hence, it is more difficult to identify the species of wild rodents that hosted plague in the Ottoman fauna of the late medieval and early modern eras. Though scanty, there is evidence that some rodent species that once likely inhabited the area, such as jerboa, marmot, and jird, may have hosted the plague.[5]

In the context of plague's transmission to humans, commensal rodents are more important to consider. *Commensal* species (literally, species that "eat at the same table") consume the food supplies of human populations and hence live in close proximity to them. When they are affected by plague, the infection can be transferred to humans via their ectoparasites. Of all the commensal animals, the rat is the most widely distributed species across the world today.

With respect to historical pandemics of plague, two species of rats in particular come into focus. It is generally accepted that while black rats (*Rattus rattus*) were the main hosts to the infection in the First and the Second Pandemics, brown rats, or Norway rats (*Rattus norvegicus*), starred in the Third. Even though both species belong to the same genus (*Rattus*), there are some important differences between them. The black rat has a tail longer than its body, which makes it a good climber, enabling it to live in the roofs of houses, close to humans. The brown rat, in contrast, has a tail shorter than its body and is not as good a climber as the former. It prefers to live away from humans, in basements and sewers.[6] Overall, the brown rat is larger, stronger, and more ferocious than the black rat, which perhaps has helped it become the dominant rat species everywhere it has colonized since its global dispersion in the early eighteenth century.[7]

As far as the late medieval and early modern eras are concerned, the black rat was the principal species of rodent serving as a host to plague. The origins of the genus *Rattus* are traced to south Asia, with the first members

---

[5] See my "New Science and Old Sources."

[6] In addition to these differences, it has also been noted that whereas black rats are commonly found on board ships, brown rats leave ships when they sail. See Bruce Skinner, "Plague and the Geographical Distribution of Rats," *British Medical Journal* 1, no. 2314 (1905): 994–95. This author noted in 1905 that Norway (brown) rats might possibly be immune to plague, which he took as one of the reasons how it managed to replace black rats. It is interesting that this view will be taken by some historians several decades later to explain the disappearance of plague from Europe.

[7] *Rattus norvegicus* was possibly originally a native of Palearctic Asia that came to be distributed worldwide, though it is more common in cooler countries of Asia. See John Reeves Ellerman and Terence Charles Stuart Morrison-Scott, *Checklist of Palaearctic and Indian Mammals, 1758–1946* (London: Printed by order of the Trustees of the British Museum, 1951), 588; Frédérique Audoin-Rouzeau, *Les chemins de la peste: le rat, la puce et l'homme* (Rennes: Presses universitaires de Rennes, 2003), 8n1.

of the species having probably evolved around three million years ago.[8] Owing to their highly adaptive nature, black rats followed human movements and migrations to spread around the world. It has been generally accepted that black rats migrated from the Indian subcontinent to Europe, whence they dispersed to different parts of the world by means of shipping.[9] A recent global study that surveyed the mitochondrial DNA (mtDNA) of black rats has identified well-differentiated lineages of the species and confirmed its migrations and patterns of dispersal. This phylogenetic research contributes significantly to our understanding of the species from an evolutionary perspective concerning the geographic patterns of diversification of the black rat and the direction and timing of its (prehistoric, historic, and contemporary) dispersals. Furthermore, it offers new ways of understanding associations of different lineages of black rats to diseases. According to this research, *Lineage I* black rats display the broadest distribution outside of Asia, occurring in a wide range of regions, including Europe, the Americas, Africa, Australia, and the Pacific Islands. This particular lineage moved from southern India to the Middle East and from there spread independently to Madagascar and Europe, and from those points globally as part of the Columbian Exchange, mainly on board ships, thus becoming referred to as "ship rats."[10] Although there seems to be consensus about this particular trajectory of spread, that is, from India to the Middle East–Mediterranean area, the timing of this migration seems unsettled. The scattered zooarcheological evidence for the presence of black rats in Palestine and Egypt seems to date to as early as the eighth to fourth millennium BCE, though this dating has been challenged; a safer assumption is the third millennium BCE.[11] However there is no doubting its widespread occurrence in the Mediterranean basin and islands over the last two thousand years, as zooarcheological evidence demonstrates.[12]

---

[8] Aplin et al., "Evolutionary Biology of the Genus *Rattus*: Profile of an Archetypal Rodent Pest," in *Rats, Mice, and People: Rodent Biology and Management*, ed. Grant R. Singleton, Lyn A. Hinds, Charles J. Krebs, and Dave M. Spratt, 487–98 (Canberra: Australian Centre for International Agricultural Research, 2003).

[9] Philip L. Armitage, "Unwelcome Companions: Ancient Rats Reviewed," *Antiquity* 68 (June 1994): 231–40. Also, for possible scenarios of the migration patterns of commensal black rats, see Anton Ervynck, "Sedentism or Urbanism? On the Origin of the Commensal Black Rat (*Rattus rattus*)," in *Bones and the Man: Studies in Honour of Don Brothwell*, ed. Keith Dobney and Terry Patrick O'Connor, 95–109 (Oxford: Oxbow, 2002).

[10] Aplin et al., "Multiple Geographic Origins of Commensalism and Complex Dispersal History of Black Rats," *PLoS One* 6, no. 11 (2011): e26357.

[11] Ervynck, "Sedentism or Urbanism?," esp. 100–104.

[12] Lise Ruffino and Eric Vidal, "Early Colonization of Mediterranean Islands by *Rattus rattus*: A Review of Zooarcheological Data," *Biological Invasions* 12 (2010): 2389–94; Robert Sallares, "Ecology, Evolution, and Epidemiology of Plague," in *Plague and the End of Antiquity: The Pandemic of 541–750*, ed. Lester Little (Cambridge: Cambridge University Press, 2007), 268. Also see Hans Zinsser's classic book for a brief account of rats in the Near East during antiquity: *Rats, Lice, and History* (New Brunswick, N.J.: Transaction,

When and to what extent black rats colonized Anatolia and the Balkans, as well as other parts of the Near East, are not well known. After the introduction of the species to the Mediterranean basin, there is no clear evidence about its presence in what later became the core areas of the Ottoman Empire. On the basis of the general tendency of the species to be dispersed through the movements of ships, it seems plausible to assume that it spread into this area following maritime links. Thus we may hypothesize that the black rat first gained a foothold on the coast, then spread farther inland, into the interior of Anatolia and the Balkans. Zooarcheological evidence from Continental Europe cautions us that during the first millennium, black rats mainly inhabited coastal and riverside towns and villages and almost always lead a commensal existence.[13] However, things started to change for black rats in Europe from the eleventh century onward. Zooarcheological evidence strongly suggests a substantially increased rat population in Europe between the eleventh and thirteenth centuries, spread across major trade routes.[14] Evidence from northwestern Russia also seems to support this pattern of spread.[15]

Unfortunately, we do not have comparable data for the core Ottoman areas in Anatolia and the Balkans for the late medieval and early modern eras. Indeed, very little is known about the historical presence of black rats in this region. According to zooarcheologists, this lack of information largely results from the fact that the bones are not collected from historic layers in archeological excavations. Even when they are collected, this is done by hand, whereas small bones, such as those of *R. rattus*, can only be retrieved through sieving. This makes it difficult to have a healthy set of data even for advancing most basic assumptions about the black rat's spread.[16] In the absence of zooarcheological findings, our understanding of past geographical distribution and populations of black rats in areas where the Ottomans came to rule has to draw from their distribution records in more recent times. The few twentieth-century distribution records available identify the black rat as a wide-ranging species but suggest that its presence across Anatolia,

2008), 193–94. For the late antiquity, the presence of black rats has been demonstrated on the basis of textual evidence in Lawrence Conrad, "The Plague in the Early Medieval Near East" (PhD diss., Princeton University, 1981), 402–12.

[13] Ruffino and Vidal, "Early Colonization of Mediterranean Islands by *Rattus rattus*," 2392.

[14] Audoin-Rouzeau, "Le rat noir (*Rattus rattus*) et la peste dans l'occident antique et médiéval," *Bulletin de la Société de Pathologie Exotique* 92 (1999): 424–25.

[15] A. B. Savinetsky and O. A. Krylovich, "On the History of the Spread of the Black Rat (*Rattus rattus* L., 1758) in Northwestern Russia," *Biology Bulletin* 38, no. 2 (2011): 203–7. The authors believe that black rats came to northwestern Russia from the west via trade routes.

[16] On the basis of personal communication with zooarcheologist Canan Çakırlar of the University of Groningen, the Netherlands, March 28, 2013.

Syria, and the eastern Mediterranean varied greatly.[17] Today, the largest population of black rats can be found in Thrace, the Black Sea region, and western Anatolia, as well as in Anatolia littoral, the eastern Mediterranean, the Nile Valley, and the Balkan Peninsula. Current distribution of black rats varies greatly depending on altitude and climate, showing considerable variation in different physiogeographic settings.[18] Even though this may not necessarily reflect the black rat's past geographic spread, it gives at least some insight into its uneven distribution and diversity.

Similar to human populations, rat populations also change over time. Both commensal and wild rats are subjected to environmental and climatic conditions that have an impact on their survival. Any major changes in their natural habitat or their built environment can increase or decrease their population. For example, earthquakes and floods affect wild rodents by damaging their underground burrows and forcing them to move elsewhere, and commensal rats by changing their built environment. Similarly, epizootics are important for causing changes in rat populations.[19]

It is important to address the question whether commensal rodents, especially *R. rattus* colonies, are capable of sustaining plague over a prolonged period of time. There is greater emphasis in the ecological scholarship on the ground-burrowing wild rodents' role in sustaining the infection, but commensal rodents' ability to function in the same manner has not been sufficiently explored. However, important studies suggest that plague can be maintained over long periods of time in small commensal rat subpopulations without any contact with wild rodents. For example, plague has been

---

[17] Bathscheba Aharoni, *Die Muriden von Palästina und Syrien* (Lucka (Bez. Leipzig): Druck von Reinhold Berger, 1932), 177–82; Gabriele Neuhäuser, *Die Muriden von Kleinasien* (Lucka (Bez. Leipzig): Druck von Reinhold Berger, 1936), 173–74, 209. In the early 1930s, Neuhäuser caught no rats in Konya (in central Anatolia) and did not catch any black rat within the city of Zonguldak (on the Black Sea coast). He observed that the black rat has not filled in its available habitat and thus suggested that its presence in most Anatolian towns does not go back very long. Similarly, Misonne reports an absolute absence of black rats in southeastern Turkey and northern Syria in 1955. See Xavier Misonne, "Mammifères de la Turquie sud-orientale et du nord de la Syrie," *Mammalia* 21, no. 1 (1957): 53–68; Robert T. Hatt, *The Mammals of Iraq* (Ann Arbor: University of Michigan Press, 1959), 85.

[18] David T. Dennis, Kenneth L. Gage, Norman Gratz, Jack D. Poland, and Evgueni Tikhomirov, "Plague Manual: Epidemiology, Distribution, Surveillance and Control," report WHO/CDS/CSR/EDC/99.2 (Geneva, Switzerland: WHO, 1999); Nuri Yiğit et al., "A Study on the Geographic Distribution along with Habitat Aspects of Rodent Species in Turkey," *Bonner Zoologische Beiträge* 50, no. 4 (2003): 355–68; Nuri Yiğit et al., "Contribution to the Geographic Distribution of Rodent Species and Ecological Analyses of Their Habitats in Asiatic Turkey," *Turkish Journal of Biology* 22, no. 4 (1998): 435–46. Unfortunately, these studies focus on rodents in rural areas and offer limited insight into the historical distributions and populations of commensal black rats in urban areas.

[19] For a treatment of how epizootics correspond spatially, chronologically, and quantitatively to epidemics, see Audoin-Rouzeau, *Les chemins de la peste*, 42–45.

calculated to persist for one hundred years in a commensal rat population of sixty thousand without importations of new infection.[20] Hence, even if a certain rat population were killed, the infection could still be kept alive over a long time. This research has tremendous implications for explaining the historical persistence of plague in urban centers. It suggests that the disease could persist in an urban area, even if quarantine measures were in place, as long as there was a sufficient commensal rat population. Hence those towns would have served as self-perpetuating engines of epidemic activity or plague foci.

Rats are generally described as opportunistic creatures, and their populations grow as long as there is food to support them. In an urban setting, for example, the opportunities to obtain food from garbage and other sources support the growth of rat colonies. Regardless, it is difficult to estimate the density of rat populations in cities, not only in the past but also today. Studies show that the population density of rats in different patches exhibits great variation even within a given city.[21] The primary reason for this is that rats do not move much, unless they are forced to migrate. Normally, when black rats leave their location in search of food, they only move within a very limited radius. This explains why rat colonies in modern cities live in patches, usually around a row of houses or a neighborhood block, separated by man-made obstacles, such as wide roads, that inhibit their movement. Some areas in a premodern city, such as garbage disposal areas, places where waste accumulated, grain and cotton warehouses, and slaughterhouses, were most likely favored by rats. Moreover, the close proximity of houses, narrow and unpaved streets, and easy access to garbage and other food sources in a premodern city could help rat colonies prosper. Early modern Ottoman cities were no exception to this.[22]

We do not lack evidence for the presence of rats in early modern Ottoman cities. The seventeenth-century traveler Evliya Çelebi presents ample evidence that rats were common throughout Ottoman towns and cities. His account seems to suggest a distinction between commensal rats (in this case,

---

[20] Gage and Kosoy, "Natural History of Plague"; M. J. Keeling and C. A. Gilligan, "Bubonic Plague: A Metapopulation Model of a Zoonosis," *Proceedings of the Royal Society of London, Series B* 267, no. 1458 (2000): 2219–30; Keeling and Gilligan, "Metapopulation Dynamics of Bubonic Plague," *Nature* 407, no. 6806 (2000): 903–6.

[21] Doris Traweger et al., "Habitat Preferences and Distribution of the Brown Rat (*Rattus norvegicus* Berk.) in the City of Salzburg (Austria): Implications for an Urban Rat Management," *Journal of Pest Science* 79, no. 3 (2006): 113–25. Even though this study is on brown rats, it gives a fair idea about patterns of urban distribution.

[22] On the basis of the available evidence, some continuity can be presumed between Byzantine Constantinople and Ottoman Istanbul as regards the density and distribution of rat populations. Arguably, it worsened in the Ottoman era, as a result of fewer restrictive blocks than the Roman model of urban planning used and because of increased density of population and housing. See Michael McCormick, "Rats, Communications, and Plague: Toward an Ecological History," *The Journal of Interdisciplinary History* 34, no. 1 (2003): 1–25.

presumably the black rat) and wild rodents.[23] During his long travels, Evliya Çelebi did not fail to note places that had an excessive number of rats. For example, he mentions the Kurdish village Bekufar (he translates as the "rats-village" in the Kurdish language) as having many rats.[24] In a similar vein, he wrote that the castle of Pontikos/Pondikoz (Pontiko-Kastro in Greece) was full of rats that were sometimes "as big as cats."[25] For other towns, he comments on the surprising rarity or even the total absence of rats. For example, he writes that the town of Muş in eastern Anatolia had no rats because it was protected by a spell.[26] Similarly, he commented on the rarity of rats in the town of Sarajevo (Bosnasaray), also protected by a spell.[27] About the Hungarian castle of Košice (Kaşa), he remarks on the absolute absence of rats and any other pests, which he explains by spells made by one of the apostles of Jesus being still extant.[28] The absence of rats and other pests in a city had to be seen as an anomaly, and perhaps it took a supernatural power to keep pests away from towns. Judging from this account, it may be assumed that rats were accepted as a common pest in the urban texture of early modern cities. That this may be so in the case of Istanbul can be evidenced in his praise of weavers (esnâf-ı örücüyân) skilled in repairing textiles gnawed by rats.[29]

---

[23] Even though the term rat (sıçan) was used as a general taxonomic caterogy comprising many rodent species in Ottoman Turkish, there seems to be a distinction between commensal and wild species depending on their denomination with their natural habitat. For an example of how Evliya Çelebi clarified his terminology, see Evliya Çelebi, Seyahatnâme, 5:211: "fâre, ya'nî kesegen, Türkçe sıçan dedikleri muzırr." In other instances, he uses the term muş. For wild rodents, he uses terms such as yer sıçanı, Erdebil sıçanı, and pündika. Even though it is difficult to know what species these terms exactly referred to, there is some evidence about their use in the nineteenth century. The Redhouse dictionary lists the following terms and the corresponding species: orman sıçanı (the short-tailed field mouse, Arvicola arvalis); çöl sıçanı (the jerboa, Dipus aegyptius); su sıçanı (the water vole, Arvicola amphibius); dağ sıçanı (the marmot, Arclomys marmotta); yaban sıçanı (the lemming, Myodes lemmus); yer sıçanı (the bank vole). Alexander Russell also names different species of rodents occurring in eighteenth-century Aleppo, along with their names in Arabic and Latin. See Alexander Russell and Patrick Russell, The Natural History of Aleppo: Containing a Description of the City, and the Principal Natural Productions in Its Neighbourhood: Together with an Account of the Climate, Inhabitants, and Diseases, Particularly of the Plague (London: Printed for G. G. and J. Robinson, 1794), 2:180–82. Needless to say, further research is needed to clarify the taxonomy of rodents in the Ottoman landscape.

[24] Evliya Çelebi, Seyahatnâme, 4:289.

[25] Ibid., 8:129.

[26] Ibid., 3:132.

[27] Ibid., 5:211.

[28] Ibid., 6:21. The example of the fortress of Košice (Kaşa) is also interesting because Evliya Çelebi mentions the absence of rats as well as the lack of plague in that town, without necessarily establishing a connection between the absence of the two.

[29] Ibid., 1:303: "bir Kişmîrî şâl ve dülbend ve atlas ve hârâ ve ihrâm makûlesi eşyâları sıçan delse veyâhûd bir gûne âfet etse bunlar ol rahnedâr olan yerleri örüp ga'ib ederler, aslâ ma'lûm olmaz, musanna' kârdır."

With the abundance of rats, people tried to control their numbers by killing them, possibly with traps or rat poison. There do not seem to be professional rat catchers in the early modern Ottoman Empire organized in a guild, either because this was a service performed by another group of professionals or more likely because this was something done by individuals.[30] Incidentally, we find anecdotal evidence in one of Evliya Çelebi's stories of the use of rat poison. Even though we do not know exactly what substance was used, it might have been a mixture of arsenic and oxymel (probably to give substance to powder arsenic and attract rats to the poison by its sweet smell).[31] Other sources support this claim and indeed point to the fairly common use of rat poison in Ottoman lands. For example, according to the sixteenth-century probate registers, rat poison was sold in the apothecary shops in Edirne.[32] Sources mention different substances used as rat poison. For example, the seventeenth-century mystic Niyazi-i Mısri believed that he had been poisoned by rat poison (*sıçan otu*, "arsenic") but also noted that there was another kind of poison, known as *sülümen*, which was more effective and could easily be found in apothecary shops.[33] It seems that both *sıçan otu* and *ak sülümen* – the colloquial form of *süleymani* (a white powder of mercuric chloride) – were sold at these shops.[34] Evidence for the use of these substances by physicians and apothecaries points to the circulation of the substance in the Ottoman markets.[35] In eighteenth-century Aleppo, using arsenic to poison rats was common enough to cause accidents, and care was

---

[30] No guild of rat catchers is listed in the processions of guilds in the sixteenth and seventeenth centuries. See Eunjeong Yi, *Guild Dynamics in Seventeenth-century Istanbul: Fluidity and Leverage* (Leiden: Brill, 2004), appendices. Professional rat catchers were known in Europe. For an illustration of a "fully equipped" rat catcher, see Werner Schreiber, *Infectio: Infectious Diseases in the History of Medicine* (Basel: Roche, 1987), 28.

[31] Evliya Çelebi, *Seyahatnâme*, 6:130. Cf. Kari Konkola, "More Than a Coincidence? The Arrival of Arsenic and the Disappearance of Plague in Early Modern Europe," *JHMAS* 47, no. 2 (1992): 186–209.

[32] Ömer Lütfi Barkan, "Edirne Askerî Kassamı'na Âit *Tereke Defterleri* (1545–1659)," *Türk Tarih Belgeleri Dergisi* 3, nos. 5–6 (1966): 104.

[33] [Niyazî-i Mısrî, *Mecmua-i Kelimat-ı Kudsiyye-i Hazret-i Mısrî*, Bursa Eski Eserler Kütüphanesi, MS Orhan 690, 9a], cited in İsmail Hakkı Altuntaş, *Niyazi-i Mısri Divan-ı İlahiyyat ve Açıklaması* (n.p., 2010), 1:86.

[34] Turhan Baytop, "Aktarlar," in *Dünden Bugüne İstanbul Ansiklopedisi* (Istanbul: Tarih Vakfı, 1993–95), 1:172.

[35] Coşkun Yılmaz and Necdet Yılmaz, eds., *Osmanlılarda Sağlık* [Health in the Ottomans] (Istanbul: Biofarma, 2006), e.g., see the probate record of a fifteenth-century physician (2:21, doc. 2); the inventory of a late-eighteenth-century shop (presumably an apothecary shop) differentiated between *taş zırnıh* (most probably, realgar) and *zırnıh-ı meshuk* (most probably, orpiment) (2:344–46, doc. 773). Even though these documents do not tell us about the uses of the substance, some medicinal uses should account partially for their availability and circulation. Also see note 75 for its use for depilatory purposes.

taken not to use it in households where there were children. Instead, most people simply relied on cats to catch rats.[36]

It should not come as a surprise that most historical accounts on rats occur in contexts other than plague. We, as moderns, expect to see evidence of rat mortality in an account of plague, but the link between rats and plague was not scientifically demonstrated until the end of the nineteenth century. As we shall see later, it was not until the Third Pandemic that the Swiss-born French bacteriologist Alexandre Yersin of the Pasteur Institute successfully isolated the pathogen causing the plague and observed that rats were primary hosts for it. Following this, the French biologist Paul-Louis Simond, also of the Pasteur Institute, demonstrated that fleas were instrumental in communicating the disease from rodent hosts to humans. In the absence of a known link between plague and rats, it was not uncommon for premodern observers to see rats, and even dead rats, during a plague epidemic and not take note of it.[37] Nonetheless, we are fortunate to find such references on a few occasions. For example, one of these references comes from Byzantine Constantinople during the Black Death and may be taken as evidence for the presence of black rats in the city before the Ottoman conquest. As an eyewitness to the plague, the Byzantine historian Nicephorus Gregoras left a brief description of the epidemic in which he noted the dead rats. He wrote: "The calamity did not destroy men only, but many animals living with and domesticated by men. I speak of dogs and horses and all the species of birds, even the rats that happened to live within the walls of the houses."[38] This seems to be a clear reference to an epizootic among the black rats of the city. Even though it may be a literary motif borrowed from the ancient Greek tradition, we may nevertheless assume that it was an acute observation.[39] Another piece of evidence for rat mortality during a plague epidemic in Istanbul comes from a late-sixteenth-century traveler's account. Michael Heberer von Bretten, a southern German traveler who witnessed a plague outbreak in Istanbul in the early months of 1588, noted dead rats, horses, and dogs left lying in the alleys. He described the streets of the city

---

[36] Russell and Russell, *Natural History of Aleppo*, 2:180–81. Also see Maurits van den Boogert, *Aleppo Observed: Ottoman Syria through the Eyes of Two Scottish Doctors, Alexander and Patrick Russell* (Oxford: Oxford University Press, 2010), 164.

[37] The scarcity of references to rats in historical sources was taken by some historians as evidence for the rejection of bubonic plague as the cause of the Black Death. For an insightful criticism of these "heretical" views, see Sallares, "Ecology, Evolution, and Epidemiology," 269–70.

[38] Christos S. Bartsocas, "Two Fourteenth Century Greek Descriptions of the 'Black Death,'" *JHMAS* 21, no. 4 (1966): 395; also reprinted in John Aberth, ed., *The Black Death: The Great Mortality of 1348–1350: A Brief History with Documents* (Boston: Bedford/St. Martin's, 2005), 15–16.

[39] According to Bartsocas, rats were considered to be related to epidemics in Greek mythology. See ibid., 399.

as filthy, which he thought was the cause of the pestilence.[40] This piece of evidence not only indicates rat mortality but also suggests an overpopulation of rats, which may cause rats to leave their safe location indoors and die on the streets.

For the most part, however, the references in the historical sources are too few and too scanty to draw healthy conclusions about epizootics and to establish their links to changes in rat populations. It is generally accepted that there is a threshold, a *critical density*, of the rat population to sustain an epizootic, and that when the number of rats exceeds that threshold, epizootics occur; conversely, when populations fall below the threshold, then epizootics recede.[41] Changes in rat populations also depend on the season, which relates the seasonality of human plague to that of the breeding patterns of rats. For example, in Istanbul, the disease manifested itself in its bubonic form typically from mid-spring to late summer or early fall, owing to the particular climatic conditions that favored the reproduction of rats and their fleas. Yet these conditions suggest only indirectly that rat populations were sometimes above the critical threshold level in Ottoman cities to sustain plague epidemics. Given the limitations of our current state of knowledge on this issue, it is nearly impossible to establish a direct relationship between plague and black rats in Ottoman cities and rural areas. Neither can such a relationship be supported by the present state of the zooarcheological data at hand. Zooarcheologists caution us that because rats live by burrowing, taphonomic analysis and dating would be necessary to check its association with the historic layer under question. Therefore, to talk about the rat-plague relationship with confidence, large, multilayer samples are necessary to study population boom and depletion around the investigated time period, rather than absence-presence surveys for the period of interest.[42] It seems that until more research is done in this area, it will be difficult to relate plague to black rats in the Ottoman landscape with any confidence.

The Vectors

Even though more than eighty species of fleas are known to have the ability to transmit plague at varying degrees of efficiency, the rat flea (especially the Oriental rat flea, *Xenopsylla cheopis*) has received the greatest attention

---

[40] Johann Michael Heberer, *Aegyptiaca servitus* (Graz: Akademische Druck und Verlag-sanstalt, 1967), 303; Metin And, *16. Yüzyılda İstanbul: Kent, Saray, Günlük Yaşam* (Istanbul: Yapı Kredi Yayınları, 2009), 90.

[41] Konkola, "More Than a Coincidence?," 204–5.

[42] Based on personal communication with zooarcheologist Canan Çakırlar of the University of Groningen, the Netherlands (March 28, 2013). I would like to thank Canan Çakırlar and Scott Redford for their invaluable assistance with this issue.

in both the scientific and historical scholarship since the Third Pandemic.[43] During his investigations of the plague in India, Paul-Louis Simond noticed that fleas were the essential vectors for transmitting the disease between rats as well as from rats to humans.[44] Even though his observations and the experiments he conducted to demonstrate the role of fleas as plague vectors were initially received with skepticism in the academic community, later research confirmed his findings.[45] In the early twentieth century, the process by which X. *cheopis* transmitted the plague was clearly identified: when X. *cheopis* fed on the blood of an infected host, plague bacteria multiplied in its gut, causing a blockage in its digestive system, urging it frantically to feed again and again. When the blocked flea bit a new host to feed, it regurgitated the multiplied bacteria, which entered the blood stream of the new host. It was this process of blockage, along with other factors, that made X. *cheopis* recognizable as the champion of plague vectors.[46] Unlike most other flea species, X. *cheopis* is not host-specific, that is, it can live and feed on different species, which makes it an important link between wild and commensal rodents and between rodents and humans, as well as a critical medium of transmission locally and over long distances. Moreover, X. *cheopis* can live in off-host environments, such as in fur, woolen cloth, grain debris, dead hosts, and the soil, even while infected with Y. *pestis*.[47]

---

[43] Anisimov, Lindler, and Pier, "Intraspecific Diversity of *Yersinia pestis*"; Rebecca J. Eisen, Lars Eisen, and Kenneth L. Gage, "Studies of Vector Competency and Efficiency of North American Fleas for *Yersinia pestis*: State of the Field and Future Research Needs," *Journal of Medical Entomology* 46, no. 4 (2009): 737–44; Carmichael, "Plague Persistence in Western Europe."

[44] Simond's observations and experiments on the mechanisms of plague transmission were published in 1898. See Paul-Louis Simond, "La propagation de la peste," *Annales de l'Institut Pasteur* 12, no. 10 (1898): 625–87. The role of fleas was also simultaneously observed by the Japanese investigator Masanori Ogata of the Hygiene Institute in Tokyo. For a detailed discussion of these discoveries, see Ann G. Carmichael, "Plague, Historical," in *Encyclopedia of Microbiology*, vol. 4, ed. Moselio Schaechter, 58–72 (Oxford: Elsevier, 2009).

[45] See M. Simond, M. L. Godley, and P. D. Mouriquand, "Paul-Louis Simond and His Discovery of Plague Transmission by Rat Fleas: A Centenary," *Journal of the Royal Society of Medicine* 91, no. 2 (1998): 101–4. Later on, Paul-Louis Simond was to serve as the director of the Ottoman Bacteriology Institute in Istanbul between 1911 and 1913. See Şeref Etker, "Paul-Louis Simond ve Bakteriyolojihane-i Osmani'nin Çemberlitaş'ta açılışı (21 Eylül 1911)," *Osmanlı Bilimi Araştırmaları* 10, no. 2 (2009): 13–33.

[46] A. W. Bacot and C. J. Martin, "Observations on the Mechanism of the Transmission of Plague by Fleas," *Journal of Hygiene* 13 (Suppl. III) (1914): 423–39.

[47] Distinguishing between *fur fleas* and *nest fleas*, historian Ole Jørgen Benedictow puts forward that X. *cheopis* is a typical fur flea because of its ability to move along with its hosts. He suggests that the human flea (*P. irritans*) is a typical nest flea, which does not move along with its human hosts, nor does it remain in the clothing; instead, it prefers to nest in or near bedding. See Benedictow, *Black Death*, 19–21.

Hence, infected fleas can carry the disease from one place to another and from one season to the next.[48]

Particular environmental and climatic conditions seem to favor the survival and reproduction of fleas, as their number fluctuates by the season (lower flea density in lower temperatures and cooler season to higher density in mild temperatures or warmer season). Temperatures between 24 and 27 degrees Celsius are ideal for most epidemic activity.[49] Temperature is also important for sustaining a successful blockage in *X. cheopis* to guarantee the transmission of the infection. In their classic 1914 study, Bacot and Martin observed that infected "fleas lived as long as 50 days at from 10°C to 15°C and 23 days at 27°C, and died infected."[50] Research in tropical medicine in the 1960s and 1970s further confirmed the critical importance of temperature. For example, it was demonstrated that the transmission rate fell in infected fleas in temperatures higher than 27.5 degrees Celsius. Another experiment showed that when temperature increased from 23.5 to 29.5 degrees Celsius, clearing of the infection increased more than ten times, and blockage rates fell more than 50 percent.[51] In addition to temperature, humidity is also an important factor. Humidity greater than 40 percent is critical for the survival of fleas and flea larvae.[52] All of this has great significance for our understanding of the *seasonal signature* of plague in a given locality.

Nonetheless, the leap of the infection to humans takes place as the result of bites by fleas. Classical plague studies demonstrated that when an infected rat died, this was detected by its fleas because of the drop in the body temperature of their host, which forced them to seek other hosts. If humans are present in close proximity, then fleas bite and infect them. Most human infections take place when large numbers of rats die from an epizootic, increasing the possibility of encounters with rat carcasses and their fleas in search of new hosts. The fact that *X. cheopis* is a highly efficient vector of transmission means that its capacity to infect new hosts is very high. This also means that the number of fleas per host does not need to be high to maintain epidemic conditions. On the contrary, it has been shown that the ratio of *X. cheopis* per host can be quite low to maintain transmission cycles.[53]

Most of this body of knowledge regarding *X. cheopis* and the mechanisms by which it transmits infection to humans is drawn from the twentieth-century ecological context of South Asia. The particular model of flea-borne

---

[48] Gage and Kosoy, "Natural History of Plague," 517–18.
[49] Rebecca J. Eisen and Kenneth L. Gage, "Transmission of Flea-Borne Zoonotic Agents," *Annual Review of Entomology* 57, no. 1 (2012): 64.
[50] Bacot and Martin, "Transmission of Plague by Fleas," 437.
[51] Gage and Kosoy, "Natural History of Plague," 516.
[52] Audoin-Rouzeau, *Les chemins de la peste*, 47.
[53] Eisen and Gage, "Transmission of Flea-Borne Zoonotic Agents," 62, 69.

plague transmission as a result of blockage has long been accepted as the dominant paradigm. However, recent research has shown that transmission could take place as a result of other processes, such as mechanical or early-phase transmission. In the meantime, other flea species, such as cat fleas (*Ctenocephalides felis*), Asiatic/northern rat fleas (*Nosopsyllus fasciatus*), and human fleas (*Pulex irritans*) are recognized as vectors.[54] Likewise, the question about the ability of human ectoparasites to transmit the infection between humans has long intrigued the scientific community. On the basis of research in Morocco in the 1940s, Blanc and Baltazard posited the human (head and body) louse as a potential plague vector. Similar observations with respect to the role of human ectoparasites were made in the 1950s based on cases of plague in Iran, Syria, and Turkey, in the absence of domestic rats.[55] Even though the findings of this research remained controversial for many decades, there seems to be a renewed interest in the role of human ectoparasites in plague transmission.[56] Most recently, promising steps have been taken to investigate the role of the human louse (*Pediculus humanus*) in the transmission of plague, both in field observations and in laboratory experiments. According to this, human lice can become infected with Y. *pestis* after one blood meal from an infected host, and as few as ten lice may be sufficient to infect a new host.[57] All this reminds us that different species of fleas and lice could have worked as plague vectors in different ecological settings.

54 Gage and Kosoy, "Natural History of Plague"; Eisen and Gage, "Transmission of Flea-Borne Zoonotic Agents." For a detailed discussion of the vector capacity of different flea species, see Audoin-Rouzeau, *Les chemins de la peste*, 59–83.

55 G. Blanc and M. Baltazard, "Rôle des ectoparasites humains dans la transmission de la peste," *Bulletin de l'Académie nationale de médecine* 126 (1942): 446; M. Baltazard, "New Data in the Interhuman Transmission of Plague," *Bulletin de l'Académie nationale de médecine* 143 (1959): 517–22.

56 Benedictow, for example, is very critical of this research. See Benedictow, *Black Death*, 17–19. Alternatively, also see Michel Drancourt, Linda Houhamdi, and Didier Raoult, "*Yersinia pestis* as a Telluric, Human Ectoparasite-borne Organism," *The Lancet Infectious Diseases* 6, no. 4 (2006): 234–41. On the reception of Blanc and Baltazard's position, see Audoin-Rouzeau, *Les chemins de la peste*, 97–101.

57 Renaud Piarroux et al., "Plague Epidemics and Lice, Democratic Republic of the Congo," *Emerging Infectious Diseases* 19, no. 3 (2013): 505–6; S. Badiaga and P. Brouqui, "Human Louse–Transmitted Infectious Diseases," *Clinical Microbiology and Infection: The Official Publication of the European Society of Clinical Microbiology and Infectious Diseases* 18, no. 4 (2012): 332–37; Saravanan Ayyadurai et al., "Body Lice, *Yersinia pestis* Orientalis, and Black Death," *Emerging Infectious Diseases* 16, no. 5 (2010): 892–893 (experimentally demonstrated that only Y. *pestis* Orientalis could be transmitted via human body lice); Thi-Nguyen-Ny Tran et al., "Brief Communication: Co-detection of *Bartonella quintana* and *Yersinia pestis* in an 11th–15th Burial Site in Bondy, France," *American Journal of Physical Anthropology* 145, no. 3 (2011): 489–94; Linda Houhamdi et al., "Experimental Model to Evaluate the Human Body Louse as a Vector of Plague," *Journal of Infectious Diseases* 194, no. 11 (2006): 1589–96.

Fleas and lice were abundant in Ottoman society, as they were in other premodern societies, though it is difficult to determine exactly what species they were. Our sources do not make a clear distinction between the types of ectoparatises, even though some species were clearly known to all. As with rats, we encounter the problem of taxonomy, as both lice (head and body lice) and fleas were used as generic categories in premodern Ottoman society. For example, the term used in reference to lice (*bit*, "louse") was also used for other insects, such as bedbugs (*tahta biti*). In the absence of archeoentomological evidence, it is nearly impossible to establish what flea species lived in the Ottoman landscape. It would be tempting to assume the historical presence of X. *cheopis* in this area owing to the occurrence of their black rat hosts. However, even though it is possible to assume that this flea species arrived to the Mediterranean basin along with their rodent hosts (*R. rattus*), some scholars suggest that X. *cheopis* previously lived in the Nile Valley on other hosts and that it adapted to *R. rattus* only after the latter's arrival to the area.[58] This does not rule out the possibility that other flea and lice species were common in the Ottoman landscape, given that humans are only incidental hosts to rat fleas.

The abundance of fleas in premodern societies may be attributed to poor hygienic practices. In the absence of modern standards of hygiene, houses could be a breeding ground for rats and fleas. Especially wooden houses favored the survival of the latter, as small crevices in the wood provided the ideal niche for the survival of flea eggs; however, sources also report their abundance in stone structures. European travelers to the Ottoman Empire often complained about rats, fleas, and other pests. For example, Hans Dernschwam, who traveled with the Habsburg ambassadorial mission to the Ottoman Empire in the mid-sixteenth century, commented on the abundance of pests in the rooms of stone buildings and noted how, in the summer months, the locals ate, relaxed, and slept outdoors on the elevated patio of a caravanserai in Istanbul to avoid pests, such as insects, mice, lizards, and snakes.[59] Similarly, Salomon Schweigger, the preacher in the retinue of the Habsburg ambassador, commented on the abundance of fleas, lice, bedbugs, mice, rats, weasels, and other pests in their ambassadorial residence

---

[58] Eva Panagiotakopulu, "Pharaonic Egypt and the Origins of Plague," *Journal of Biogeography* 31, no. 2 (2004): 269–75. Paleoentomological research suggests that the historical distribution of ectoparasites does not necessarily coincide with the patterns of migration of their current hosts. For example, it is possible that human fleas (*P. irritans*) were spread via other species before they adjusted to humans. See Paul C. Buckland and Jon P. Sadler, "A Biogeography of the Human Flea, *Pulex irritans* L. (Siphonaptera: Pulicidae)," *Journal of Biogeography* 16, no. 2 (1989): 115–20. About the Egyptian origins of X. *cheopis*, also see Robert Traub, "The Fleas of Egypt: Two New Fleas of the Genus *Nosopsyllus* Jordan, 1933," *Proceedings of the Entomological Society of Washington* 65, no. 2 (1963): 96.

[59] Hans Dernschwam, *İstanbul ve Anadolu'ya Seyahat Günlüğü*, trans. Yaşar Önen (Ankara: Kültür ve Turizm Bakanlığı, 1987), 61–62.

in Istanbul in the late sixteenth century.[60] Dark houses, with no direct sunlight, favored the survival of fleas indoors; rugs and woolen bedding material made the perfect hiding place, and fur and woolen clothes provided a good shelter. Infrequent washing of clothes could preserve the fleas, even if one's body was clean.

Items of clothing were expensive and changed hands rather frequently. Sometimes family members inherited them; other times, they were sold after one's death. In Ottoman cities, secondhand clothing items were sold in the appropriately named flea markets (*bit pazarı*). Istanbul's notorious flea market and its brokers have been described by contemporary sources. For example, historian Mustafa Ali's *Cami' ü'l-buhur der mecalis-i sur* (Gatherer of the Seas in the Gatherings of the Festival) mentions these merchants (*bit pazarı halkı*) in the description of the procession of the guilds in Istanbul in 1582. He wrote elsewhere that the brokers of the flea market made at least a hundred gold pieces every year, and most more.[61] Evliya Çelebi also seems to be suspicious of their trade, as he labeled them treacherous (*ehl-i hilekar, bitbazarı*). He reports there being four hundred shops and seven hundred dealers, larger than many other groups in the textile trade.[62] The trade was a profitable one, which resisted the attempts of the Ottoman administration to regulate it in the late-sixteenth century by issuing a series of orders for that purpose. For example, a *mühimme* order of 1581 refers to an earlier prohibition of the trade within the walled area of Istanbul, which clearly was not honored.[63]

Several European observers of the Ottoman Empire believed that selling secondhand clothes in the flea markets was instrumental in spreading plague. For example, the French physician François Pouqueville (d. 1838) observed that the fur clothes of deceased plague victims, harboring *miasma*, were sold in flea markets, and the market was a plague focus.[64] A. Brayer, a French

---

[60] Salomon Schweigger, *Sultanlar Kentine Yolculuk, 1578–1581*, trans. S. Türkis Noyan (Istanbul: Kitap Yayınevi, 2004), 57. Before him, Stephan Gerlach had also written that there were scorpions, lizards, mice, and insects crawling around in the very same ambassadorial residence. Stephan Gerlach, *Türkiye Günlüğü* (Kitap Yayınevi, 2007), 1:77.

[61] Yi, *Guild Dynamics*, Appendix B, 255; Mustafa Ali, *Câmi'u'l-Buhûr Der Mecâlis-i Sûr*, ed. Ali Öztekin (Ankara: TTK, 1996), 154–55; Mustafa Ali, *Mustafā Ali's Counsel for Sultans of 1581*, ed. Andreas Tietze (Vienna: Österreichischen Akademie der Wissenschaften, 1979), 57.

[62] Evliya Çelebi, *Seyahatnâme*, 1:316; for the flea market in Edirne, see 3:241; in Tokat, 5:35. It appears that the number of shops in the flea market was much smaller in the late fifteenth century. See Çiğdem Kafescioğlu, *Constantinopolis/Istanbul: Cultural Encounter, Imperial Vision, and the Construction of the Ottoman Capital* (University Park: Penn State University Press, 2009), 40.

[63] MD 42/276/851, 27 Ca 989/June 29, 1581.

[64] François-Charles-Hugues-Laurent Pouqueville, *Voyage en Morée, à Constantinople, en Albanie, et dans plusieurs autres parties de l'Empire othoman, pendant les années 1798, 1799, 1800 et 1801* (Paris, 1805), 2:109–11.

physician who lived in Istanbul for nine years in the early nineteenth century, remarked that the secondhand clothing trade was a deadly business because the personal belongings of the deceased, including those who died of plague, accumulated in the shops of the flea market and produced "pestilential miasmas." Like Pouqueville, Brayer singled out the Jews as those who bought the items of clothing and bedding from the houses of the deceased, including plague victims. Claiming that the personal belongings of the 150,000 plague victims of the 1812 outbreak ended up in the flea market, he exclaimed, "What a focus of pestilential miasma!"[65] Likewise, Helmuth von Moltke (d. 1891), a German military officer who served as adviser for the Ottoman Empire in 1830s, commented on the role of used items of clothing and linens in spreading the plague. Moltke noted that some of these items were sold in the streets by itinerant Jewish merchants.[66] Panzac also discussed this as one of the social practices that contributed to plague's dissemination in late Ottoman society. He suggested that the circulation of cotton, wool, and fur clothing items was instrumental in spreading plague.[67]

Evliya Çelebi makes clear that having lice or fleas on one's body was accepted in Ottoman society as the norm. Not having any lice or fleas or having too many was considered inappropriate. In his travel account, he mentions peoples who had too many of them (including on their body, hair, beard, and even nose and ear hair) or those who did not have them at all. He notes that the absence of fleas and lice was commonly attributed to foul smells on one's body or to leprosy. He adds, "The louse is of delicate nature, it likes clean places, does not like the leper body."[68] This seems to be a common belief in Ottoman society, so much so that having lice could be taken as evidence that one was not a leper. The famous story of the grand vizier Rüstem Pasha's louse illustrates the case. According to the story, when Süleyman was about to marry his daughter Mihrimah off to Rüstem, he heard rumors that Rüstem suffered from leprosy. So he sent one of the court physicians to Diyarbakır, where Rüstem was a governor, to examine the latter's body and clothes. If the physician were to find a louse, then the rumors of leprosy would be proven wrong and Rüstem

---

[65] A. Brayer, *Neuf années à Constantinople, observations sur la topographie de cette capitale, l'hygiène et les mœurs de ses habitants, l'islamisme et son influence: la peste . . . les quarantaines et les lazarets . . .* (Paris: Bellizard, 1836), 2:354–56; quote on 355.

[66] Helmuth Karl Bernhard von Moltke, *Türkiye'deki Durum ve Olaylar Üzerine Mektuplar (1835–1839)* (Ankara: TTK, 1960), 89.

[67] Panzac, *La peste*, 176. Even though this seems to have provided some local circulation of the disease, it may be worth considering what species of fleas would move with used clothing. According to Benedictow, human fleas did not move with clothing, but rat fleas did. See note 47.

[68] "Kehle nâzük tabî'atdır, pâk yeri sever ve cüzâm vücûdu sevmez. Ve cüzâm ve miskîn âdemde kehle olmaz. Olmamak ve çok olmak dahi fenâdır." Evliya Çelebi, *Seyahatnâme*, 4:48; 7:303–4; quote on 304.

would be allowed to marry the princess. Upon finding a louse, the doctor confirmed that the latter was not a leper, and Süleyman let him marry his daughter.[69] As someone who speedily rose through the ranks of the Ottoman administration, Rüstem Pasha was perceived by his contemporaries with suspicion and contempt. Hence, this story circulated to emphasize that even his louse brought him good fortune (*kehle-i ikbal*). Whether true or not, the story might be taken as an indication of how common ectoparasites were in early modern Ottoman society, even among the elite.[70] Further testimony for fleas being a commonly occurring nuisance in Aleppo comes from the eighteenth-century Scottish physician Alexander Russell. According to him, it was "impossible to walk about without collecting a colony," and even bathing was "no remedy against fleas."[71]

It was not only the Ottoman urban population who suffered from ectoparasites. Fleas were as much a part of Ottoman sedentary life as they were of the nomadic, so much so that the beginning of warmer seasons, marked by a proliferation of fleas, meant that it was time to move to highland pastures (*yayla*). For Anatolian nomads (*yürük*), the winter quarters becoming flea ridden or full of vermin (*pirelendi*) marked the time to move to cooler temperatures.[72] For example, Dernschwam noted, while traveling to Amasya in the early days of April 1555, that the seminomadic pastoralists of Anatolia were busy leaving their residences in low-lying villages to move to the mountains for the summer months. This move, he claimed, was mainly to avoid fleas and other pests that bred in their houses over the summer months.[73]

When fleas and lice were so abundant, people often had to delouse themselves or each other. This could be done simply by hand. A more radical solution against lice and flea infestation was to shave off hair and beard completely, a practice reserved for slaves in Ottoman society for the most part.[74] Depilating body hair, however, was common both among men and women because it was believed to prevent such infestations.[75] Also, fragrant

---

69 Mustafa Ali, *Künhü'l-ahbâr: dördüncü rükn, Osmanlı tarihi* (Ankara: TTK, 2009), 358b. For rumors about Rüstem's indisposition, also see Bernardo Navagero, "Relazione dell'impero ottomano del clarissimo Bernardo Navagero stato Bailo a Costantinopoli fatta in pregadi nel mese di febbraio de 1553," in *Relazioni degli ambasciatori Veneti al Senato*, series III, ed. Eugenio Albèri (Florence, 1840), 1:99. I am grateful to Zahit Atcıl for his help on the stories of Rüstem Pasha's louse.

70 For an account of how common ectoparasites were among the members of European nobility in the same era, see Audoin-Rouzeau, *Les chemins de la peste*, 242–43.

71 Russell and Russell, *Natural History of Aleppo*, 2:225–26.

72 Fernand Braudel, *The Mediterranean and the Mediterranean World in the Age of Philip II* (Berkeley: University of California Press, 1995), 1:97.

73 Dernschwam, *Seyahat Günlüğü*, 265, 298, 300–302; for the same in the Balkans, 337, 342.

74 Gerlach, *Türkiye Günlüğü*, 2:794; Schweigger, *Sultanlar Kentine Yolculuk*, 109.

75 Brayer, *Neuf années à Constantinople*, 1:162. In the mid-sixteenth century, Dernschwam described the use of a powder in the bathhouses for depilatory purposes. According to his

oils (or grease) could be used for repelling fleas and lice. For example, Evliya Çelebi mentions the use of clarified butter (*say yağı*) by locals of the Nile Valley, who rubbed it on their bodies.[76] Some essential oils were much praised in plague treatises because they were believed to clear the miasma and keep plague away, without any mention of their flea-repellent properties. For example, the sixteenth-century Sephardic convert physician İlyas bin İbrahim recommended the use of almond oil and violet oil to preserve health in times of plague, as well as chamomile oil and rose oil in preparing ointments for the treatment of plague buboes.[77]

Similar to the case with rats, the connection between plague and fleas and lice was not noted by premodern observers. In the absence of knowledge of plague vectors, even when an association was observed, the authors did not think of a causal relationship; rather, they attributed the association to larger natural or supernatural factors. This is perhaps most remarkably illustrated in the case of William Quacquelben, the physician in the Habsburg ambassadorial mission to the Ottoman Empire in the mid-sixteenth century. On account of his doctor's death of plague, the Habsburg ambassador Busbecq mentioned the discovery of fleabites on the former's body, which was soon followed by death. He wrote, "He [William Quacquelben] himself noticed on his body, when it was stripped, a purple spot, which they declared was a flea-bite. However, seeing more and larger spots, he exclaimed, 'These are no flea-bites, but a warning that death is at hand.'"[78] Neither the physician himself, nor anyone else suspected that the fleabites had anything to do with his affliction. A similar example comes from Evliya Çelebi, who noted the absence of plague in places where he also noted the absence of rats and fleas, though making nothing of the connection. Rather, he attributed their absence to the power of spells or talismans, as we have seen earlier. The eighteenth-century Scottish physicians Alexander and Patrick Russell also observed fleabites on the bodies of plague patients in Aleppo but failed to make the connection.[79] By the same token, later accounts of Pouqueville and

account, one unit of *zırnık* was to be mixed with two units of quicklime and with water into a thick paste. This paste was to be applied to the skin where unwanted hair grew and washed away with water shortly afterward. For this purpose either the black or the yellow *zırnık* was used, which could be found everywhere in Istanbul. See Dernschwam, *Seyahat Günlüğü*, 80–81, 185–86. Schweigger also mentioned that both men and women in Istanbul used a powder in bathhouses to rid themselves of body hair. See Schweigger, *Sultanlar Kentine Yolculuk*, 131.

[76] Evliya Çelebi, *Seyahatnâme*, 10:435.
[77] İlyas bin İbrahim, *Majannah al-ta'un wa al-waba'*. Süleymaniye Library, ms. Esad Efendi 2484/3, 28–42ff.; İlyas, *Tevfikatü'l-hamidiyye fi def'i'l-emrazi'l-veba'iyye*, trans. Ahmedü'ş-Şami Ömeri, Istanbul University Cerrahpaşa History of Medicine Library, ms. 105, 42, 45–47.
[78] Ogier Ghiselin de Busbecq, *The Turkish Letters of Ogier Ghiselin de Busbecq* (Baton Rouge: Louisiana State University Press, 2005), 185.
[79] van den Boogert, *Aleppo Observed*, 166.

Brayer attributed plague etiology to climatic and environmental factors. In the absence of the knowledge of vectors, Brayer comes close to identifying the problem by talking about the trade of secondhand clothes and other personal items of plague victims being a channel for the distribution of the disease, not only locally but also over long distances.[80] As for Pouqueville, he dismisses all evidence believed by locals to be signs of plague outbreaks. Among them, he mentions epizootics that took place concurrently, insects, and the presence of oil stains on walls (clear reference to traces left behind by rats), but dismisses them all.[81]

As a final point, some animals could have served a secondary role as transitory hosts to vectors, that is, plague-infected fleas. These can be wild or commensal rodents or other mammals that can transmit the disease. In particular, the role of carnivores, such as hyenas and weasels, feeding on infested rodents may be taken into consideration in this process.[82] For example, the Habsburg ambassador Busbecq mentioned hyenas that dug up human bodies from graves in sixteenth-century Anatolia and noted that people placed heavy stones on top of graves to protect them from hyenas.[83] Similarly, the fifteenth-century account of Pero Tafur commented on the abundance of weasels in Damietta both in the streets and in the houses.[84] More or less limited to local transmission, such activities would take place alongside other means of transmission and thus may be difficult to trace. However, one type of such transitory host deserves more careful consideration because of its potential to transmit the disease over long distances and cause metastatic leaps. Predator birds that fed on dead rodents, especially migratory birds, may be significant in the dissemination of infected fleas.[85] Sixteenth-century Ottoman plague treatises loosely observed a connection between the behavior of migratory birds and epidemics. For example, İlyas bin İbrahim mentioned that outbreaks of disease were preceded by certain environmental events, including the flight of certain animals and birds.[86] For some, the arrival of migratory birds, especially the white stork, was seen as a sign of a coming plague. The sixteenth-century theologian and biographer Ahmed Taşköprizade (d. 1561) mentions this in his comprehensive plague treatise. The appearance of certain species of insects and animals, such as

---

[80] Brayer, *Neuf années à Constantinople*, 2:354–56.
[81] Pouqueville, *Voyage en Morée*, 1:408.
[82] Ruth I. Meserve, "Striped Hyenas and 'Were-Hyenas' in Central Eurasia," in *Archivum Eurasiae Medii Aevi*, ed. T. T. Allsen, P. B. Golden, R. K. Kovalev, and A. P. Martinez (Wiesbaden: Harrassowitz, 2012), 199–220. I am grateful to Ann G. Carmichael for bringing this piece to my attention.
[83] Busbecq, *Turkish Letters*, 48–49.
[84] Pero Tafur, *Travels and Adventures, 1435–1439*, ed. Malcolm Letts (New York: Harper, 1926), 68.
[85] Benedictow, *Black Death*, 47.
[86] *Tevfikāt*, 28.

the white stork, was considered, according to Taşköprizade, as a precursor of plague.[87] This association between the arrival of migratory birds and that of the plague may have been based on coincidental seasonality, in the absence of knowledge about plague vectors. White storks (*Ciconia ciconia*) are predatory birds that feed on insects as well as small rodents, such as voles and possibly rats. Some of the practices of the white stork, such as feeding at garbage dumps and nesting at roofs, poles, and straw stacks, make them a prime candidate for carrying diseases.[88] Research has shown their role in carrying and spreading diseases, such as the West Nile virus.[89] It is suggested that migratory birds can be a factor in disseminating fleas infected by plague.[90] Interestingly, the migratory route followed by the white stork, from Europe to southeast Africa, crisscrossed the Ottoman lands from northwest to southeast and largely corresponded to the pilgrimage route in the eastern Mediterranean before crossing over the Sinai Peninsula to Egypt, Sudan, and farther south into Africa.[91] This trajectory also corresponded, as we shall we, with one of the major trade routes of the empire, and not surprisingly with one of the plague routes as well.[92]

The Pathogen

The pathogen causing plague is *Yersinia pestis*, a gram-negative bacillus that belongs to the group of enteric bacteria – the kind of pathogens that develop in the intestines of a host organism and spread through contaminated food

---

[87]   Ahmed Taşköprizade, *Risalah al-shifa' li-adwa' al-waba'* ([Cairo]: al-Matbaʻah al-Wahbiyah, 1875); Süheyl Ünver, "Türkiye'de veba tarihçesi üzerine," *Tedavi Kliniği ve Laboratuvarı Mecmuası* 5 (1935): 70–71.

[88]   Willem van den Bossche, Peter Berthold, Michael Kaatz, Eugeniusz Nowak, and Ulrich Querner, *Eastern European White Stork Populations: Migration Studies and Elaboration of Conservation Measures* (Bonn: Bundesamt für Naturschutz (BfN)/German Federal Agency for Nature Conservation, 2002); Zdenek Hubálek, "An Annotated Checklist of Pathogenic Microorganisms Associated with Migratory Birds," *Journal of Wildlife Diseases* 40, no. 4 (2004): 639–59.

[89]   Mertyn Malkinson et al., "Intercontinental Transmission of West Nile Virus by Migrating White Storks," *Emerging Infectious Diseases* 7, no. 3(suppl.) (2001): 540; Mertyn Malkinson et al., "Introduction of West Nile Virus in the Middle East by Migrating White Storks," *Emerging Infectious Diseases* 8, no. 4 (2002): 392–97.

[90]   Lise Heier et al., "Emergence, Spread, Persistence and Fade-out of Sylvatic Plague in Kazakhstan," *Proceedings of the Royal Society, Series B* 278, no. 1720 (2011): 2915–23.

[91]   van den Bossche et al., *Eastern European White Stork Populations*. Incidentally, this migratory route went right over Istanbul, across the Bosphorus. Historical sources sometimes mention the sight of flocks of storks. For example, Dernschwam noted seeing flocks of thousands of storks near Edirne ([August 19, 1553]). See Dernschwam, *Seyahat Günlüğü*, 44.

[92]   For a discussion of the implications of transitory hosts of vectors, such as hyenas and white storks, to the spread of plague in the Ottoman context, see my "New Science and Old Sources," 213–16.

and water – though *Y. pestis* is quite atypical in its choice of host environment (blood) and the method of transmission (vector borne). Our knowledge of this pathogen is about 120 years old, even though it has been around for at least fifteen hundred years, and quite likely much longer. *Y. pestis* was first isolated in 1894 by Alexandre Yersin in Hong Kong during the Third Pandemic.[93] For most of the twentieth century, the body of scientific knowledge on the pathogen (*Pasteurella pestis*, later recognized as *Y. pestis*) came from scientific observations drawn from South Asia. However, the last decade witnessed revolutionary changes in *Y. pestis* research. The recent work of geneticists, especially from the perspective of evolutionary biology, has improved our understanding of this pathogen considerably. For example, we now know that *Y. pestis* did not exist from time immemorial, as it was once believed, but that it evolved from *Y. pseudotuberculosis*, another enteric bacterium, about fifteen hundred to twenty thousand years ago.[94] Hence, it is considered to be a young bacterium, with surprisingly limited genetic diversity, which makes it a model organism for studying bacterial virulence.

This new understanding of the recent evolution of the bacterium triggered further research efforts in the scientific community, resulting in the sequencing of the genome of *Y. pestis* for the first time. In 2001, a group of English scientists declared the triumphant significance of their effort as follows: "*Y. pestis* is a pathogen that has undergone large-scale genetic flux and provides a unique insight into the ways in which new and highly virulent pathogens evolve."[95] Continued efforts of biological archeologists and geneticists culminated ten years later in the reconstruction of the full genome of *Y. pestis* entirely from aDNA recovered from the remains of fourteenth-century plague victims buried in East Smithfield Cemetery in London.[96] Both molecular archeology and genetics research have contributed massively to our understanding of the evolutionary history of the pathogen and its adaptations to different environments. Every time *Y. pestis* acquires new genes

---

[93] Alexandre Yersin, "La peste bubonique à Hong-Kong," *Annales de l'Institut Pasteur* 8 (1894): 662–67. A near-simultaneous discovery was realized by the Japanese physician and bacteriologist Shibasaburo Kitasato, a former student of Robert Koch.

[94] Mark Achtman et al., "*Yersinia pestis*, the Cause of Plague, Is a Recently Emerged Clone of *Yersinia pseudotuberculosis*," *PNAS* 96, no. 24 (1999): 14043–48. More recent estimates project a slightly older date for the evolution of *Y. pestis*, e.g., see Yanjun Li et al., "Genotyping and Phylogenetic Analysis of *Yersinia pestis* by MLVA: Insights into the Worldwide Expansion of Central Asia Plague Foci," *PLoS ONE* 4, no. 6 (2009): e6000; Yujun Cui et al., "Historical Variations in Mutation Rate in an Epidemic Pathogen, *Yersinia pestis*," *PNAS* 110, no. 2 (2013): 577–82.

[95] J. Parkhill et al., "Genome Sequence of *Yersinia pestis*, the Causative Agent of Plague," *Nature* 413, no. 6855 (2001): 523–27, quote on 523.

[96] Kirsten I. Bos et al., "A Draft Genome of *Yersinia pestis* from Victims of the Black Death," *Nature* 478, no. 7370 (2011): 506–10.

and loses others, these changes indicate important genetic events in its environment, host susceptibility, or vector dynamics. It was demonstrated, for example, that at some point during its evolution, *Y. pestis* adapted to the flea environment and began to be transmitted by fleas efficiently.[97] This meant that *Y. pestis* first acquired the critical ability to colonize the flea so as to be transmitted as a flea-borne septicemic disease of limited transmissibility. From the vantage point of the bacterium, this transition would diminish its evolutionary chances of survival. It was only later, as a result of the acquisition of new genes, that *Y. pestis* obtained the bubonic form and hence increased its capacity for epidemic spread.[98] Questions of the bacterium's evolutionary history were accompanied by questions of its origin. Even though where *Y. pestis* first originated exactly is still contentious, most recent research suggests its origins to be "in or near the Qinghai-Tibet Plateau," followed by its distribution to other areas as a result of rodent and human migration and travel.[99] Historically, this spread is believed to have taken place across three pandemics.[100]

In the mid-twentieth century, it was proposed that *Y. pestis* had three biovars or biotypes (Antiqua, Medievalis, and Orientalis), assumed to have caused the First, Second, and Third pandemic, respectively.[101] This typology – which was produced on the basis of the bacillus's nutritional properties, more specifically, its ability to ferment glycerol and reduce nitrate – was widely accepted in the scientific community and remained as the dominant paradigm of its classification until recently. In this scheme, the evolutionary context of these differences between *Y. pestis* biovars went largely unnoticed.[102] New research grew critical with this typology and taxonomy of *Y. pestis* on grounds that the differentiation of the three biotypes could

---

[97] Unlike *Y. pestis*, *Y. pseudotuberculosis* is orally toxic to fleas, which suggests evolutionary changes between the pathogen and the vector. David L. Erickson et al., "Acute Oral Toxicity of *Yersinia pseudotuberculosis* to Fleas: Implications for the Evolution of Vector-borne Transmission of Plague," *Cellular Microbiology* 9, no. 11 (2007): 2658–66; B. J. Hinnebusch, "The Evolution of Flea-Borne Transmission in *Yersinia pestis*," *Current Issues in Molecular Biology* 7 (2005): 197–212.

[98] Florent Sebbane et al., "Role of the *Yersinia pestis* Plasminogen Activator in the Incidence of Distinct Septicemic and Bubonic Forms of Flea-borne Plague," *PNAS* 103, no. 14 (2006): 5526–30.

[99] Cui et al., "Historical Variations."

[100] For the periodization of plague pandemics, see the introduction.

[101] R. Devignat, "Variétés de l'espèce *Pasteurella pestis*: nouvelle hypothèse," *Bulletin of the World Health Organization* 4, no. 2 (1951): 247–63.

[102] An exception to this was John Norris's suggestion that adaptation to different rodent species may have been responsible for biochemical differences of *Y. pestis* biovars. See Norris, "East or West? The Geographic Origin of the Black Death," *Bulletin of the History of Medicine* 51, no. 1 (1977): 22–24. This point is also highlighted in George D. Sussman, "Was the Black Death in India and China?," *Bulletin of the History of Medicine* 85, no. 3 (2011): 331.

not be translated into genetic changes in the pathogen's history. In a pioneering article that came out in 2004, an international group of researchers rejected the use of biovars for evolutionary or taxonomic purposes. Instead, they proposed that *Y. pestis* be subdivided into populations based on molecular groupings.[103] Even though some early efforts within the scientific community tried to refute the hypothesis of matching the three biovars with the three pandemics,[104] the methods used were not accepted as sound.[105] Because of the limited pool of modern *Y. pestis* strains (most isolated in the second half of the twentieth century) and even a smaller sample of aDNA fragments, the scientific community had to wait for more aDNA evidence from past pandemics and for better means of analysis before an association between modern molecular groupings and premodern pandemics could be confidently advanced.[106] More robust studies, using a much greater pool of *Y. pestis* isolates and more rigorous methods of analysis, only started to come about toward the end of the decade. Hence, in 2009, an international team of researchers firmly rejected the position that the Orientalis biovar could have been responsible for all three pandemics.[107] This was followed, the next year, by another authoritative phylogenetic study based on a broad spectrum of *Y. pestis* aDNA recovered from plague pits throughout Europe (dated to the Black Death and its successive waves). This team declared, "The strains causing mass deaths were unrelated to either Medievalis or Orientalis biovars."[108] The scientific community seemed to have left behind the use of biovars for purposes of taxonomic and genetic classification.

Questions of transmission also seem to have benefited from phylogenetic methods. A nuanced analysis of variations in *Y. pestis*'s evolution may offer invaluable insights for historical pandemics. The evolution of *Y. pestis* in times of epidemics and epizootics seems to be much faster than in enzootic periods of inactivity because of the higher rates of bacterial replication involved. This means that demographic changes can affect the pathogen's speed of evolution, which has tremendous implications for understanding

---

[103] Mark Achtman et al., "Microevolution and History of the Plague Bacillus, *Yersinia pestis*," *PNAS* 101, no. 51 (2004): 17837–42.

[104] Michel Drancourt et al., "Genotyping, Orientalis-like *Yersinia pestis*, and Plague Pandemics," *Emerging Infectious Diseases* 10, no. 9 (2004): 1585–92.

[105] For a summary account of why this finding was criticized and how it was refuted, see Michaela Harbeck et al., "*Yersinia pestis* DNA from Skeletal Remains from the 6th Century AD Reveals Insights into Justinianic Plague," *PLoS Pathogens* 9, no. 5 (2013): e1003349.

[106] In 2007, some French researchers triumphantly announced that all three historical pandemics were caused by the Orientalis biovar. See Michel Drancourt et al., "*Yersinia pestis* Orientalis in Remains of Ancient Plague Patients," *Emerging Infectious Diseases* 13, no. 2 (2007): 332–33. This was once again followed by a round of stern criticism. See Harbeck et al., "*Yersinia pestis* DNA from Skeletal Remains."

[107] Li et al., "Genotyping and Phylogenetic Analysis of *Yersinia pestis* by MLVA."

[108] Stephanie Haensch et al., "Distinct Clones of *Yersinia pestis* Caused the Black Death," *PLoS Pathogens* 6, no. 10 (2010): e1001134; quote on 2.

historical pandemics. It follows that a greater number of hosts would mean a faster rate of bacterial replication and thus would imply the possibility of faster evolution. In other words, large colonies of ground-burrowing or commensal rodents or, alternatively, crowded urban areas might have been instrumental in the process of the emergence of different *Y. pestis* populations and lineages. In fact, researchers suspect that this is exactly what happened during the Black Death. Nonetheless, they do not rule out the involvement of other factors, such as variations in host density, that may result from climatic and environmental changes.[109]

Biologists caution us that more than one strain of a pathogen might be at work in a given epidemic or pandemic. They argue that "at least two related but distinct genotypes of *Y. pestis* were responsible for the Black Death and suggest that distinct bacterial populations spread throughout Europe in the 14th century."[110] Another team of researchers further supported this conclusion by demonstrating that several *Y. pestis* genotypes circulated in medieval Europe.[111] The fact that distinct bacterial populations were circulating in a given epidemic may suggest that these distinct entities came from different places, along different routes, and/or at different times.

Scientific studies in plague research continue at full pace. What has become clear is that the implications of this new body of scholarship for studying past pandemics can no longer be ignored by historians. Tracing the movements of different populations of *Y. pestis* and correlating them to different historical periods has tremendous implications for the temporal and spatial identification of *Y. pestis* in the historical study of plague pandemics. Thus, genetic changes of the pathogen serve as markers of temporal and spatial spread of historical pandemics. In the light of this body of research and its implications, it should be possible to make new historical suggestions. Nevertheless, despite the vast array of research on *Y. pestis* and the many questions addressed by plague scientists, it is still difficult to nail down some of our immediate historical questions. For example, were the Ottoman areas visited by the same strain of *Y. pestis* as those in other parts of Eurasia? How many different strains of the bacterium circulated in the Ottoman Empire throughout the early modern era? Which plague foci were the source of these strains in this era? Answers to these questions require collaboration between bioarcheologists and geneticists. Currently no archeological dig from the Ottoman period has aimed to find evidence of *Y. pestis* in the aDNA of the remains of suspected plague victims. We can only hope for such evidence to be revealed in the future. For now, we are not in a position to answer most of these questions with clarity. Nevertheless, the evidence drawn from digs in Europe may shed some light

[109] Cui et al., "Historical Variations."
[110] Haensch et al., "Distinct Clones of *Yersinia pestis*," 4.
[111] Tran et al., "Brief Communication."

on our concerns, especially when combined with the available historical evidence.[112]

Alternatively, it is also possible to draw from modern Y. pestis isolates that were collected from former Ottoman areas (including Turkey, northern Iraq, and western Iran) and included in recent phylogenetic analyses. These studies shed some light on where these strains originated with respect to the evolutionary subdivisions of Y. pestis.[113] An article published in Turkey in 1952 presented four Y. pestis isolates that were preserved in Refik Saydam Institute in Ankara, three of which were defined as biotype Orientalis.[114] Of the four isolates, three were not clearly identified as to when or where they were isolated. The authors believe they were isolated in Istanbul and Antalya. One isolate was known to have been isolated in a human case of plague in the Akçakale (Urfa) outbreak of 1947. This was a small outbreak of plague – in February and March, a total of thirteen deaths took place out of a total of eighteen cases affected – in two Turkish villages on the Syrian border where bubonic cases were identified. In the absence of recent plague outbreaks in Turkish port cities prior to it, this outbreak puzzled the authors, who personally observed the epidemic in the field. The presence of an excess of number of fleas was reported in the dwellings, which the authors believed was responsible for transmitting the disease from person to person. Where the epidemic took place, house mice were observed in great numbers, but not a single rat was found, which led the authors to believe that humans were accidentally infected by a plague of sylvatic character.[115] The 1947 outbreak appears to be the last recorded outbreak of plague in Turkey, with no record of further human cases.

Humans

Despite being only accidental hosts to plague, humans have been perhaps the most important of all protagonists in shaping the natural history of this disease. How did human agency make a difference in spreading or containing

---

[112] For a more detailed discussion of the growing imbalance between the "new science" and the historical sources in the study of plague in the Ottoman Empire, see my "New Science and Old Sources."

[113] 2.MED1, isolated from this region, evolved more than 235 years ago (in 2010), which places it before 1775, i.e., before the Third Pandemic. Similarly, 1.ORI3 is thought to have come from Madagascar during the Third Pandemic, most probably via the pilgrimage route. See Giovanna Morelli et al., "Yersinia pestis Genome Sequencing Identifies Patterns of Global Phylogenetic Diversity," Nature Genetics 42, no. 12 (2010): 1140–43.

[114] Bilal Golem and Kemal Özsan, "Türk Veba Suşlarında Biyoşimik Karakter Farkları," Türk İjiyen ve Tecrübi Biyoloji Dergisi 12, no. 1 (1952): 29–51.

[115] The same observation regarding the absolute absence of rats in the area was further confirmed in 1955 by Xavier Misonne. Xavier Misonne, "Mammifères de la Turquie sud-orientale et du nord de la Syrie," 53–68.

the disease or in changing its course?[116] The human actors come into play in different capacities. For example, as hosts to plague, infected individuals can directly infect other human beings, which is known to happen in the pneumonic form of the disease. Humans can also alter the course of an epidemic by efforts at controlling, containing, and now treating the disease (with antibiotics). However, most important, humans can (inadvertently) facilitate the movement of plague hosts and vectors beyond the natural abilities of these agents and carry the disease over long distances as a result of their own movements. Hence, they provide enhanced means of mobility to plague hosts and vectors that have limited ability to move. In other words, the long distance spread of *Y. pestis* is mostly owed to human agency in moving infected rodents and/or vectors from one place to another. This could happen in different forms and through varying activities involved in human mobility, such as travel, migration, or transportation of goods. As we shall see in more detail, all of these human activities have contributed to circulating the plague within the Ottoman domains and beyond.

Among various forms of mobility, warfare is long known to affect the spread of epidemics, perhaps must notably in the dissemination of the plague out of the Genoese colony of Caffa at Crimea, besieged by a Mongol army in 1346.[117] Warfare certainly contributed to both the local and long-distance spread of the disease. The movement of large numbers of people, close army encampments, and the lack of hygienic conditions have been associated with outbreaks since the ancient period and elaborated in the *miasma* paradigm. According to this paradigm, the stench and putrid vapors rising from rotting corpses of soldiers fallen dead on the battlefield could contaminate the air and produce miasma, considered to be the cause of epidemics.

As we shall see in greater detail in Part II, we do not lack examples in late medieval and early modern Ottoman history to link the spread of plague to warfare. The fourteenth through seventeenth centuries were marked by intense military activity in Ottoman history, in which massive territorial expansion took place, accompanied by the simultaneous expansion of plague. Some military practices used by the Ottomans, such as digging

---

[116] For a comprehensive overview of the human experience with epidemic infectious diseases, including the plague, see Ann G. Carmichael, "Infectious Disease and Human Agency: An Historical Overview," in *Interactions between Global Change and Human Health*, 3–46 (Vatican City: Pontificia Academia Scientiarum, 2006).

[117] Friedrich Prinzing, *Epidemics Resulting from Wars* (Oxford: Clarendon Press, 1916). Even though the Italian chroniclers of the Black Death have claimed that the disease was transmitted to the Genoese as a result of the plague corpses being catapulted and thrown at them, modern epidemiological knowledge does not support such a method of transmission. Instead, it has been proposed that infected rodents from the army encampments must have found their way of introducing the infection to the commensal rodents of the town. For a detailed analysis for why the catapulting story does not work, see Benedictow, *Black Death*, 52–53.

underground tunnels during sieges, may have added the additional risk of exposing soldiers to rodents' burrows and possibly to the pathogen kept alive in the soil or in the dead tissues of rodents. The zigzagging underground tunnels the Ottomans used for sieges were fittingly known as *sıçan yolları* (rat tunnels).[118]

Other forms of human mobilities may be worth considering in this context. Among them, pilgrimage involved the movement of large numbers of people across long distances. Even though we do not know the precise number of people traveling to and from the Muslim holy cities of Mecca and Medina every year, the figures were significant enough in premodern standards of long-distance travel. Pilgrims who sometimes traveled and camped in poor hygienic conditions were also prime candidates for local outbreaks and to some extent can be associated with the movement of diseases. This is especially significant for the era of focus here. As we shall see, when the Ottomans took over the pilgrimage routes, they took measures to improve the safety of the journey, which resulted in an even greater number of pilgrims.[119]

Migration constituted another such form of human mobility in Ottoman society. *Sürgün* and *şenlendirme*, policies of resettlement used by the

---

[118] Even though there is no direct bioarcheological evidence at hand to support this from the Ottoman areas, it may be possible to draw analogies from studies conducted elsewhere. For example, recent research has confirmed cases of coinfection of louse-borne trench fever (*Bartonella quintana*) and plague (*Y. pestis*) in a late medieval mass burial site in France. See Tran et al., "Brief Communication." For associations to epidemic typhus (*Rickettsia prowazekii*) and other louse-borne infections, see Didier Raoult et al., "Evidence for Louse-Transmitted Diseases in Soldiers of Napoleon's Grand Army in Vilnius," *Journal of Infectious Diseases* 193, no. 1 (2006): 112–20; Tung Nguyen-Hieu et al., "Evidence of a Louse-Borne Outbreak Involving Typhus in Douai, 1710–1712 during the War of Spanish Succession," *PLoS ONE* 5, no. 10 (2010): e15405. Considering the louse-borne nature of these infections and evidence for their occurrence, especially in soldiers, it should be possible to seek further links to occurrences of plague. For plague transmission via lice, also see note 57. Given the notorious threat of epidemic typhus in Hungary – known as *morbus hungaricus* – in the early modern era, especially for soldiers, there may be further reason to explore such links. See Gábor Ágoston, "Where Environmental and Frontier Studies Meet: Rivers, Forests, Marshes and Forts along the Ottoman–Hapsburg Frontier in Hungary," in *The Frontiers of the Ottoman World*, ed. A. C. S. Peacock (Oxford: Oxford University Press, 2009), 78.

[119] Ottoman pilgrimage routes are explored in conjunction with plague in Chapter 5. Bruce Masters, "Hajj," in *Encyclopedia of the Ottoman Empire*, ed. Gábor Ágoston and Bruce Alan Masters, 246–48 (New York: Facts on File, 2009); Suraiya Faroqhi, *Pilgrims and Sultans: The Hajj under the Ottomans, 1517–1683* (London: I. B. Tauris, 1994). Also see Richard Blackburn, ed. and trans., *Journey to the Sublime Porte: The Arabic Memoir of a Sharifian Agent's Diplomatic Mission to the Ottoman Imperial Court in the Era of Suleyman the Magnificent* (Beirut: Orient-Institut, 2005). The connection between pilgrimage and epidemic diseases has been better explored for the late Ottoman era. See, e.g., Michael Christopher Low, "Empire and the Hajj: Pilgrims, Plagues, and Pan-Islam under British Surveillance, 1865–1908," *IJMES* 40, no. 2 (2008): 269–90.

Ottoman administration involving forced relocation of entire populations, were most rigorously pursued by Mehmed II (r. 1451–81) as a tool of demographic engineering. These policies were sometimes used to secure underpopulated frontier areas. It was also at times an important concern for Ottoman rule to populate newly conquered areas by Muslim subjects or to relocate the landed aristocracy of a conquered area to limit their power.[120] Even though this was an older practice used by the Byzantines for repopulating imperial domains, and most significantly enforced in the wake of epidemic outbreaks, the Ottomans have pursued such policies thoroughly.[121] As such, population policies intimately linked demographic losses caused by plague in the cities to those of their hinterlands.

The policies of forced migration were also accompanied by voluntary immigration, which constantly increased the Ottoman urban population, most prominently in the sixteenth century. Generally speaking, the fifteenth and sixteenth centuries witnessed the rise and development of many new urban clusters throughout the Ottoman realm. The process of urbanization, however slow in the beginning, took a definitive character in the sixteenth century, when several villages in Anatolia grew into new towns and undistinguished cities developed into thriving metropolises.[122] Such urban clusters with dense populations where people lived in close proximity provided the best environment for the local and regional spread of diseases. As we shall see in greater detail, there was an intimate link between the intensification of urbanization and plague epidemics in early modern Ottoman history.[123]

Moreover, there were mass population movements in this period. For example, an estimated fifteen thousand to twenty thousand Iberian Jews

120 See e.g., Halil İnalcık, *An Economic and Social History of the Ottoman Empire. Vol. I: 1300–1600* (Cambridge: Cambridge Univerity Press, 1994), 167–71; Cengiz Orhonlu, *Osmanlı İmparatorluğu'nda Aşiretlerin İskanı* (Istanbul: Eren, 1987); İbrabim Solak, "Anadolu'da Nüfus Hareketleri ve Osmanlı Devleti'nin İskan Politikası," *Türk Dünyası Araştırmaları* 127 (2000): 157–92.

121 Following an epidemic, in 754–55 CE, large numbers of people from the Greek peninsula and islands and the Peloponnese were sent to the capital to repopulate it. See Stathakopoulos, *Famine and Pestilence*, 385. Cf. Kritovolus's description of Mehmed's policy of population management in *History of Mehmed the Conqueror* (Princeton, NJ: Princeton University Press, 1954).

122 For the rise and development of urban centers in the sixteenth century, see Suraiya Faroqhi, *Towns and Townsmen of Ottoman Anatolia: Trade, Crafts and Food Production in an Urban Setting, 1520–1650* (Cambridge: Cambridge University Press, 1984); Ronald C. Jennings, "Urban Population in Anatolia in the Sixteenth Century: A Study of Kayseri, Karaman, Amasya, Trabzon, and Erzurum," *IJMES* 7, no. 1 (1976): 21–57.

123 This connection is more thoroughly explored in Chapter 4, in the examples of Bursa, Edirne, and Istanbul in the fifteenth and sixteenth centuries. In Europe, it has been observed that certain professionals, such as bakers, butchers, leather/tannery workers, and artisans handling fabric and paper, were at greater risk of infection at times of plague. See Audoin-Rouzeau, *Les chemins de la peste*, 233–38.

arrived in Ottoman lands toward the end of the fifteenth century.[124] Similarly, seasonal migration of various communities should be taken into account. Pastoralist nomads of Anatolia and the Balkans moved between their summer pastures and winter encampments, between highlands and lowlands. Seasonal workers sought employment in other places. As much as it is difficult to quantify these movements, the seasonality and trajectories of such movements can be established in the sources.[125] In addition to these forms of movement and migration, it should be possible to add the travel of couriers, administrators, officials, and so on. As Ottoman power grew and expanded, and centralization took hold, a growing number of officials were appointed to different locations, where they traveled with their staffs and households. When one takes into account that these officials held appointments for short durations, the number of people who traveled on state duty alone seems to add up to a substantial figure.[126]

Among all forms of human mobility, trade and the transportation of goods are perhaps the most significant. Trade made it possible for people, rats, and fleas to move over considerable distances. Maritime trade in this period was of tremendous importance. Ships were known to transport rats in addition to humans and cargo. A sixteenth-century testimony makes clear that this was known and that precautions were taken against these unwelcome passengers accordingly. Salomon Schweigger wrote that the Ottomans had the habit of carrying weasels or cats on board ships expressly for the purpose of "rat control."[127] Even though all forms of trade could facilitate the metastatic growth of the disease, maritime trade was ideal because of its greater pace and the possibility for rats to travel along in vessels. For example, grain trade almost guaranteed the movement of plague. Grain warehouses attracted rats and provided a suitable habitat in which fleas could live. Shipping grain would almost guarantee shipping rats and fleas along with it.[128] Like grain, other trade items, such as wool, woolen cloths,

[124] Benjamin Braude, "The Rise and Fall of Salonica Woollens, 1500–1650: Technology Transfer and Western Competition," *Mediterranean Historical Review* 6, no. 2 (1991): 218.

[125] For a detailed discussion of the connections between plague and higher altitudes, as well the implications of this research on the movement of pastoralist nomads in the Ottoman landscape, see Chapter 3.

[126] For the growing number of appointees in the Ottoman system of provincial administration, the short term of service, considerable retinues and soldiers, and continuous reshuffling, the classic study is Metin I. Kunt, *The Sultan's Servants: The Transformation of Ottoman Provincial Government, 1550–1650* (New York: Columbia University Press, 1983). More recently, a concise overview of provincial administration was offered in Colin Imber, *The Ottoman Empire, 1300–1650: The Structure of Power* (Houndmills, UK: Palgrave, 2002), 177–215. For a call to a more nuanced vision, with respect to regional variations, see Gábor Ágoston, "A Flexible Empire: Authority and Its Limits on the Ottoman Frontiers," *International Journal of Turkish Studies* 9, nos. 1–2 (2003): 15–31.

[127] Schweigger, *Sultanlar Kentine Yolculuk*, 115.

[128] McCormick, "Rats, Communications, and Plague."

hides, and fur, could also shelter fleas, if not rats, for several weeks and even months.

It is argued in this book that the process of empire building in the long sixteenth century contributed significantly to increased human mobility. Even though it is difficult to trace and quantify these forms of mobility temporally and spatially, it should be plausible to conceive their contribution to the increased pace and scope of epidemiological activity. Needless to say, more research is needed to explore the various links between empire building and disease ecologies in the early modern Ottoman case.

The Environment

It should be remembered that the etiology of plague involves a complex system of entanglements in which every agent (such as host, vector, and pathogen) is in constant interaction with others as well as with the greater environment around it. As such, the environment is one of the main protagonists of plague etiology because of its tremendous capacity to trigger, sustain, or diminish plague activity; any slight change in the environment can cause a series of changes in the entire complex. Today there is a fairly well established body of knowledge, regarding the behavior of the pathogen, its relationship with its hosts and vectors, and how it adapts to new environments. Nevertheless, we also know that experiences of plague may change from one place to another because of differences in disease ecologies. In other words, the knowledge of plague etiology cannot be applied universally; because plague behaves differently in different environments, its etiology is more like a guideline that should be read in conjunction with specific local conditions.

From the vantage point of plague, there are two different environments. One is the natural environment, the other the built environment of human settlements, towns, and cities. Historically speaking, during the long stretch of plague out of its place of origin in Asia, the disease was spread to numerous regions by different hosts, vectors, or the mediation of humans. Once introduced to a new area, if the pathogen found a favorable ecosystem for its survival, it lived among the wild rodents. In other words, it became enzootic among rodents susceptible to the disease but generally resistant to the infection. These places became reservoirs or plague foci, in which the disease was kept in naturally occurring cycles of activity and nonactivity.[129] As long as

---

[129] In addition to living in wild rodent hosts, there is also some evidence that *Y. pestis* survives in flea feces, in postmortem rodent hosts, in soil, and in plants. See Gage and Kosoy, "Natural History of Plague"; W. Ryan Easterday et al., "An Additional Step in the Transmission of *Yersinia pestis*?," *ISME Journal* 6, no. 2 (2012): 231–36; Drancourt et al., "*Yersinia pestis* as a Telluric, Human Ectoparasite-Borne Organism"; Saravanan Ayyadurai et al., "Long-Term Persistence of Virulent *Yersinia pestis* in Soil," *Microbiology* 154,

the disease is not transmitted to humans, it is difficult to know much about its enzootic (sylvatic) existence.

According to the World Health Organization (WHO), plague foci fall, for the most part, between the 55 degrees north and 40 degrees south parallels. Some of these foci extend over substantial areas in the western United States, the Russian Federation, China, Mongolia, and southern Africa. For our more immediate area of concern, the plague foci in or around Ottoman areas are known to be located in Libya, Yemen, Iran, the Transcaucasian, and the northwest Caspian regions.[130] These plague foci were active in the Third Pandemic, and perhaps even before. They were identified in the second half of the twentieth century, and there is no precise information as to how old they are. Some of these foci are believed to be older than others. For example, historian William McNeill claimed in the 1970s that while the foci in central Africa and the Himalayan foothills were older, the steppe foci across Eurasia were formed not before the fourteenth century.[131] Chinese epidemiologist Wu Lien-Teh suggested in the 1920s that twelve plague foci antedated the Third Pandemic: two in Africa, ten in Asia (including the Assyr in the western Arabian Peninsula and the highlands of what is today southeast Turkey, northern Iraq, and western Iran).[132] According to Daniel Panzac, some of these foci can be traced as far back as the eighteenth century. Distinguishing between permanent and temporary plague foci in the Ottoman Empire, Panzac claims that the highlands between western Iran, northern Iraq, and southeastern Turkey as well as the mountainous areas of Hijaz and Yemen were permanent foci that supplanted the infection in the eighteenth and nineteenth centuries. Among the temporary foci, he listed the western Balkans focus, Moldavia and Wallachia, Istanbul, the Anatolian peninsula, and Egypt.[133]

Identifying plague foci of the earlier Ottoman eras may be challenging. It may be erroneous to assume that current or recent foci existed long before. It should be remembered that enzootic foci are dynamic complexes. One needs to use caution in making assumptions about the presence and/or function

no. 9 (2008): 2865–71; Rebecca J. Eisen et al., "Persistence of *Yersinia pestis* in Soil Under Natural Conditions," *Emerging Infectious Diseases* 14, no. 6 (2008): 941–43. For a study of *Y. pestis*'s survival in water, see David R. Pawlowski et al., "Entry of *Yersinia pestis* into the Viable but Nonculturable State in a Low-Temperature Tap Water Microcosm," *PLoS ONE* 6, no. 3 (2011): e17585.

[130] David T. Dennis, Kenneth L. Gage, Norman Gratz, Jack D. Poland, and Evgueni Tikhomirov, "Plague Manual: Epidemiology, Distribution, Surveillance and Control," WHO/CDS/CSR/EDC/99.2 (Geneva, Switzerland: WHO, 1999); Anisimov, Lindler, and Pier, "Intraspecific Diversity of *Yersinia pestis.*"

[131] William McNeill, *Plagues and Peoples* (Garden City, NY: Anchor Press, 1976), 137–40.

[132] Wu Lien-Teh, "The Original Home of Plague," in *Far Eastern Association of Tropical Medicine, Transactions of the Fifth Biennial Congress Held at Singapore, 1923*, ed. A. L. Hoops and J. W. Scharff, 286–304 (London: John Bale/Danielsson, 1924).

[133] Panzac, *La peste*, 105–33.

of a present plague focus in the past. It is difficult to know how old each of these foci is and how long it has remained active. Although under favorable climatic and environmental conditions, plague may seem to remain enzootic indefinitely, myriad changes – ranging from an increase or decrease in the number of predators of wild rodents to rodent migration, from climate to changes in the use of landscape – can make a difference. An old plague focus can shrink or even disappear, and new ones can emerge. Hence, a current plague focus does not guarantee its presence and function in the same manner in the past. While studying the natural history of plague in the Ottoman areas, one needs to take into account where the plague foci were, when they were formed, and how they were connected to the more densely populated human areas to replenish new epidemic outbreaks.

This difficulty in identifying the plague foci of the early modern Ottoman era largely arises from the imprecise and lacunous nature of the sources. Only rarely do early modern accounts specify where plague came from in a manner that would allow tracing the area of known (or suspected) origin. Even then, this reflects rumors or hearsay of the locals about it. By the same token, the importation of the infection to port cities by means of maritime contacts with other infected cities makes it difficult to trace the origins of an outbreak to a particular plague focus. This is further complicated by the possibility of the infection being introduced from multiple foci and/or via multiple channels. For any given past outbreak, it is possible that we are looking at multiple strains of the pathogen circulating through different trajectories. Unfortunately, the available sources do not allow making such micro-scale observations. What can be more confidently ascertained is that some Ottoman cities or areas seem to have been continuously affected by plague in the sixteenth century, first and foremost among them Istanbul, whose emergence as a plague hub is examined in detail here.[134] Similarly, Egypt, Syria, and several cities of coastal Anatolia and the Balkans are documented to have witnessed numerous waves of plague in the early modern era. Despite the unremitting presence of plague in these areas, it is difficult to know whether the infection was introduced each time from outside or was sustained by means of commensal rodents and/or ectoparasites from one plague season to the next, thus acting as independent urban plague foci.

Generally speaking, plague epidemics are related to a variety of environmental conditions, such as changes in climate (temperature, humidity, precipitation, and winds), changes in landscape, vegetation, and the levels of radiation. Drawing from a wealth of sources and scientific analyses, historian Bruce Campbell demonstrates how the emergence of a plague pandemic in the fourteenth century was related to global climatic and environmental conditions.[135] For the most part, though, the effort to understand and study

---

[134] See Chapter 6.
[135] Bruce M. S. Campbell, "Physical Shocks, Biological Hazards, and Human Impacts: The Crisis of the Fourteenth Century Revisited," in *Le Interazioni Fra Economia E*

the ways in which plague related to environmental changes is frustrated by the very nature of these relations. The environmental changes that can be associated with changes in plague are not easy to identify, as they do not entail direct causal links. They involve the agency of a complex series of factors and thus can be difficult to identify and study. For example, increased precipitation is generally held to bring increased plague activity. The trophic cascade hypothesis can help relate increased precipitation to epizootics in a chain reaction in natural foci (increased precipitation → increased plant size → increased food supply for rodents → increased rodent population → critical threshold exceeded → epizootic).[136] In the Ottoman context, such connections need to be explored especially with respect to the impact of the Little Ice Age on Ottoman plagues in the early modern era. The northern hemispheric cooling starting in the second half of the sixteenth century seems to have adversely affected the plague activity of the region owing to a combination of reasons related to changes in flora and fauna biodiversity, habitat destruction of rodents, and changes in uses of landscape.[137]

In an urban context, increased precipitation may entail a different set of relations between hosts, vectors, and humans. For example, changes in temperature do not seem to affect commensal rats directly in an urban context. Black rats that live indoors have relatively stable living conditions, such as access to food and regulated temperatures of homes.[138] In a similar vein, a study conducted in Egypt in the 1990s found no significant variations of the rat population throughout the year; seasons did not seem to make a major difference.[139] Nevertheless, in rainy seasons, when outdoor humidity is high, rats prefer to stay in indoor human environments, where there is stored food. Humans are also more likely to stay indoors in the rainy season, which may increase the potential physical proximity between commensal rats and humans.[140] Temperature and humidity seem to matter

Ambiente Biologico nell'Europa Preindustriale. Secc. XIII–XVIII (Economic and Biological Interactions in Pre-Industrial Europe from the 13th to the 18th Centuries), ed. Simonetta Cavaciocchi (Florence: Firenze University Press, 2010): 13–32.

[136] R. R. Parmenter et al., "Incidence of Plague Associated with Increased Winter-Spring Precipitation in New Mexico," *American Journal of Tropical Medicine and Hygiene* 61, no. 5 (1999): 814–21.

[137] Geoffrey Parker, *Global Crisis: War, Climate Change and Catastrophe in the Seventeenth Century* (New Haven, CT: Yale University Press, 2013). For the Ottoman case, see White, *Climate of Rebellion in the Early Modern Ottoman Empire*; White, "The Little Ice Age Crisis of the Ottoman Empire: A Conjuncture in Middle East Environmental History," in *Water on Sand*, ed. Alan Mikhail, 71–90; Faruk Tabak, *The Waning of the Mediterranean, 1550–1870: A Geohistorical Approach* (Baltimore: Johns Hopkins University Press, 2008).

[138] J. E. Brooks and F. P. Rowe, *Commensal Rodent Control* (Geneva, Switzerland: WHO, Vector Biology and Control Division, 1987), 13–14.

[139] S. Soliman et al., "Seasonal Studies on Commensal Rats and Their Ectoparasites in a Rural Area of Egypt: The Relationship of Ectoparasites to the Species, Locality, and Relative Abundance of the Host," *Journal of Parasitology* 87, no. 3 (2001): 545–53.

[140] Jacques M. May, "Map of the World Distribution of Plague," *Geographical Review* 42, no. 4 (1952): 629.

even more for plague vectors because of the nature of the flea's life cycle. Favorable climatic conditions are critical for flea eggs to hatch into larvae and eventually become adult fleas, the only form in which they perform their function as vectors.

Evidently, aside from climatic factors, other changes in the natural or built environment can alter plague etiology, though we do not know as much about the exact mechanisms at work. For example, an earthquake may dislocate ground-burrowing wild rodents from their natural habitat and force them to migrate elsewhere.[141] Similarly, floods can force such dislocations.[142] Such migrations, because they may bring wild rodents into contact with commensal rodents and/or humans, may lead to a plague epidemic. In fact, early modern observers have identified some of these associations that related plague to a larger environmental context. The dominant plague etiology that emphasized miasma had close ties to changes in climate, cosmic, and celestial phenomena that were believed to affect the quality of the air. The sources have often presumed a link between plague and unusual celestial phenomena, such as comets, lunar and solar eclipses, and the like. In that paradigm, the links between epidemic disease and changes in the greater environment have been commonly observed. I shall limit myself to two examples here drawn from late medieval and early modern Ottoman witnesses to plague. First, the aforementioned plague treatise of İlyas bin İbrahim insisted that plagues break out after earthquakes. He claims to draw this view from Aristotle, who posited that during earthquakes, poisonous underground vapors are unleashed to the surface of the earth and, while rising through the air, corrupt the substance of the air and form miasma, leading to epidemics. In fact, İlyas claims to have written his plague treatise following a big earthquake in Istanbul so as to offer means of prevention from the disease and methods of treatment.[143] Second, writing in the second half of the fifteenth century, the Greek historian Kritovoulos of Imbros commented on the unusual celestial phenomena observed before the appearance of plague in 1467. He wrote that a sudden and bright light appeared in the sky, which he did not know whether was a comet or a star. He certainly

---

[141] See Tsiamis et al., "Earthquakes and Plague during Byzantine Times: Can Lessons from the Past Improve Epidemic Preparedness?," *Acta Medico-Historica Adriatica* 11, no. 1 (2013): 55–64.

[142] An example for excess rain and flooding leading to plague, possibly as a result of forcing dislocation of rats, can be seen in the outbreak of 1791 in Egypt. For a detailed account of this outbreak, see Alan Mikhail, "The Nature of Plague in Late Eighteenth-Century Egypt," *Bulletin of the History of Medicine* 82, no. 2 (2008): 249–75; Mikhail, "Plague and Environment in Late Ottoman Egypt," in *Water on Sand*, 111–31.

[143] İlyas, *Tevfīkāt*. This was a common view in Europe in the seventeenth century. See Daniel Gordon, "Confrontations with the Plague in Eighteenth-Century France," in *Dreadful Visitations: Confronting Natural Catastrophe in the Age of Enlightenment*, ed. Alessa Johns (New York: Routledge, 1999), 6.

interpreted this as a bad omen that would be succeeded by a disaster or calamity, in this case a portent of the devastating plague outbreak in Istanbul.[144] The association between comets and outbreaks of plague was a widely maintained one in early modern Ottoman society, as was most famously illustrated in the closing down of the Ottoman observatory in Istanbul. When plague broke out following the appearance of a comet in Istanbul's skies in 1577, the observatory was closed down on grounds that it was inauspicious.[145]

Conclusion

This chapter has offered an overview of the natural history of plague to better understand the Ottoman experience of this disease in the late medieval and early modern eras. It draws from scientific and historical scholarship, with a view to bringing this body of knowledge in dialogue with the evidence found in Ottoman historical sources. Such an effort requires adopting a multilayered outlook, as it seeks to engage with multiple actors and agencies – especially cumbersome in dealing with nonhuman agencies, a direction that the Ottomanist historiography has only recently begun to pursue more thoroughly. Thus, owing to the complex etiological nature of the disease, the chapter surveys the protagonists of Ottoman plagues in separate sections devoted to hosts (rodents in particular, among various species of mammals), vectors (fleas and lice in particular, among other arthropods), the pathogen (*Y. pestis*), the humans, and the environment. Moreover, each of these protagonists is intimately linked to the others; establishing these connections is essential to fully comprehending the complex of plague.

The chapter has presented scientific and historical evidence about the presence of a number of wild and commensal rodent species in the Ottoman domains that may be associated with plague. In particular, it has emphasized the importance of commensal rodents for sustaining epidemics in urban areas. The analysis of historical sources suggests that the Ottomans did not observe direct links between rodents and plague outbreaks, even though they sometimes made indirect associations. In doing so, the Ottomans were not alone; this association was not identified until the end of the nineteenth century. It appears that the Ottoman urban population saw rats and mice as common pests and used rat poison and other means to exterminate them.

Similarly, vectors of plague (fleas and lice) in the historical and scientific sources are presented here in detail. It appears that such ectoparasites were common in Ottoman society, including among the elite, much like

---

[144] Kritovoulos, *History of Mehmed the Conqueror*, 217.

[145] For a discussion of the observatory in historical context, see Avner Ben-Zaken, *Cross-Cultural Scientific Exchanges in the Eastern Mediterranean, 1560–1660* (Baltimore: Johns Hopkins University Press, 2010), 8–47.

other contemporary societies. To a certain extent, such pests were culturally acceptable, even though Ottoman urban populations frequently resorted to hygienic practices to rid themselves of the pests, such as removing body hair, bathing, and using aromatic oils, while nomadic populations moved to higher altitudes to that end. Early modern observers evidently noticed fleabites on the bodies of plague victims but did not link these to the disease. The discovery of fleas as vectors of plague had to wait until the close of the nineteenth century. Drawing from sources of the Ottoman experience of plague, the chapter underlined the transitory role played by some animals in carrying infected vectors locally (predators of rodents, e.g., hyenas or weasels) or over long distances (migratory birds, e.g., white stork).

The discussion of the plague pathogen (*Y. pestis*) almost entirely draws from research from non-Ottoman experiences, owing to a lack of bioarcheological data from Ottoman cases of plague. At present, there is no aDNA evidence of *Y. pestis* recovered from former Ottoman areas. Such studies are much awaited for confirming the presence of the pathogen in this area. The only exception is the availability of modern *Y. pestis* isolates from former Ottoman areas (Turkey, northern Iraq, and western Iran) that have been included in recent phylogenetic analyses of the pathogen. However, these are not very helpful for studying late medieval and early modern plagues.

As incidental hosts to the disease, the agency of the human species has been the most important of all. Humans can spread the disease much more rapidly and widely than any of the other protagonists. At the same time, however, it was the human effort that developed means of containing and treating the plague. The myriad forms of human interaction with natural and built environments had an impact on the spread of the disease. It should not come as a surprise that in an era marked by massive efforts toward empire building, such as the era studied here, human mobility should increase both spatially and temporally. How the Ottoman growth in the fifteenth and sixteenth centuries intensified various forms of human and nonhuman plague agents' mobility (warfare and conquest, urbanization, and trade) and how such mobility stimulated the plague in the Ottoman experience are analyzed in greater detail in later chapters.

Finally, this chapter highlighted the part played by environmental factors in shaping the disease. It discussed how the Ottoman plagues may be linked to the broader environment and offered possible ways of studying these connections, drawing from both scientific literature and Ottoman historical sources. The vision that placed epidemics on a larger spectrum of natural (and supernatural) causes, such as earthquakes, weather events, and cosmic influences, was familiar to the Ottomans in this era.

2

Plague in Ottomanist and Non-Ottomanist Historiography

It needs no very extensive reading or profound study to find many indications of the ever present importance of the pest from the fourteenth even to the eighteenth century. Once one begins to look for such signs, one seems to find them in almost every book on the period to which one turns.[1]

More than a decade ago, Ottomanists were warned loudly that the history of plague in the early Ottoman centuries needed urgent scholarly attention. In an article published in 2003, aptly titled "Pushing the Stone Uphill," the Ottoman historian Heath Lowry was the one to move the heavy stone from its resting place. Stating the obvious, Lowry showed how none of the standard texts of Ottoman history mentioned the subject.[2] In a fortunate coincidence, two publications followed suit immediately after that. One was Uli Schamiloglu's pioneering article on the history of the Black Death in Anatolia, and the other, a lesser-known work, was Orhan Kılıç's book on epidemics in the Ottoman Empire.[3] From that time, students of Ottoman history started showing a greater interest in this subject, which resulted in a growing pool of scholarship in the area.

Notwithstanding this fresh burst of scholarly interest, the observation made by both Lowry and Schamiloglu more than a decade ago that plague

---

[1] Lynn Thorndike, "The Blight of Pestilence on Early Modern Civilization," *The American Historical Review* 32, no. 3 (1927): 455–74, quote on 455.

[2] Heath W. Lowry, "Pushing the Stone Uphill: The Impact of Bubonic Plague on Ottoman Urban Society in the Fifteenth and Sixteenth Centuries," *Osmanlı Araştırmaları* 23 (2003): 93–132.

[3] Uli Schamiloglu, "The Rise of the Ottoman Empire: The Black Death in Medieval Anatolia and Its Impact on Turkish Civilization," in *Views from the Edge: Essays in Honor of Richard W. Bulliet*, ed. Neguin Yavari, Lawrence G. Potter, and Jean-Marc Ran Oppenheim, 255–79 (New York: Columbia University Press, 2004); Orhan Kılıç, *Eskiçağdan Yakınçağa Genel Hatlarıyla Dünyada ve Osmanlı Devletinde Salgın Hastalıklar* (Elazığ: Fırat Üniversitesi Rektörlüğü, 2004).

was absent in the contemporary Ottomanist historiography still holds true to a large extent, especially for the early Ottoman centuries. The particular set of circumstances for this silence is very telling in itself. Indeed, it is no coincidence that the history of early modern Ottoman plague has been mostly unexplored. For reasons discussed later, it would be unthinkable to expect otherwise. To historicize this silence, this chapter reviews the state of the field in plague research in Ottomanist studies with respect to the complex meshwork of historical and historiographical factors that played a role in the development of such inquiries, wherever there is such development. To disentangle this complex problem, first, I offer a critical review of the scholarship on epidemic disease in Ottoman history. Second, I explore the development of historiographical trends in both the Ottomanist and non-Ottomanist scholarship with a view to identifying the misconceptions about Ottoman history of plague. Finally, I challenge the current misconceptions and offer a line of resituating the Ottoman experience of plague in a larger historical context.

The State of the Field in Plague Research in Ottomanist Studies

Over the last decade, Ottoman plague studies have received an unusual level of interest, opening the field to a host of research questions, new types of sources, and innovative methodologies. Collectively, these efforts offer promising prospects for the future of the field.[4] Generally speaking, these studies have benefited from a parallel awakening in allied fields wherein

---

[4] Oya Dağlar, *War, Epidemics and Medicine in the Late Ottoman Empire (1912–1918)* (Haarlem: SOTA, 2008); Mikhail, "Nature of Plague in Late Eighteenth-Century Egypt," 249–75; Mikhail, "Plague and Environment in Late Ottoman Egypt," 111–31; Aaron Shakow, "Marks of Contagion: The Plague, the Bourse, the Word and the Law in the Early Modern Mediterranean, 1720–1762," PhD diss., Harvard University, 2009; Yaron Ayalon, "Plagues, Famines, Earthquakes: The Jews of Ottoman Syria and Natural Disasters," PhD diss., Princeton University, 2009; Gisele Marien, "The Black Death in Early Ottoman Territories: 1347–1550," MA thesis, Bilkent University, 2009; Aaron Shakow, "'Oriental Plague' in the Middle Eastern Landscape: A Cautionary Tale," *IJMES* 42, no. 4 (2010): 660–62; Sam White, "Rethinking Disease in Ottoman History," *IJMES* 42, no. 4 (2010): 549–67; Andrew Robarts, "A Plague on Both Houses? Population Movements and the Spread of Disease across the Ottoman-Russian Black Sea Frontier, 1768–1830s," PhD diss., Georgetown University, 2010; Nuran Yıldırım, *A History of Healthcare in Istanbul: Health Organizations, Epidemics, Infections and Disease Control, Preventive Health Institutions, Hospitals, Medical Education* (Istanbul: Istanbul University, 2010); Nalan Turna, "İstanbul'un veba ile imtihanı: 1811–1812 veba salgını bağlamında toplum ve ekonomi," *Studies of the Ottoman Domain* 1, no. 1 (2011): 23–58; Nükhet Varlık, "Conquest, Urbanization, and Plague Networks in the Ottoman Empire, 1453–1600," in *The Ottoman World*, ed. Christine Woodhead, 251–63 (New York: Routledge, 2012); Varlık, "Tâun" [Plague], in *TDVİA*; Varlık, "From 'Bête Noire' to 'le Mal de Constantinople': Plagues, Medicine, and the Early Modern Ottoman State," *Journal of World History* 24, no. 4 (2013): 741–70; Varlık, "Plague, Conflict, and Negotiation: The Jewish Broadcloth Weavers of Salonica and the Ottoman Central Administration in the Late Sixteenth Century," *Jewish History* 28, nos. 3–4 (2014): 261–88; Miri Shefer-Mossensohn, "Communicable Disease in Ottoman Palestine: Local Thoughts and

a novel interest in the history of environment, climate, and animal studies has come to fruition, not only in Ottomanist studies but also in Middle East studies more generally.[5] Informed by a historiographical tradition that acknowledges the role of nonhuman agents in history, there seems to be a growing awareness among the Ottomanists today that the environment, animals, and microorganisms have been important actors of Ottoman history. Despite the breadth and scope of this body of burgeoning scholarship, however, there are still many questions that remain to be addressed. To have a more accurate picture of the state of the field in plague research in the Ottomanist scholarship, it may be useful to offer a critical review of the development of the field.

Writing the History of Ottoman Epidemics: Breaks and Continuities

The interest in the history of epidemic diseases of the Ottoman Empire can be traced to the early decades of the Turkish republic, if not earlier.[6] With a growing concern to turn its impoverished and disease-ridden population into

Actions," *Korot* 21 (2012): 19–49; Birsen Bulmuş, *Plague, Quarantines, and Geopolitics in the Ottoman Empire* (Edinburgh: Edinburgh University Press, 2012); and most recently Yaron Ayalon, *Natural Disasters in the Ottoman Empire: Plague, Famine, and Other Misfortunes* (Cambridge: Cambridge University Press, 2014), which was published during the production of this book; unfortunately it was not possible to integrate it into the discussion here. Also relating to disease, see Amy Singer, "Ottoman Palestine (1516–1800): Health, Disease, and Historical Sources," in *Health and Disease in the Holy Land: Studies in the History and Sociology of Medicine from Ancient Times to the Present*, ed. Manfred Waserman and Samuel S. Kottek, 189–206 (Lewiston, NY: Edwin Mellen Press, 1996); Colin Heywood, "Sickness and Death in an Ill Climate: The Detention of the Blackham Galley at Izmir 1697–8," in *Ottoman Izmir Studies in Honour of Alexander H. de Groot*, ed. Maurits H. van den Boogert, 53–74 (Leiden: Nederlands Instituut voor het Nabije Oosten, 2007).

5 See, e.g., Tabak, *Waning of the Mediterranean*; Mehmet Erler, *Osmanlı Devleti'nde Kuraklık, 1800–1880* (Istanbul: Libra Kitap, 2010); Suraiya Faroqhi, *Animals and People in the Ottoman Empire* (Istanbul: Eren, 2010); Alan Mikhail, "An Irrigated Empire: The View from Ottoman Fayyum," *IJMES* 42, no. 4 (2010): 569–90; Mikhail, *Nature and Empire in Ottoman Egypt: An Environmental History* (Cambridge: Cambridge University Press, 2011); Mikhail, *Water on Sand*; Mikhail, *The Animal in Ottoman Egypt* (Oxford: Oxford University Press, 2013); Edmund Burke III, "Pastoralism and the Mediterranean Environment," *IJMES* 42, no. 4 (2010): 663–65; Richard Bulliet, "The Camel and the Watermill," *IJMES* 42, no. 4 (2010): 666–68; Giancarlo Casale, "The 'Environmental Turn': A Teaching Perspective," *IJMES* 42, no. 4 (2010): 669–71; White, *Climate of Rebellion*; Onur İnal, "Environmental History as an Emerging Field in Ottoman Studies: An Historiographical Overview," *Osmanlı Araştırmaları* 38 (2011): 1–25; H-Environment Discussion Network, *Roundtable Reviews* 3, no. 8 (2013): 1–26, http://www.h-net.org/~environ/roundtables/env-roundtable-3-8.pdf.

6 Galib Ata, "İstanbul'da veba salgınları," *Tıp Fakültesi Mecmuası* 3 (1918): 189. Ata gave a brief summary list of plague epidemics in Istanbul from the sixth century to the mid-nineteenth. He suggested that there was no record of plague in the fifteenth century in Ottoman-controlled areas, whereas outbreaks were rampant in Europe. He pointed out seven outbreaks for the sixteenth century, that of 1591–92 being especially serious.

healthy and able-bodied citizens of the new nation-state, the early Turkish republic launched a rigorous campaign to survey, identify, and eradicate prevalent infectious diseases, especially malaria, syphilis, trachoma, and tuberculosis.[7] These efforts included the establishment of modern public health institutions, the training of new medical professionals, implementation of programs for educating the public, and mass vaccination campaigns. While taking an active part in these efforts, some Turkish physicians also nurtured a keen interest in the nation's Ottoman past and produced the first works about its history of medicine and science.[8] This era also coincides with the founding of medical history programs in universities and the establishment of the Turkish Society for the History of Medicine (Türk Tıp Tarihi Kurumu). The pioneering efforts of these physicians and scholars were instrumental in establishing a tradition of scholarship in Turkey, which still continues to this day, with a quite substantial number of scholars housed in medical schools.

Taken as a whole, this tradition of scholarship has largely epitomized two important caveats: first, it has been (and to a certain extent still is) largely *iatrocentric* in nature, that is, a kind of internalist history written by medical professionals for other medical professionals.[9] Almost exclusively produced by scholars trained in the medical sciences, this body of scholarship has shown disproportionately heavy interest in subjects such as the history of medical and pharmaceutical sciences, medical institutions, biographies, and the history of medical education.[10] Second, this body of scholarship is dominated by an unmistakably nationalist overtone, which envisions an unchanging – hence, timeless – *Turkish* tradition in the history of medicine. Such an approach becomes especially transparent in a selective approach to Ottoman history, a typical example of which can be observed in modern

---

7 Kyle T. Evered and Emine Ö. Evered, "Governing Population, Public Health, and Malaria in the Early Turkish Republic," *Journal of Historical Geography* 37, no. 4 (2011): 470–82; Evered and Evered, "State, Peasant, Mosquito: The Biopolitics of Public Health Education and Malaria in Early Republican Turkey," *Political Geography* 31, no. 5 (2012): 311–23; Evered and Evered, "Syphilis and Prostitution in the Socio-medical Geographies of Turkey's Early Republican Provinces," *Health and Place* 18, no. 3 (2012): 528–35; Evered and Evered, "Sex and the Capital City: The Political Framing of Syphilis and Prostitution in Early Republican Ankara," *JHMAS* 68, no. 2 (2013): 266–99.

8 Abdülhak Adnan Adıvar (d. 1955), Besim Ömer Akalın (d. 1940), Galib Ata (Ataç) (d. 1947), Akil Muhtar Özden (d. 1949), Osman Şevki Uludağ (d. 1964), Feridun Nafiz Uzluk (d. 1974), and Süheyl Ünver (d. 1986) can be mentioned among the most prominent representatives of this tradition.

9 For a critical assessment of this tradition of scholarship, see Miri Shefer Mossensohn, "A Tale of Two Discourses: The Historiography of Ottoman-Muslim Medicine," *Social History of Medicine* 21, no. 1 (2008): 1–12.

10 A quick glance at the subjects covered in the scholarship produced between 1973 and 2002 reveals this. Zuhal Özaydın and H. Hüsrev Hâtemî, *Türk Tıp Tarihi Araştırmalarının Son 30 Yılda (1970–2002) Yönelişleri ve Bir Bibliografya Denemesi* (Istanbul: Cerrahpaşa Tıp Fakültesi Vakfı, 2002), esp. 311–14.

scholarly efforts to translate, edit, and publish medical works composed in the vernacular Turkish, as opposed to a large medical corpus in the Arabic language that remains mostly unexplored.[11] Both of these factors have further implications for studying Ottoman plagues. In a nutshell, until plague became medicalized in Ottoman society – I contend that this does not occur until the latter part of the sixteenth century (see Chapter 7) – the disease was not seen as a medical phenomenon per se, which, as a subject of inquiry, would leave it outside the radar of an iatrocentric scholarship. It is not until it comes to be defined as a medical phenomenon, which could be managed, if not treated, by the medical enterprise, that it comes to be seen as a subject worthy of historical examination. After all, it could not be a coincidence that most of what has been written on Ottoman history of plague (and other epidemic diseases) deals with the nineteenth century, especially with the establishment of the institution of quarantine.[12]

The significant contributions of this scholarship remain to be acknowledged. Most prominently, the pioneering work of Süheyl Ünver in the Ottoman history of plagues is outstanding. In a series of articles from the 1930s through the 1970s, Ünver published on different aspects of plague in Ottoman history. A tremendously prolific writer with a multitude of interests, Ünver seems to have maintained a lasting passion for the subject, which is also evidenced in his unpublished notes and files.[13] In an early article published in 1935, for example, Ünver provided a brief history of

[11] The effort to publish medical manuscripts has demonstrated an unmistakable preference for works composed in Turkish. To cite but a few examples, Celâlüddin Hızır (Hacı Paşa), *Müntahab-ı Şifâ*, ed. Zafer Önler (Ankara: Türk Dil Kurumu, 1990); Şerefeddin Sabuncuoğlu, *Cerrâḥiyyetü'l-Ḫâniyye*, ed. İlter Uzel, 2 vols. (Ankara: TTK, 1992); İbn-i Şerîf, *Yâdigâr: 15. Yüzyıl Türkçe Tıp Kitabı*, ed. Ayten Altıntaş, 2 vols. (Istanbul: Merkez Efendi ve Halk Hekimliği Derneği, 2003–4); Abdülvehhâb bin Yûsuf ibn-i Ahmed el-Mârdânî, *Kitâbu'l-Müntehab fî't-Tıb: inceleme, metin, dizin, sadeleştirme, tıpkıbasım*, ed. Ali Haydar Bayat (Istanbul: Merkezefendi Geleneksel Tıp Derneği, 2005).

[12] These studies include Bedi Şehsuvaroğlu, "Karantina Tarihi," PhD diss., Istanbul University, 1956; Gülden Sarıyıldız, "Karantina Teşkilatının Kuruluşu ve Faaliyetleri (1838–1876)," MA thesis, Istanbul University, 1986; Sarıyıldız, "Karantina Meclisi'nin Kuruluşu ve Faaliyetleri," *Belleten* 58, no. 222 (1994): 329–76; Sarıyıldız, *Hicaz Karantina Teşkilatı (1865–1914)* (Ankara: TTK, 1996).

[13] Süheyl Ünver's unpublished notes on plague are kept in the Süleymaniye Library collection in Istanbul. See Süheyl Ünver, ms. 662, Süleymaniye Library. Some of his published work on plague include Ünver, "Türkiyede Veba (Taun) Tarihçesi Üzerine," *Tedavi Kliniği ve Laboratuvarı Mecmuası* 5 (1935): 70–88; "İstanbul Halkının Ölüm Karşısındaki Duyguları," *Yeni Türk* 68 (1938): 312–21; "Romanya Tıb Tarihine Ait Bir Vesika," *Türk Tıp Tarihi Arkivi* 9 (1938): 25–27; "Türk Tıb Tarihinde Veba Hastalığına Karşı Kına Tatbiki," *Türk Tıp Tarihi Arkivi* 7 (1938): 82–85; "Buğdan Voyvodası Oğlunun Vebadan Ölümü," *Türk Tıp Tarihi Arkivi* 12 (1939): 147–50; "Mezar Taşlarında Veba ve Tauna Ait Kayıtlar," *Dirim* 11–12 (1965): 268–72; "Les épidémies de choléra dans les terres balkaniques aux XVIIIe et XIXe siècles," *Études Balkaniques (Sofia)* 4 (1973): 89–97; "Taun Nedir? Veba Nedir?," *Dirim* 3–4 (1978): 363–66.

Ottoman plagues, discussed issues of terminology, and introduced the most important sources to guide future studies.[14] To this day, this article stands as the single most important piece for the student of early Ottoman plagues. Equally important is the work of Sırrı Akıncı, another Turkish medical historian whose contribution to Ottoman historiography of plague needs to be recognized. In the preface of his 1969 dissertation, Akıncı observed that publications of physicians' biographies were numerous in Turkish medical history scholarship, and yet there was very little on the history of diseases.[15] Nevertheless, this scholarship remained largely underutilized; the efforts to identify the outbreaks of plague in Ottoman history and the sources that are brought to attention in these works were not followed up in the later scholarship.[16]

The lack of interest in Ottoman history of disease on the part of medical historians was to be compensated by newly arising historiographical sensitivities in the Ottomanist field from the 1970s onward. Ottoman social and economic historians recognized the importance of epidemic disease as an important force in the history of the empire.[17] In line with this new outlook, the late Daniel Panzac focused his attention on plague in the Ottoman Empire and produced a valuable corpus on the subject. His 1985 *La peste dans l'empire ottoman* was a great contribution to the plague studies of the 1970s and 1980s, prominently represented by historians, such as Jean-Noël Biraben, Michael Dols, and Lawrence Conrad. Panzac's meticulous work based on diplomatic correspondences and ambassadorial dispatches still remains the most comprehensive and authoritative study devoted to the history of plague in the Ottoman Empire focused between 1700 and 1850.[18]

[14] Ünver, "Türkiyede Veba (Taun) Tarihçesi Üzerine"; also published in French as "Sur l'histoire de la peste en Turquie," presented at the 9ᵉ Congrès International d'Histoire de la Medicine in Bucarest, September 1932. It may be useful to remember that the recurrent waves of the Third Plague Pandemic still continued in many parts of the world through the first half of the twentieth century, including minor outbreaks in Turkey (e.g., the plague of Akçakale, Urfa, in 1947). It was not until 1960 that the WHO declared the end of the pandemic.

[15] Sırrı Akıncı, "Osmanlı İmparatorluğunda Veba (Taun) Salgınları ve Yorumlanması," PhD diss., Istanbul University, 1969, preface. Also see Sırrı Akıncı, "Tarih Boyunca Veba" *Tarih Mecmuası* 6 (1973): 32–37.

[16] Scholars such as Panzac and Dols used some of Ünver's articles published in French. The important work of Akıncı remained practically unknown in the scholarship – in Turkish and unpublished – though Panzac listed it in the bibliography of his 1985 book.

[17] Social and economic historians of the Ottoman Empire have long entertained an interest on the subject and emphasized its importance, even if they themselves did not write on it. For example, Halil İnalcık listed epidemics in the history of Ottoman Istanbul, based on primary sources. See Halil İnalcık, "İstanbul," *EI²*.

[18] Panzac, *La peste*; Daniel Panzac, *Osmanlı İmparatorluğu'nda Veba: 1700–1850* (Istanbul: Türkiye Ekonomik Toplumsal Tarih Vakfı, 1997). Panzac also authored a number of works devoted to plague, sanitary regulations, and health in eighteenth- and nineteenth-century Ottoman society. See, e.g., "La peste à Smyrne au XVIIIᵉ siècle," *Annales: Économies,*

His works seem to have inspired further interest in the subject among the Ottomanists.[19] Environmental history, climatic history, and social history of medicine are among the fields that are currently budding in Ottomanist studies. As fruits of these recent interests, there has been a renewed incentive to consider the question of disease in Ottoman history. There has also been a significant effort in the non-Ottomanist scholarship for studying history of epidemics in former Ottoman lands.[20] Regardless, it may be worth asking why the earlier plagues in Ottoman history have not been as thoroughly explored as those of the eighteenth and nineteenth centuries. Was this merely because of the availability of sources on the latter era? Or are there other historical

---

Sociétés, Civilisations 28, no. 4 (1973): 1071–93; *Quarantaines et lazarets: l'Europe et la peste d'Orient, XVIIe–XXe siècles* (Aix-en-Provence: Édisud, 1986); "Alexandrie: peste et croissance urbaine (XVIIe-XIXe siècles)," *Revue de l'Occident musulman et de la Méditerranée* 46, no. 1 (1987): 81–90; "Mourir à Alep au XVIIIe siècle," *Revue du monde musulman et de la Méditerranée* 62, no. 1 (1991): 111–22; "Wabā'," *EI²*; "Plague," in Ágoston and Masters, *Encyclopedia of the Ottoman Empire*, 462–63; "Population," in Ágoston and Masters, *Encyclopedia of the Ottoman Empire*, 467–69. For a full bibliography of Panzac, see Colette Establet Vernin, "Daniel Panzac (1933–2012)," *Revue des mondes musulmans et de la Méditerranée*, no. 134 (2013): 307–14.

[19] See, e.g., Feda Şamil Arık, "Selçuklular Zamanında Anadolu'da Veba Salgınları," *Tarih Araştırmaları Dergisi* 15, no. 26 (1991): 27–57; Ronald C. Jennings, "Plague in Trabzon and Reactions to It According to Local Juridical Registers," in *Humanist and Scholar: Essays in Honor of Andreas Tietze*, ed. Heath W. Lowry and Donald Quataert, 27–36 (Istanbul: Isis Press, 1993); Necdet Sakaoğlu, "Osmanlı'da Salgınlar," *Toplumsal Tarih* 22 (1995): 23–25; Nuran Yıldırım, "Salgınlar," *Dünden Bugüne İstanbul Ansiklopedisi*, 6:423–25; Nükhet Varlık, "The Study of a Plague Treatise 'Tevfikatü'l-Hamidiyye fi Def'i'l-Emrazi'l-Veba'iyye,'" MA thesis, Boğaziçi University, 2000; Varlık, "Attitudes toward Plague Epidemics in Ottoman Society of the Nineteenth Century," *Proceedings of the International Congress for the History of Medicine*, Galveston, TX, 2002, 359–64; A. Latif Armağan, "XVII. Yüzyılın Sonu ile XVIII. Yüzyılın Başlarında Batı Anadolu ve Balkanlarda Görülen Veba Salgınlarının Sosyo-Ekonomik Etkileri Üzerine Bir Araştırma," in *Proceedings of the 38th International Congress on the History of Medicine*, ed. Nil Sarı et al. (Ankara, 2005), 3:907–14; Ömür Ceylan, "Ölümün unutulan adı: veba," *Dergâh* 15, no. 182 (2005): 20–21; Mehmet Ali Beyhan, "1811–1812 İstanbul Veba Salgını, Etkileri ve Alınan Tedbirler," in *1. Uluslararası Türk Tıp Tarihi Kongresi/10. Ulusal Türk Tıp Tarihi Kongresi Bildiri Kitabı (20–24 May 2008)*, ed. Ayşegül Demirhan Erdemir (Konya: TTK, 2008), 2:1029–36; Said Öztürk, ed., *Afetlerin gölgesinde İstanbul: tarih boyunca İstanbul ve çevresini etkileyen afetler* (Istanbul: İstanbul Büyükşehir Belediyesi, 2009).

[20] Bogumil Hrabak, "Kuga u balkanskim zemljama pod Turcima od 1450 do 1600 godine," *Istoriski glasnik* 1–2 (1957): 19–37; B. Krekic, "Europe centrale et balkanique," *Annales: Économies, Sociétés, Civilisations* 18, no. 3 (1963): 594–95; Kōstas Kōstēs, *Ston kairo tēs panōlēs: eikones apo tis koinōnies tēs Hellēnikēs chersonēsou, 140s-190s aiōnas* (Hērakleio: Panepistēmiakes Ekdoseis Krētēs, 1995); Nadja I Manolova-Nikolova, *Čumavite vremena: (1700–1850)* (Sofia: IF-94, 2004); Stuart J. Borsch, *The Black Death in Egypt and England: A Comparative Study* (Austin: University of Texas Press, 2005); Costas Tsiamis et al., "Epidemic Waves of the Black Death in the Byzantine Empire (1347–1453 AD)," *Le Infezioni in Medicina: Rivista Periodica Di Eziologia, Epidemiologia, Diagnostica, Clinica E Terapia Delle Patologie Infettive* 19, no. 3 (2011): 194–201.

and historiographical reasons that can help us explain the trends in the scholarship?

To this end, it may be worthwhile to consider the complex interlacing of historical and historiographical factors that affected the development (or lack thereof) of such inquiries. This problem seems partly to stem from presentist conceptions of past epidemics. In the modern view, epidemic diseases evoke a sentiment of poor health standards and inadequate health organization of the state. In premodern contexts, however, conceptualizing the presence or absence of epidemics "as a measure of civilization" may lead to anachronistic interpretations. One such elucidation that has inevitably shaped the Ottomanist studies of plagues (and of other epidemic diseases) seems to be a certain association between epidemics and the state. The conventional conceptualization of Ottoman history and the periodization that stems from it had lasting implications for this subject. It was long imagined that the Ottomans reached the apex of their history in the sixteenth century, during the reign of Sultan Süleyman, a "golden age" that was followed by a long "decline." It goes without saying that modernist (and anachronistic) conceptions of plagues could not be associated with the "golden age," when the Ottomans were at the height of their power. In this historical imagination, plagues only belonged in the historical narrative of the age of "decline" – something that would justify the decline, if not explain it. This vision of Ottoman history is no longer acceptable today.[21] Nevertheless, traces of its effects are still discernible in the Ottomanist studies of plagues, with an almost exclusive focus on late Ottoman history at the expense of earlier eras.

This vision of past epidemics is further complicated by certain historical assumptions. For reasons that we discuss in detail in the following pages, epidemics of pre-1700 Ottoman history and their effects are still largely unknown. The lacunae in our knowledge leave the subject open for assumptions such as that there were no major epidemics in early Ottoman centuries. In other words, the absence of (known) evidence for plague is accepted as evidence for its absence. Hence, it was suggested that the Ottoman society was mostly free from plague epidemics during the sixteenth century, while the earlier centuries of Ottoman history were largely ignored.[22] No historical explanation is offered to account for the absence of plague during the sixteenth century and earlier, not least for its presence in the later centuries. It is

---

[21] For a recent overview of the decline paradigm and its critiques, see Dana Sajdi, "Decline, Its Discontents and Ottoman Cultural History: By Way of Introduction," in *Ottoman Tulips, Ottoman Coffee: Leisure and Lifestyle in the Eighteenth Century*, ed. Dana Sajdi, 1–40 (London: Tauris Academic Studies, 2007).

[22] Panzac, "Wabā'," 4. Panzac argues that the plague was only seen between 1572 and 1589 in the sixteenth century. Michael W. Dols, "The Second Plague Pandemic and Its Recurrences in the Middle East: 1347–1894," *JESHO* 22, no. 2 (1979): 176. The work of Uli Shamiloglu (2004) is an exception to this trend. See note 3.

equally unclear how such an absence can be assumed for the Ottoman landscape, while all the surrounding areas were repeatedly affected by waves of plague in the very same period. Moreover, the fact that the sixteenth century was an era marked by acute population growth and thus was characterized by an absence of plague may not always be true, as is discussed later.

Plague in Ottoman Chronicles

The chapter epigraph comes from a 1927 article by the historian of medieval science Lynn Thorndike, in which he suggested that the student of European history of pestilence had to turn "to local histories of towns or provinces, to the records of schools and individuals, not to mention the history of medicine," to find evidence.[23] Indeed, students of European history did go on to exploit a host of written and nonwritten sources to study past plagues and their effects on European society, which generated a rich and powerful body of scholarship.[24] Unfortunately, the same cannot be said for the current state of Ottomanist plague studies of the late medieval and early modern eras, where silence prevails.

The silence is partly due to a lack of detailed Ottoman primary sources offering narrative accounts of the plague. Scholars working on the late fifteenth and sixteenth centuries have relied heavily on narratives supplied by the chronicles. Interestingly enough, the absence of plague in the contemporary Ottomanist historiography of the first centuries of Ottoman history can be traced to the absence of plague as a topos in the early chronicles. The Ottoman chronicles of the fifteenth and sixteenth centuries mention plague rarely, if ever. Stated differently, because the early chronicles did not talk about plague, modern Ottomanist scholarship that has drawn from them has also failed to consider the importance of plague in these centuries.[25] Establishing the proper relationship between sources and plagues remains critical to overcoming the difficulties in the study of this subject. Clearly, utilizing these sources simply for the purpose of mining for information does not meet the challenge. It is necessary to attune the methods of inquiry closer to the sources. In fact, a close reading of contemporaneous chronicles may offer more than they reveal. For example, why something is recounted, the context in which it is told, and why something is omitted can be equally

---

[23] Thorndike, "Blight of Pestilence," 455.

[24] The scholarship on plague in European history is simply too extensive to be listed here. By way of introduction, a concise bibliography can be found in Paul Slack, *Plague: A Very Short Introduction* (Oxford: Oxford University Press, 2012), 127–32. For a more extensive bibliography, I refer the reader to the following volume: Vivian Nutton, ed., *Pestilential Complexities: Understanding Medieval Plague*, Medical History 27 (London: Wellcome Trust Centre for the History of Medicine at UCL, 2008).

[25] E.g., Panzac is very critical about the value of Ottoman chronicles for supplying information on the history of the plague. See Panzac, *La peste*, 18–19.

telling in approaching a question at hand. Hence, instead of accepting the absence of plague in these accounts as a one-to-one reflection of historical reality, it is imperative to question why the early Ottoman chronicles did or did not mention plagues.

Then, why did the early Ottoman chronicles fail to mention plagues? Were the chroniclers not keen observers of their era? How could they have failed to write about such important phenomena as epidemic diseases with disastrous consequences? Before addressing these questions, it may be necessary to reflect on the (distrustful and presentist) assumptions lying behind them. It is tempting to presume that important events had to be recorded by those who wrote such accounts in the past. The fact that a certain event, person, or place is mentioned in a chronicle, for example, can be taken as evidence for the significance of that element for the narrator. By the same token, the fact that something is not mentioned at all can be evidence of its nonexistence or its ephemeral status. Nonetheless, expecting the chronicles to be a direct reflection of historical reality is naive, to say the least. As shown in the pages to come, plague outbreaks became increasingly frequent in Ottoman cities through the fifteenth and sixteenth centuries, and yet this is not easily discernible from the chronicles. In this context, it may be useful to remember that chronicles, like other forms of narratives, are reconstructions of historical "reality" within their own spatial and temporal relativity. A full correspondence between the scale and rhythm of the narrative, on one hand, and the historical sequence, on the other, is not to be expected. The narrative, as a product of selective reconstruction of the past, may include events or omit them, may adopt a slower tempo in the narration of certain events or accelerate in other cases, or change the order of events altogether. All such techniques were used by Ottoman chroniclers to reconstruct the past in their narratives, especially in writing about the distant past. For example, it has been long noticed that there is a gaping hole in the narrative of events in early Ottoman chronicles; the course of events from roughly the 1330s to the 1350s is missing for the most part.[26] Surprisingly, this silence happens to coincide with the appearance of the plague. One wonders why we do not hear about the course of events, for instance, between the time of the Black Death and the Ottomans' crossing over the Dardanelles? Why is this piece missing in the narrative? Is it possible that this was precisely because there was a major break in life? Or alternatively, was it because the chain of transmission, either in written form or more likely in oral testimonies, was broken as a result of the epidemic and mortality? Is it possible that for those chroniclers writing in the fifteenth century, their ties to the pre–Black Death Ottoman histories were largely or entirely lost, so much so that they had

[26]   Joseph von Hammer-Purgstall, *Histoire de l'empire ottoman depuis son origine jusqu'à nos jours* (Paris: Bellizard, Barthès, Dufour, et Lowell, 1835), 1:162. For Hammer, this silence resulted from Ottomans' friendly relations with their neighbors around that time.

to reconstruct that past haphazardly? Needless to say, these questions are hypothetical in nature and cannot be addressed effectively with the evidence at hand. Yet, the effects of the Black Death and its successive waves on the early Ottoman chronicle-writing tradition deserve to be explored further.

Regardless, it should be possible to offer some relevant insights about why plague does not figure (or is simply mentioned as an ephemeral theme) in the early Ottoman chronicles. One of the earliest of Ottoman histories was Ahmedi's *Tevārīh-i Mülūk-i Āl-i ʿOsmān* (History of the Kings of the Ottoman Lineage). Born around 1334, Ahmedi very likely witnessed the Black Death as a child. Yet, except for a few scattered allusions to plague, mostly in the metaphoric sense, Ahmedi's epic history of the House of Osman does not talk openly about it. Even though he does not give an account of the plague in the form of historical narrative, the manner in which plague appears in his poetry and the tone of its usage conjure up a general sense of familiarity with it.[27] It has been suggested that the effects of the plague are revealed in the language of religiosity he uses.[28]

Toward the end of the fifteenth century, the first signs of plague start to surface in the Ottoman chronicle genre, but even then, these barely go beyond brisk references. Generally speaking, the earlier Ottoman chronicles, which are written at the end of the fifteenth and the beginning of the sixteenth century, such as the works of Aşıkpaşazade and Neşri, chronicled events using a simple language. These works are histories of the House of Osman, whose narrative is dominated by a series of military and political events, with scarce references to plague. For example, both Aşıkpaşazade and Neşri mention the plague in one instance, on the occasion of the death of the prince of Karesi.[29] As we shall see in the next chapter, this is evidence of prime importance for the presence of the Black Death in Ottoman Bursa, but it does not tell much about the plague itself. Surely the said Karesi prince was not the only one to die of plague in Bursa. Even though the historical significance of an isolated reference cannot be overestimated, it would be foolish to believe that only one person died of plague at the time. It follows that many others must have died of it as well, possibly including members of the Ottoman elite. If so, then it may be worthwhile to question why the chroniclers only mention the death of the Karesi prince as a result of plague

---

[27] Ahmedî, *Divan*, ed., Yaşar Akdoğan ([Ankara]: T.C. Kültür ve Turizm Bakanlığı Yayınları, 1999). E.g., see 13 (V/13) *"Dünyî hevâsı aslı vebâdur suyı maraz/Olmasun aldaya seni bu âb u bu hevâ"*; 60 (XXII/23) *Peleng zahmına bevl eyledügi muş nedür/ Vebâya oldugı yâkût dâfi'-i âsâr."*

[28] Ahmedi, *History of the Kings of the Ottoman Lineage and Their Holy Raids against the Infidels*, ed. Kemal Sılay (Cambridge, MA: Department of Near Eastern Languages and Literatures, Harvard University, 2004).

[29] *Aşıkpaşaoğlu Tarihi*, 44. Mehmed Neşri, *Kitab-ı Cihan-Nüma = Neşrî Tarihi*, Faik Reşit Unat and Mehmed A. Köymen (Ankara: TTK, 1995), 1:166–67. See Chapter 3 for more details on this reference.

but not that of others. Was it because this was believed to be a punishment proper to a prince whose dominions were conquered – a fate befitting a fallen rival prince? The death of the said prince from plague was perhaps judged as being worthy of mention for rhetorical reasons. The enemy suffering a well-deserved death could solidify the righteous and divinely favored Ottoman cause – a cause that a chronicler of the House of Osman would not miss using as an ideological tool.[30] This brings to mind Ahmedi's poetical usage of plague in conjunction with Prince Süleyman's rivals for the throne in the interregnum years.[31] Whereas in the beginning of the fourteenth century, Ahmedi saw the plague as a punishment fit for the rivals of the Ottoman throne within the House of Osman, at the end of the century, Aşıkpaşazade used it more cautiously. Clearly no longer deemed a fitting punishment for the Ottomans themselves, it was projected only to those who rivaled them.[32] Needless to say, when the latter composed his work, fortunes had favored the Ottomans far away from the anxieties of the interregnum era.

Leaving aside this isolated and heavily ideological reference to a past plague, it may be worthwhile to consider the chroniclers' attitude toward writing about the outbreaks of their own time. Not unlike their failure to write about past outbreaks, they neglected to write about outbreaks that took place during their own lifetimes. For example, whereas there is no reference in Aşıkpaşazade's chronicle to the outbreaks of 1455–56 or 1466–67 – both took place during his lifetime – Neşri only mentions the latter, in the context of military events. As is discussed at length in Chapter 4, Neşri wrote that when Mehmed II was returning from the Albanian campaign with his army, he moved to the Black Sea coast to avoid the plague. In this narrative, plague seems to be mentioned only by virtue of its effect on the sultan and the army. Neşri's account makes no other mention of other outbreaks, despite their repeated occurrence. Another contemporary chronicler, Tursun Bey, does not mention plague at all. For instance, when telling the story of Mehmed's second campaign to Albania, he simply writes that the sultan returned to Istanbul with glory.[33] As histories of the Ottoman

---

[30] The chronicle of Oruç, even though it overlaps with that of Aşıkpaşazade in most instances, is silent on the death of this aforementioned prince. See Oruç Beğ, *Oruç Beğ Tarihi: Giriş, Metin, Kronoloji, Dizin, Tıpkıbasım*, ed. Necdet Öztürk (Istanbul: Çamlıca Basım Yayın, 2007), 18. Oruç mentions the conquest and then moves on to talk about the conquest of Thrace, skipping about a decade in the account of events. He mentions the conquest of the Karesi dominions, including Balıkesir, Bergama, Edremid, and Ulubad, but does not talk about the death of the said prince. Neither the bringing of the prince to Bursa nor his death of bubonic plague is included in Oruç's account.

[31] Ahmedî, *Divan*, 87 (XXX/26) "*Bu tâhûn-ı felek altında hışmı / İricek hasma tâ'ûn ı vebâdur*" [Der-medh-i Emir Sülman].

[32] Written in 1490, Kemal's account is exceptional in mentioning the death of the members of the Ottoman dynasty as a result of plague – something we do not see in other chronicles. Kemal, *Selâtîn-Nâme (1299–1490)* (Ankara: TTK, 2001), 135.

[33] Tursun Bey, *Fatih'in Tarihi*, ed. Mertol Tulum (Istanbul, 1977), 125.

dynasty, these chronicles were dominated by a narrative of political and military events and did not have a topos for the discussion events like plagues. In other words, the genre only discussed events deemed commensurate with their significance to the dynasty. Under such circumstances, plague was generally not brought up, unless it was seen as affecting the House of Osman directly.

In comparison with the earlier examples of the genre, chronicles composed in the sixteenth century are more elaborate works of history, expressed in more sophisticated language. In these chronicles one may expect to find references to plague, though those mostly appear in brief. For example, Hoca Saadeddin's (d. 1599) *Tacü't-Tevarih* mentions plague only in a few instances, such as those in 1467–68, 1491, and 1495–96. In most cases, outbreaks are mentioned because they cause the sultan to stay in a different place.[34] One of the most refined products of Ottoman history writing in the sixteenth century, Mustafa Ali's (d. 1600) *Künhü'l-Ahbar* has scattered references to plague.[35] Another work of the late sixteenth century, Selaniki Mustafa Efendi's (d. [1600]) *Selaniki Tarihi*, has abundant references to plague alongside other such events, like fires, earthquakes, and floods in Istanbul.[36]

There were important changes in Ottoman chronicle writing from the late fifteenth to the late sixteenth century. Whereas plague was barely mentioned in the works of the former era, it figured more often and in greater detail in the works of the latter. It may be tempting to explain this change by increased frequency of plague. Nevertheless, the reasons for the increased visibility of plagues in the narratives may need to be sought in other historical processes, such as the development of an urban context in the Ottoman chronicle-writing tradition, the articulation of a certain meaning of plague, and the changes in the conceptualization and writing of history.

First, narratives of plague, much like accounts of earthquakes, fires, and other similar events, typically required an urban context. In narratives of plague of the late medieval and early modern eras in both Europe and the Middle East, the urban setting is easily recognizable. Urban plagues are much better recorded, studied, and known than those in rural areas. This is because their effects are felt and observed more dramatically in cities where people live in close proximity, in contrast with effects in rural settlements, where population density is relatively scarce. In other words, the urban context is what makes plague observable, and thus memorable. This may have been one of the factors determining why plague is not a topos in early

---

34 E.g., see Hoca Saadettin Efendi, *Tacü't-tevarih* (Istanbul: Milli Eğitim Basımevi, 1979), 3:93–94, 269–70.

35 Mustafa bin Ahmet Âli, *Künhü'l-ahbâr: dördüncü rükn, Osmanlı tarihi* (Ankara: TTK, 2009).

36 Selânikî Mustafa Efendi, *Tarih-i Selânikî*, ed. Mehmet İpşirli (Ankara: TTK, 1999).

Ottoman chronicles, where such an urban context was largely lacking. In the works of the latter era, when the urban context was fully developed, the effects of the plague became more dramatically visible.

Second, the absence of plague in these texts does not mean a real absence of plague as an event to be narrated. It can be conceived as the absence of meaning itself.[37] The lack of plague in these texts should be "read" in conjunction with the perception of the disease. In other words, the ways in which plague was understood by the chroniclers are essential in understanding its presence or absence in the narrative. Plague epidemics are only reflected in the sources to the extent that they were perceived by their contemporaries and narrated within the available means of expression. As Chapter 7 shows in more detail, plague may have been like a black hole, devoid of meaning until the sixteenth century, when a set of beliefs, principles, and knowledge emerged. It was a bête noire, a foreign experience that the Ottomans were not sure how to write about. Plague only acquired a certain meaning as the forms along which it could be understood developed, multiplied, and circulated; in this manner the black hole was filled.[38] Plague came to be identified and written about. Both scholarly and popular works bear witness to this process. For example, medical works described its causes and symptoms and offered means of prevention from and treatment of it. Works of hagiography utilized it in stories of miraculous individual and communal cures. State documents mentioned plague as they related troubles it caused in communities as well as the response of the Ottoman central administration. This emergent body of writing in reference to plague testifies to this process, with a host of images, metaphors, and meanings that were crafted in due course. This wealth of added meaning unfolded in the legacy of post-1600 plague writing, not only in the genre of Ottoman chronicles, but in other forms of writing as well. Starting in the seventeenth century, the Ottoman historians inherited a certain form and context in which they could construct narratives of plague. In other words, plague came to be a legitimate topos they could use. Perhaps this explains why we start seeing increasing numbers of references to plague in the works of Ottoman chroniclers starting in the seventeenth century, and not because this marks the beginning of plague epidemics.

Third, the increased visibility of plague in the chronicles also reflected more substantial changes in the conception and writing of history. The concerns, language, and historical consciousness of the chroniclers changed remarkably from the fifteenth through the sixteenth centuries. As the genre

---

[37] For a discussion of meaning and narrativity in history writing, see e.g., Hayden White, "The Value of Narrativity in the Representation of Reality," *Critical Inquiry* 7, no. 1 (1980): 5–27.

[38] I discuss this change at length elsewhere. See my "From '*Bête Noire*' to '*le Mal de* Constantinople,'" 741–70.

developed, plague came to be perceived as a proper subject of historical writing, a discursive theme integrated into the Ottoman history-writing tradition, even if it lacked models or templates with which to frame it.[39] In the absence of available models to emulate, late-sixteenth-century Ottoman historians, such as Ali or Selaniki, experimented in crafting a basic template for plague narratives. For instance, whereas Ali included some basic information, such as an epidemic's place of origin, area of coverage, and death toll, Selaniki added a fair amount of detail, such as the increase or decrease in the death toll within a single outbreak and how people responded to it. As such, these accounts constituted a model that later historians could – and did – draw from, starting in the seventeenth century.[40] It is easier to find references to plague in Ottoman historical literature beginning in the seventeenth century, as these historians had inherited a model of plague narratives. In this manner, plague came to be integrated into the mainstream history-writing tradition around the turn of the seventeenth century. Thus, it may be possible to observe that these changes were correlative with the evolution of conceptualization of an urban context, changes in the genre of chronicle writing, and perhaps in the broader sweep of Ottoman history, to the articulation of a refined imperial ideology. The development of plague as a topos in this genre and its emerging discursivity went hand in hand with

[39] As a point of comparison, the Byzantine history-writing tradition possessed such models or templates to draw from. For example, both Procopius's description of the Plague of Justinian and Cantacuzenos's account of the Black Death are based on the model of Thucydides's narrative of the Plague of Athens. See Christos S. Bartsocas, "Two Fourteenth Century Greek Descriptions of the 'Black Death,'" *JHMAS* 21, no. 4 (1966): 394–400; T. S. Miller, "The Plague in John VI Cantacuzenus and Thucydides," *Greek, Roman and Byzantine Studies* 17, no. 4 (1976): 385–95; Stathakopoulos, *Famine and Pestilence*, 135–43. Similarly, Kritovoulos, as heir to Byzantine traditions of historiography, produced an account of the plague of 1467 based on older models. See Pierre Villard, "Constantinople et la peste (1467). (Critoboulos, V, 17)," in *Histoire et société: La mémoire, l'écriture et l'histoire*, ed. Georges Duby, 143–50 (Aix-en-Provence: Université de Provence, 1992).

[40] E.g., seventeenth-century historian Solakzade's treatment of plague is clearly written on the basis of Selâniki's. See Solakzade, *Solakzâde Tarihi* (Istanbul, 1880), 303–5, 318–19. A slightly later example is the work of Müneccimbaşı Ahmed Dede (d. 1702), the chief court astrologer of Mehmed IV (r. 1648–87), known as Müneccimbaşı Tarihi, whose references to plague seem to rely on earlier accounts, especially those by Ali and Hoca Saadeddin. See Müneccimbaşı Ahmed bin Lütfullah, *Müneccimbaşı Tarihi*, trans. İsmail Erünsal ([Istanbul]: Tercüman, [197–]). A case in point is the example of the 1429–30 plague outbreak in Bursa. This outbreak, which was noted in some detail in a fifteenth-century calendar, was used by later chronicles and even found its way into modern scholarship. As such, this is a good example for a successful transmission of a recorded plague in the Ottoman chronicle-writing tradition. Had there been better recording of the plague in the earlier Ottoman accounts by its contemporaries and near-contemporaries, then perhaps the later accounts could have transmitted the information in this manner. For this particular outbreak, see, e.g., Müneccimbaşı Ahmed bin Lütfullah, *Müneccimbaşı Tarihi*, 1:218; Evliya Çelebi, *Seyahatnâme*, 2:30–32; İsmail Hakkı Uzunçarşılı, *Osmanlı Devletinin Saray Teşkilâtı* (Ankara: TTK, 1988), 136–37; Schamiloglu, "Black Death in Medieval Anatolia," 266.

changes in social consciousness, medical knowledge, and governmental regulations about epidemics as well as changes in the perception of the body and health.

This takes us to the question of why the chroniclers mentioned plagues when they did. In what contexts did they write about plague? What was the purpose or function of such accounts in their broader narrative? For example, whereas most fifteenth-century chroniclers did not even mention plague, others, such as Oruç, sparingly recorded epidemics, earthquakes, and other catastrophes. As is discussed at length in Chapter 7, the framework of apocalyptic beliefs in the fifteenth-century Ottoman world seems to account for the emphasis given to plagues and other such phenomena in his narrative. After all, if the end was imminent, the historian's task was to chronicle the events that could be seen as the signs of an impending apocalypse. There are similar examples of such efforts in other chronicle-writing traditions outside the Ottoman context. For example, it has been suggested that the Byzantine chronicles used motifs such as plagues, earthquakes, famines, and wars in support of their beliefs in the impending apocalypse.[41] A similar case is made for the Chinese chronicle-writing tradition, which typically recorded epidemics to argue for the fall of dynasties and change of fortunes.[42]

Non-Ottomanist Plague Scholarship

Although it is certainly true that the Ottomanist study of plague has been shaped by the internal dynamics of its own field, plague studies in the non-Ottomanist scholarship have also been equally influential. Since the 1970s, a significant body of scholarship on plague took hold, studying the experience of plague in both Europe and in non-Western contexts. One of the fundamental problems for this scholarship was to offer an explanation for the differences in the epidemiological experiences of the post–Black Death Mediterranean. While plague gradually receded from western Europe, eighteenth century onward, it lingered longer in the Ottoman-controlled areas. For the European observers, plague's persistence in this region led to enduring associations between the disease and the Ottomans from the eighteenth century on. As a result, Europe came to see the empire as a plague exporter, against which it strove to protect itself by implementing quarantine measures and establishing cordons sanitaires. Looking to offer an explanation for the differences in the plague experiences, the scholarship since the 1970s has approached the Mediterranean world with an assumed epidemiological

---

[41] Dionysios Stathakopoulos, "Crime and Punishment: The Plague in the Byzantine Empire, 541–749," in *Plague and the End of Antiquity: The Pandemic of 541–750*, ed. Lester K. Little (Cambridge: Cambridge University Press, 2007), 99–118; Paul Magdalino, "The History of the Future and Its Uses: Prophecy, Policy and Propaganda," in *The Making of Byzantine History. Studies Dedicated to Donald M. Nicol on His Seventieth Birthday*, ed. Roderick Beaton and Charlotte Roueché (Aldershot, UK: Variorum, 1993), 3–34.

[42] Paul D. Buell, "Qubilai and the Rats," *Sudhoffs Archiv* 96, no. 2 (2012): 136–37.

division by producing binary oppositions, such as Christian versus Muslim or Oriental versus Occidental. Those invisible divisions of the epidemiological experience have created the boundaries in plague scholarship, hence producing separate histories of plague in Europe and the Middle East–Islamic world.[43] Even for studies that maintained a unified Mediterranean vision, those divisions played an important role in explaining (in fact, rather, justifying) the very differences in the spread of plague and the responses it stirred. For example, in his authoritative work on the history of plague in France, Europe, and the Mediterranean, Jean-Noël Biraben brings forth an epidemiological divide between regions he calls *nord-occidental* and *sud-oriental*.[44] He accounts for this bipartite view of the Mediterranean in terms of differences in climate, fauna, and attitudes toward disease. However, a close analysis of his division clearly suggests a construct of epidemiological zones, where religion is the single most dividing factor. Emerging in this general framework of the bipartite epidemiological vision, the historians of the Ottoman Empire also seem to have adopted a similar tone. For example, Panzac's 1985 study situates the empire as a plague exporter to Europe during the eighteenth and nineteenth centuries, while not fully addressing the roots of the historical divergence in their epidemiological experience. In brief, the dichotomies of the Mediterranean disease zone and the underlying essentialist assumptions of differences not only bind the scholarly analyses to reductionist perceptions of past societies but also produce a rather thin sense of the historicity of plague. It may be more fruitful to adopt a perspective that would focus on the commonalities, at least for studying the late medieval and early modern periods. Until the eighteenth century or so, the plague experiences of Europe and the Ottoman world shared many similar features, as these regions belonged to a unified microbial zone of the Mediterranean.[45] It was not only the germs and the disease environment that were shared; the two ends of the Mediterranean also shared a common heritage of medical knowledge regarding the etiology and spread of epidemic diseases.[46]

---

43 E.g., Dols, *Black Death in the Middle East*, which stops in the year 1517 (the Ottoman conquest of Syria and Egypt) – clearly not an epidemiological division. See also Lawrence Conrad, "The Plague in the Early Medieval Near East," PhD diss., Princeton University, 1981. Among them, Biraben's *Les hommes et la peste*'s area of coverage is probably the most ambitious and ambiguous: France and European and Mediterranean countries. For further discussion of these imagined epidemiological boundaries in plague scholarship, see my "New Science and Old Sources."

44 Biraben, *Les hommes et la peste*, 1:106.

45 Le Roy Ladurie, "Un concept." To what extent the Mediterranean climate, flora, and fauna favored the plague and the processes by which it became enzootic in different parts of it await future research.

46 Vivian Nutton, "The Seeds of Disease: An Explanation of Contagion and Infection from the Greeks to the Renaissance," *Medical History* 27 (1983): 1–34. A comparative study of late medieval and early modern plague treatises written in Europe and in the Ottoman Empire should reveal that they were drawing from a common body of medical knowledge.

Notwithstanding these commonalities, the plague scholarship of the 1970s and 1980s has emphasized dichotomies drawn from an early modern epidemiological orientalism.[47] The imagined differences were not epidemiological in nature; they do not offer an explanation as to which mechanisms sustained plague in one part of the Mediterranean world, whereas it did not in others. Instead, there is heavy reliance on perceived differences in attitudes toward plague, thought to be based on religious difference. An attempt to reduce perceived differences to religion does not offer an adequate and satisfactory historical explanation for the suggested differences. As recent studies have shown, religion cannot be taken as the sole determinant of a social response to an epidemic.[48] By the same token, this body of scholarship has focused on the notion of contagion as a critical concept that was imagined to have marked the boundaries of difference. What did not receive emphasis, however, is that both the acceptance of the notion of contagion and its refusal were ideas shared across religious boundaries. In other words, there were people who believed in contagion and those who rejected it, in both Christian Europe and the Muslim Middle East.[49] It should be remembered that the early modern legacy of the *fatalistic Turk* was influential in shaping retrospectively the historical discourses about Ottoman history not only in Europe; the Ottomanists themselves internalized the very same discourses. Hence, it is to the emergence of this trope that we should now turn.

Fatalistic Turk

What did I mean and whither did I think of flying? Did I not know that pestilence is God's arrow, which does not miss its appointed mark? Where could I hide so as to

---

[47] I propose using *epidemiological orientalism*, drawing from the recent work of environmental historians of the Middle East and North Africa (MENA) and their use of the term *environmental orientalism*. See Diana K. Davis, "Introduction: Imperialism, Orientalism, and the Environment in the Middle East: History, Policy, Power, and Practice," in *Environmental Imaginaries of the Middle East and North Africa*, ed. Diana K. Davis and Edmund Burke III, 1–22 (Athens: Ohio University Press, 2011).

[48] Paul Slack, introduction to *Epidemics and Ideas: Essays on the Historical Perception of Pestilence*, ed. Terence Ranger and Paul Slack (Cambridge: Cambridge University Press, 1992), 17–18; Justin Stearns, "New Directions in the Study of Religious Responses to the Black Death," *History Compass* 7, no. 5 (2009): 1363–75.

[49] For a thoughtful discussion of how ideas of "miasma" and "contagion" were simultaneously present in early modern German imperial towns and how they were mobilized on the basis of conflicting interests of different segments of the society, see Annemarie Kinzelbach, "Infection, Contagion, and Public Health in Late Medieval and Early Modern German Imperial Towns," *JHMAS* 61, no. 3 (2006): 369–89. Also see Justin K. Stearns, *Infectious Ideas* (Baltimore: Johns Hopkins University Press, 2011); Irmeli Perho, *The Prophet's Medicine: A Creation of the Muslim Traditionalist Scholars* (Helsinki: Finnish Oriental Society, 1995); Sheldon J. Watts, *Epidemics and History: Disease, Power, and Imperialism* (New Haven, CT: Yale University Press, 1997).

be outside its range? If He wished me to be smitten, no flight or hiding-place could avail me; it was useless to avoid inevitable fate. His own house at the moment was not free from plague; yet he remained there. I likewise should do better to remain where I was.[50]

Such, allegedly, were the words of the Ottoman sultan Süleyman (r. 1520–66), reported by his grand vizier Rüstem Pasha to Ogier Ghiselin de Busbecq (d. 1592), in response to his inquiry about leaving his quarters in Istanbul on account of a raging plague in the city in 1561. Busbecq, the Habsburg ambassador to the Sublime Porte between 1554 and 1562, lost his doctor, William Quacquelben, and other members of his household to the plague.[51] His observations about the indifference of the *Turks*[52] declared unambiguously:

The Turks hold an opinion which makes them indifferent to, though not safe from, the plague. They are persuaded that the time and manner of each man's death is inscribed by God upon his forehead; if, therefore, he is destined to die, it is useless for him to try to avert fate; if he is not so destined, he is foolish to be afraid... "If," they say, "it is God's will that I should die, then die I must; if not, it can do me no harm." Thus contagion is spread far and wide, and sometimes whole families are exterminated.[53]

Upon returning to Europe, Busbecq published his memoirs, first in the original Latin in the 1580s. The work became so successful that several editions and translations into a number of European languages were subsequently published. The preceding excerpts are possibly among the most influential passages to shape European perceptions of the Ottomans' attitudes in the face of plague.

This episode has often been interpreted as the pinnacle of Ottoman fatalism in the face of plague, not only by early modern Europeans, but also by the modern scholarship. Scholars used Busbecq's account to confirm the apparent differences between the European and Ottoman experiences of plague. Perhaps the following passage from William McNeill's influential *Plagues and Peoples* (1976) will suffice to illustrate the case. McNeill wrote:

Moslem response to plague was (or became) passive... By the sixteenth century, when Christian rules of quarantine and other prophylactic measures against plague had attained firm definition, Moslem views hardened against efforts to escape the will of Allah. This is well illustrated by the Ottoman Sultan's response to a request from

50 Busbecq, *Turkish Letters*, 182–83.
51 For this outbreak, see Chapter 5. For William Quacquelben, see Chapter 8.
52 In the early modern European travel literature, the term *Turk* was used to refer to the Muslim subjects of the Ottoman Empire, regardless of their ethnicity, language, or culture. In this parlance, to *turn Turk* would be understood as conversion to Islam. In this chapter, I have mostly preserved the term (*Turk* or *Turkish*) in the manner it was used in these texts for the purpose of emphasis.
53 Busbecq, *Turkish Letters*, 189.

the imperial ambassador to Constantinople for permission to change his residence because plague had broken out in the house assigned to him: "Is not the plague in my own palace, yet I do not think of moving?" Moslems regarded Christian health measures with amused disdain, and thereby exposed themselves to heavier losses from plague than prevailed among their Christian neighbors.[54]

McNeill did not single-handedly arrive at this conclusion; he used Michael Dols's 1971 dissertation and some other studies, which all seem to have supported this view.[55] Nevertheless, the direct quote from Busbecq, where we allegedly "hear" the response of Süleyman, as well as the echoes of European travel writers about putative Muslim attitudes toward plague are overwhelmingly loud.

So resilient was the view that the Muslim attitudes toward plague were – or had become, by the sixteenth century – passive that even ten years ago, a historian of the Ottoman Empire could freely use Busbecq's work as a source to approach Ottoman-Muslim attitudes in this matter. Hence, drawing from a body of scholarship that held that the Muslim attitude toward plague was fatalistic, Heath Lowry argues that Süleyman's alleged reply to Busbecq stood in clear contrast with the fifteenth-century flight behavior of Mehmed II, a transition he explains as resulting from the gradual acceptance of the Muslim orthodoxy that developed after the conquest of the former Mamluk landholdings in 1516–17. Taking the preceding passage at its face value, it would perhaps be possible to arrive at the same conclusion that "Süleyman's fatalistic statements" indicated the Ottoman attitudes that ridiculed flight and rejected the concept of contagion.[56] However, we have good reason to believe that this was not the case. Sources suggest that flight was one of the responses the early modern Ottomans resorted to at times of plagues.[57] Moreover, the sixteenth century saw a conscious effort to make this practice compatible with Muslim religious law. In addition, the notion of contagion was not entirely foreign to the members of early modern Ottoman society; both scholarly and popular works made use of this notion with reference to disease transmission.[58] With this in view, a literal reading of this passage does a great disservice to understanding the Ottoman attitudes toward plague. Indeed, this is a fairly rhetorical passage that begs for further consideration.

In the light of recent scholarship on European travel writing and its reception, as well as how the genre contributed to the European imagination of its

---

[54] McNeill, *Plagues and Peoples*, 198–99.

[55] Ibid.; also 333–36.

[56] Lowry, "Pushing the Stone Uphill."

[57] A quick glance at the archival documents discussed in Chapter 6, especially the cases of flight as evidenced in *mühimme* registers testifies that this was fairly common in Ottoman society. These cases however do not allow us to speculate about who, when, and why individuals decided to flee.

[58] For a detailed discussion of flight and contagion, see Chapter 7.

difference, it may be useful to revisit the Busbecq episode with a fresh eye.[59] Considering the larger political context in which this episode took place, one cannot but note the significant exchange of rhetoric here. Political discourses featuring imperial rivalry and competing claims to universal sovereignty held by the Ottomans and the Habsburgs, for example, have been shown to be very lively in that era.[60] In their dealings with the Europeans, the Ottomans deliberately deployed a distinct discourse, which manifested itself in the form of pomp and splendor to elicit awe, and of violence to elicit fear.[61] Read in this framework, the alleged words of Süleyman did not necessarily embody fatalism, as it has been suggested, but asserted a rhetoric in which he assumed a position of higher moral ground, exhibiting stoic virtues of valor and integrity and an overt contempt for the fear of plague.

Notwithstanding the influence of the passage, Busbecq was not a lone voice in using this tone in his writing, so as to emphasize *fatalism* in conjunction with plague. Along with constructs like the *Grand Turk* and the *terrible Turk*, both the figure of the *fatalistic Turk* and the alleged tendency of *Turkish fatalism* were products of the European industry of the *Turkish* episteme. In fact, this trope has been a particularly successful one that had a life of its own beyond the genre of early modern travel literature. Needless to say, the accounts of European travel writers have been largely instrumental in creating a particular image of the *Turk* in early modern European imagination.

Early modern Europeans recognized that traveling was an important part of cultivating culture and scholarship. The travel literature penned by European visitors to Ottoman lands was not only a testimony of that experience but also a step toward attaining the ranks of a learned society. As far as observations on plague go, there seems to be some stereotypical notions that travel writers used commonly. For example, they seem to agree on how the Ottomans qua Muslims did not take any precautions against plague. According to these narratives, the *Turks* did not flee the plague because they believed that their fate was already determined. It was pronounced how and when they were going to die, and so it would be pointless to try to avoid it.

---

[59] E.g., see Mary Louise Pratt, *Imperial Eyes: Travel Writing and Transculturation* (London: Routledge, 1992); Gerald M. MacLean, *The Rise of Oriental Travel: English Visitors to the Ottoman Empire, 1580–1720* (New York: Palgrave Macmillan, 2004); Sonja Brentjes, *Travellers from Europe in the Ottoman and Safavid Empires, 16th–17th Centuries: Seeking, Transforming, Discarding Knowledge* (Burlington, VT: Ashgate/Variorum, 2010).

[60] Gülru Necipoğlu, "Süleyman the Magnificent and the Representation of Power in the Context of Ottoman-Hapsburg-Papal Rivalry," *The Art Bulletin* 71, no. 3 (1989): 401–27; Cornell H. Fleischer, "The Lawgiver as Messiah: The Making of the Imperial Image in the Reign of Süleymân," in *Soliman le magnifique et son temps*, ed. Gilles Veinstein, 159–77 (Paris: La Documentation française, 1992).

[61] Özlem Kumrular, *The Ottoman World, Europe and the Mediterranean* (Istanbul: Isis Press, 2012).

If they were destined to die of plague, nothing could stop it. It followed that they were completely ignorant about the nature of the plague, indifferent to its significance, and oblivious to its consequences; they did not understand the notion of contagion. These accounts depict the *Turks* as passive and fatalistic in the face of epidemics. Indeed, this particular attitude was constructed such that it would contrast the European Christian attitude, imagined to be one of active combat with disease. This particular vision of difference has proved to be tremendously resilient so much so that even modern scholarship continues to recycle it in one form or another.

Surveying the genealogy of the trope of the *fatalistic Turk* in the European travel literature from the early modern to the modern era promises to offer a better understanding of how this trope was constructed, modified, and circulated, depending on the needs of European society. What follows is a sketch of the highlights in this genealogy, on the basis of some prominent examples of the genre, which enables us to trace the emergence and development of this stereotype, how it circulated, and how it was received, to contextualize this particular vision. This is by no means an exhaustive account of the massive corpus of *Turcica* literature produced in the early modern era. Such a study will need to await a more systematic compilation of a wide range of scattered material.

The Genealogy of a Trope in Early Modern European Travel Writing

In the early modern era, western Europeans composed a number of works based on their travel to Ottoman lands. This literature flourished significantly after the Ottoman conquest of Constantinople in the mid-fifteenth century through the heyday of the city in the sixteenth century and later. The growth of this literature was commensurate with the increasing number of European visitors and diplomatic missions that included merchants, scholars, artists, preachers, and the like. Many of those visitors certainly witnessed outbreaks of plague in Istanbul or elsewhere in Ottoman territory. If they survived, they wrote about those outbreaks in a particular, suspiciously uniform way. The rise of the printing press and increased possibilities of easy circulation of printed material certainly contributed to the process of shaping the nature of these accounts. Recent studies have taught us that the composition of these travelogues was the result of a careful process of compilation, classification, selection, and elimination of knowledge.[62]

For the European travelers to the Ottoman Empire in the late seventeenth or eighteenth centuries, plague was familiar, as outbreaks were still seen in Europe. Depending on their education or exposure, travelers may have had varying degrees of knowledge about the causes, symptoms, and prognosis of this illness as well as what to do to avoid it. They would draw from a body of knowledge and a set of norms to judge what they saw in Ottoman

---

[62] Brentjes, *Travellers*.

society. Perhaps this explains why these accounts, including those written by physicians, did not engage in lengthy comparisons of the disease itself or its effects as experienced in their homeland versus in the Ottoman areas. They clearly recognized that "European" and "Ottoman" plagues were one and the same disease, imagined as having the same effects everywhere. For them, the discordance rather lay in the attitudes and responses of people. It appears that a set of prescriptive norms to avoid *contagion* was already known to these travelers. The lack of what they typically thought was the *fear of contagion* is central to their narratives. They saw this as bizarre or irrational behavior and inevitably contrasted it to what was more familiar, that is, behaviors to *avoid contagion*, such as imposing physical barriers between the *infected* and the *uninfected*, in the form of quarantines, as much for people as for objects. Clothing, but also any item made of fabric, feather, or paper, was conceived as material that could sustain the infection (as opposed to items imagined as being contagion-free). Once suspected of being infected, these materials had to be either immersed in water or fumigated to eliminate the contagion. The absence of such practices must have been a shock to these travelers and required an explanation. The lack of quarantine measures or the absence of precautions against contagion was immediately taken as a sign of ignorance, incapacity to understand the concept of contagion, and indifference toward it. The explanation for this difference, therefore, had to be sought in religion. Hence, we see narratives of Muslim (or, for that matter, *Turkish*) *fatalism* overflowing in these travelogues.

Even though it is not easy to pinpoint precisely when the motif of *Turkish fatalism* first started to be used in conjunction with plague, it can be said that it was used to some extent in the European travelogues composed in the sixteenth century and certainly became regular in the first half of the seventeenth. An early example of the use of the trope, slightly before that of Busbecq, can be found in the writings of the French naturalist Pierre Belon (d. 1564). Belon was sent by Francis I (r. 1515–47) to the Sublime Porte to accompany a diplomatic mission. While in the Ottoman lands in the 1540s, he traveled and prepared a travel account, which was published after his return to Europe. *Les Observations de plusieurs singularitez et choses mémorables, trouvées en Grèce, Asie, Iudée, Egypte et autres pays estranges, rédigées en trois livres* (1553) was first published in Paris, followed by successive editions and translations, giving Belon great recognition. In the year 1547, while on the way to Thessaloniki, Belon heard news of a plague there, though the residents had fled the town on account of the epidemic. Belon remarks here that the Turks, of all other nations, were the least haunted by those stricken with plague.[63] He also notes elsewhere that the Turks live long lives because they are not of delicate nature, living largely

---

[63] "Les Turcs entre toutes autres nations sont les gens qui font le moins d'estime de hanter ceux qui sont frappez de peste: chose qu'auōs aperceue à Salonichi." Pierre Belon, *Les Observations de plusieures singularitez... trouvées en Grece, Asie...* (Paris, 1588), 99.

on garlic and onions, not drinking wine or drinking it rarely. And yet, at times of plagues, Belon adds solemnly, they do nothing to defend themselves, nor do they fear to catch it.[64] Belon adds these observations almost like an afterthought on both occasions, without engaging in a discussion of what this meant.

A few decades later, the Lutheran preacher Salomon Schweigger (d. 1622) made similar observations. Schweigger accompanied the Habsburg diplomatic mission to the Sublime Porte in 1577 and spent three years in Istanbul and traveling in other parts of the empire. Upon his return, he published his memoirs in Nurnberg in 1608, which underwent several later editions throughout the seventeenth century and afterward. This work was among the earliest examples of travel accounts to Ottoman lands published in the German language, which may explain its great success. Even though Schweigger's account is very useful for some observations he made about daily life, he did not have anything new to say on the subject of plague. In fact, like Belon, he merely repeated the cliché that the Turks were not afraid of contagious diseases, as they believed that one's fate was written on one's forehead and thus they did not refrain from physical contact with the sick.[65] Perhaps to solidify his account, he added that he witnessed one day the death of a poor man from plague on a street near their ambassadorial residence. Upon seeing this, people passing by stopped and surrounded the man immediately; one took his hat, others his shoes, and in this way, they undressed the man to his underwear. Finally, two men took pity and carried the body away to bury.[66]

While these accounts, alongside that of Busbecq, could be considered typical in their use of the trope of the *fatalistic Turk* for the late sixteenth century, this was something they mentioned briefly without giving much detail. As we move into accounts written in the seventeenth century, narratives of plague and the behavior depicted as fatalism become more elaborate. For example, the secondhand clothing trade becomes closely associated with contagion. In the early seventeenth century, Ottaviano Bon (d. 1623), the Venetian *bailo* in Istanbul (1604–6), described how the belongings of the dead were brought to the flea market (*bezisten/bedesten*) to be sold.[67] He noted with

---

[64] "Les Turcs sont gens qui viuent longuement: car ils son peu delicats, viuans à tous propos d'aulx & oignons, ne beuuans point de vin sinon rarement. Mais pource qu'en temps de peste ils ne se gardent de riē, & n'ont point peur de la prendre, ils y sont souuent trompez." Ibid., 402.

[65] An early version of this statement that would be familiar to the European audience can be found in Theodore Spandounes's *On the Origins of Ottoman Emperors*. See Theodōros Spandouginos, *Theodore Spandounes: On the Origins of the Ottoman Emperors*, trans. and ed. Donald M. Nicol (Cambridge: Cambridge University Press, 1997), 131.

[66] Schweigger, *Sultanlar Kentine Yolculuk*, 200. This account seems to contradict his own description of funerary rites and ceremonies practiced in Istanbul, e.g., see 199.

[67] Jérôme Maurand had already observed in 1544 that the belongings of plague victims were brought to the flea market (*basestag*) and sold outside its doors at lower prices. See Jérome

amazement that people bought these items without fear of pestilence, "as if the disease were not infectious at all." The cause of this behavior, he reasoned, was because of their belief that "their end is written in their forehead, and that it is a vain thing to think, or seek to prevent it by any human rule, or policy; as either the avoiding the company of infected persons, or the not wearing of the clothes of them that died."[68] He explained this belief in fate as follows: "at the creation of man [God] prefixed, and appointed a set time for his end, it is impossible that the wit or device of mortal man should be able to divert, or prevent it."[69] In doing so, Bon created a site for contagion that later accounts would also use: the bazaar where secondhand clothes were sold, the flea market, emerged as the site where contagion was imagined to take place.[70]

Soon after this, the account of Tommaso Alberti, a merchant from Bologna or Venice who traveled to the Ottoman Empire in the early seventeenth century, repeated the same template without even adding much detail to it. While in Istanbul, Alberti visited the grand bazaar and described the exotic goods that one could find there, including the clothes for sale. However, he added suspiciously that some of those clothes had once belonged to people who had died from plague and observed that this did not stop others from buying or handling them, "as if the plague were not contagious." Making an effort to explain this behavior (which must have seemed most bizarre to him), he commented that the *Turks* believed that one's future was written on one's forehead and that one could not do anything to avoid it.[71] It is possible that Alberti used this *fatalistic Turk* motif on the basis of his own observations or what he heard from others, yet the similarity to Bon's account is too great to miss.

By the second half of the seventeenth century, the trope of the *fatalistic Turk* already seems to be entrenched in the European imagination, so as to be mobilized as the European alterity at times of plague. For example, Maurice de Toulon, a Capuchin monk, condemned *Turkish fatalism* in the

Maurand, *Itinéraire de Jérome Maurand d'Antibes à Constantinople (1544)* (Paris: E. Leroux, 1901), 236–37.

68 Ottaviano Bon, *The Sultan's Seraglio: An Intimate Portrait of Life at the Ottoman Court: (from the Seventeenth-Century Edition of John Withers)* (London: Saqi, 1996), 86.

69 Ibid., 126.

70 For examples of European travelers' accounts that pointed out the flea market as the origin of contagion, see Chapter 1.

71 Tommaso Alberti, *Viaggio a Costantinopoli (1609–1621)* (Bologna: Romagnoli, 1889), 139: "Il ritratto delle quali robe è riportato in mano del Casnadar Bassi di dentro, Eunuco, e conservato nel Casnà; e se bene le robe sono di quelli che muoiono dalla peste, non è perciò alcuno che si astenga di comprarle e di maneggiarle, come se il male non fosse contagioso; reputando i Turchi di aver nel fronte scritto il suo line, senza poterlo per opera umana fuggire." This work remained unpublished until the late nineteenth century. For Tommasso Alberti, see Stefanos Yerasimos, "Alberti, Tommaso," *Dünden Bugüne İstanbul Ansiklopedisi*, 1:181.

face of plague to criticize his own society. The use of the alleged Turkish indifference to plague was a call to his own society to get better organized, clearly a reference that would move his audience, for they would all know what he was referring to.[72] Hence, there is good reason to believe that the trope of *Turkish fatalism*, similar to *Turkish despotism* or *tyranny*, had by then become familiar even to those in Europe who did not have direct knowledge of Ottoman society. By the mid-seventeenth century, the trope had already anchored in the European imagination.

Later in the seventeenth century, the narratives of the *fatalistic Turk* became even more elaborate. For example, Paul Rycaut's (d. 1700) well-known *The Present State of the Ottoman Empire* gives interesting details on the matter. Rycaut was sent by the English King Charles II to the Sublime Porte to accompany a diplomatic mission. After spending several years in Istanbul, he composed *The Present State* in 1665, incidentally in the same year as the Great Plague of London. The work was first published in 1668, followed by several editions, eventually becoming one of the most famed works on the Ottoman Empire in English. In his account, Rycaut starts out by describing the lack of avoidance behavior that other texts had attributed to fatalism. Once again, we hear the same story: "According to this Doctrine, none ought to avoid or fear the Infection of the Plague; Mahomets precepts being not to abandon the City-house where Infection rages, because God hath numbred their days and predestinated their fate; And upon this belief, they as familiarly attend the Beds and frequent the company of Pestilential persons."[73] Rycaut then goes on to demonstrate the disastrous consequences of not fleeing the site of pestilence; he gives examples of entire households being wiped out as a result. In doing so, he assures the reader that the *Turks* behave wrongly, with suggestions that this behavior is not only dangerous but also immoral. For example, he refers to "the custom in the Families of great men to lodge many Servants . . . in the same room, where *the diseased and healthful lie promiscuously together*, from whence it hath hapned often, that three parts of . . . two hundred men, most *youthful and lusty*, have perished in the heat of July and Augusts Pestilence."[74] Hitherto, this would

---

[72] Father Maurice de Toulon, *Le Capucin charitable, enseignant la méthode pour remédier aux grandes misères que la peste a coûtume de causer parmi les peuples* (Paris, 1662); cited in L. W. B. Brockliss and Colin Jones, *The Medical World of Early Modern France* (Oxford: Clarendon Press, 1997), 68; and Colin Jones, "Plague and Its Metaphors in Early Modern France," *Representations*, no. 53 (1996): 115.

[73] Paul Rycaut, *The Present State of the Ottoman Empire: Containing the Maxims of the Turkish Politie, the Most Material Points of the Mahometan Religion, . . . Their Military Discipline . . . : Illustrated with Divers Pieces of Sculpture Representing the Variety of Habits amongst the Turks; In 3 Books* (London: Starkey, 1670), 116. On Rycaut, also see Sonia P. Anderson, *An English Consul in Turkey: Paul Rycaut at Smyrna, 1667–1678* (Oxford: Oxford University Press, 1989).

[74] Rycaut, *Present State*, 116, emphasis mine.

not be unusual given the conventions of the genre, neither for an English audience nor for a Continental one at this time. After all, as the scholarship has convincingly demonstrated, the European readers' thirst could be quenched with a mixture of religious and sexual fantasies of the *Turk*. The early modern Republic of Letters harbored countless such examples.[75]

However, Rycaut's account presents an interesting twist at this point, where it diverges from the known trope of fatalism. After a lengthy discussion of why it is wrong not to flee, Rycaut goes on to remark that some *Turks* did actually try to avoid plagues by leaving plague-infested cities. He wrote: "But yet I have observed, in the time of an extraordinary Plague, that the Turks . . . fled to retired and private Villages, especially the Cadees and men of the Law."[76] As much as Rycaut believed in the value of this behavior, he could not refrain from voicing a cynical disapproval, because he thought that those who fled were doing it with the wrong motivations, namely, for a lack of courage. He wrote, "[Those] Turks have not confided so much to the precept of their Prophet, as to have *courage enough to withstand* the dread and terrour of that slaughter the sickness hath made; but have under other excuses fled."[77] It is interesting to read these lines by Rycaut, describing the very attitudes others had believed was caused by a *lack of fear* of contagion. Notwithstanding this subtle criticism, Rycaut's acknowledgment that people did resort to flight at times of epidemics is very valuable, something we can confirm with evidence drawn from the Ottoman sources.[78] Yet, Rycaut was not the only foreign observer to write that flight behavior could be witnessed at times of plagues in Ottoman society. Several decades before him, the Venetian *bailo* Lorenzo Bernardo (*bailo* between 1585 and 1587 and between 1591 and 1592) gave a report to the Senate in which he observed a change in Ottoman attitudes toward favoring flight. He wrote,

The belief that one's death is "written" and that one has no free will to escape dangers is declining in Turkey with each passing day. Experience teaches them the opposite when they see that a man who avoids plague victims saves his life while one who has stayed with them catches plague and dies. During my time there as bailo I even saw their mufti flee Constantinople for fear of plague and go to the garden to live, and the Grand Signor himself took care to avoid all contacts with his generals. [They] . . . learned they can escape from plagues.[79]

---

75 Alain Grosrichard, *The Sultan's Court: European Fantasies of the East* (London: Verso, 1998). On Rycaut's reference to homosexuality in his narrative, see Nabil Matar, *Turks, Moors, and Englishmen in the Age of Discovery* (New York: Columbia University Press, 2000), 117–18, 121–23.

76 Rycaut, *Present State*, 116.

77 Ibid., emphasis mine.

78 See Chapter 7 for a discussion of flight in Ottoman sources of this era.

79 Lorenzo Bernardo, 1592 "Its decline may be under way" [Alberi, III, 2:366–77], in James Cushman Davis, *Pursuit of Power: Venetian Ambassador's Reports on Spain, Turkey and France in the Age of Phillip II: 1560–1600* (New York: Harper and Row, 1970), 158.

As acute observers of Ottoman society, Venice worked as the hub of information on the Ottomans, whence it was distributed across Europe. Thus, there is good reason to believe that the observation communicated by *bailo* Bernardo – that the Ottomans started to favor flight from epidemics – would find some circulation in Venice, and possibly beyond. Yet, curiously there is no trace of it. This observation, which did not fit in the European stereotype of Muslim *fatalism*, did not seem to find acceptance in Europe. Even the Venetian *bailo* Ottaviano Bon, writing not too long after Bernardo, reverted to the old stereotypical vision of the *fatalistic Turk*. Thus, there does not seem to be any direct or indirect link between the observations of Bernardo in the late sixteenth century and those of Rycaut about three-quarters of a century later, except for what they had observed.

Despite his condescending attitude, Rycaut did point accurately to the presence of two different opinions on the issue of flight. According to his account, the opinion "most general and current with the Turks" is that one should flee plague. He referred to those of this opinion as *"Jebare."* Those holding the opposite opinion believed that one must not leave where there is plague; Rycaut referred to the latter as *"Kadere."*[80] His observation about the conflict of opinion on the issue of flight was a keen one and deserves further consideration.

Ottoman sources inform us of the presence of two camps with conflicting opinions on the issue of flight – a conflict of opinion, they claim to have existed since early Islamic times. For example, the renowned Ottoman theologian and biographer Ahmed Taşköprizade lays out the development of the conflict with proofs of the opinion of each camp.[81] Rycaut highlights in particular one group who was of this opinion, namely, the religious scholars (*ulama*). He wrote,

Especially the Cadees and men of the Law, who being commonly of more refined wits and judgments then the generality, both by reason and experience have found that a wholesome Air is a preserver of life, and that they have lived to return again to their own house in health and strength, when perhaps their next Neighbours have through their brutish ignorance been laid in the Graves.[82]

Here Rycaut suggests that the Ottoman religious scholars made learned judgments about leaving places of infection, while others became victims of their ignorance. The way he presented the proofs of the beliefs held by the religious scholars is in line with the Ottoman religious and legal understanding of this issue, as demonstrated in the plague treatise of Taşköprizade and the legal opinions issued by the Chief Jurisconsult Ebussuud Efendi (d. 1574). Given Rycaut's close personal ties with Ottoman religious scholars, it is

---

[80]   Rycaut, *Present State*, 116.
[81]   For a detailed treatment of Taşköprizade's view on this issue, see Chapter 7.
[82]   Rycaut, *Present State*, 116.

not surprising that he was cognizant of and could articulate their opinion accurately. It remains to be said that we are not well informed about which group held which opinion in seventeenth-century Ottoman society, so as to assess the merits of his assertion, though it is also possible that his suggestion spoke to an English audience, instead of being a simple reflection of historical reality in the Ottoman case.[83] Whatever the reasons for Rycaut's suggestion may have been, he made clear that fleeing plagues was commonplace at least among the Ottoman religious scholars in the second half of the seventeenth century.

With regard to the reception of Rycaut's work back in Europe, we know for a fact that Rycaut's *The Present State* quickly became a reference point for addressing all things *Turkish*. A selective reading of his ideas could serve to enable a wide range of criticisms of domestic political issues in England. He was as much read at home (e.g., there is evidence that John Locke read him) as abroad, when his works were translated. *The Present State* was translated into French in the years following its initial appearance in English. The seventeenth-century French philosopher Pierre Bayle, regarded as the forerunner of the Encyclopedists, also read Rycaut and cited him as his source for things Muslim.[84] The work was also translated into Dutch, German, Polish, Italian, and Russian. Despite the evidence in support of the wide circulation and reception of Rycaut's work, it is what he described as the Muslim doctrine on the issue of flight that survived and flourished in the European writings on the Ottomans, at the expense of his observations that the very people who were experts of that doctrine (the religious scholars) believed that it was better to flee. Curiously, the fatalistic trope triumphed over the other opinion in the European theater of the *Turk*. How are we to account for this? What were the causes for the elimination of this view in favor of the stereotypical trope of the *fatalistic Turk*?

To better understand this issue, one needs to consider the larger context for the production, circulation, and consumption of knowledge in early modern Europe, which actively shaped these travel accounts. In her comparative work on western European travelers to the Ottoman and Safavid empires

---

[83] Rycaut was very knowledgeable of the political, economic, and social aspects of Ottoman life. Yet some of his writings suggest that he was repeating some of the age-old stereotypes of that society. According to Linda T. Darling, he was using the old stereotypes for new purposes, which should be understood in the political context of seventeenth-century British history. See Darling, "Ottoman Politics through British Eyes: Paul Rycaut's *The Present State of the Ottoman Empire*," *Journal of World History* 5, no. 1 (1994): 71–97. E.g., the fact that he tried to establish clear parallels between the Ottoman views of predestination and those of the Calvinists may suggest that these remarks had further implications for an English audience.

[84] John Marshall, *John Locke, Toleration and Early Enlightenment Culture* (Cambridge: Cambridge University Press, 2006), 395. Marshall suggests that both Locke and Bayle used Rycaut's work to support their arguments of religious toleration.

in the sixteenth and seventeenth centuries, Sonja Brentjes offers invaluable insights for approaching the genre. According to Brentjes, travelers to the Ottoman Empire meticulously processed their travel notes, upon returning to their countries, by eliminating, selecting, modifying, and adapting them to what they perceived as the accepted norm in the European centers of learning. In doing this, they were informed by a body of *apodemic* literature, which, by the late sixteenth century, not only provided the travelers with tips on the travel itself but also worked as templates for how to write about their travel experiences. Travelers also consulted classical sources of learning; exchanged information, specimens, manuscripts, and the like with colleagues; and altered – when deemed necessary – their personal observations and experiences in the light of the more acceptable forms of knowledge about the very places and people they wrote about. After all, these individuals were writing these works with the expectation to advance their position or career in their home country. In this manner, the standardized narratives helped produce as much as confirm certain Western preconceptions about Muslim societies.[85]

It may be fruitful to reflect on the trope of the *fatalistic Turk* in this larger context. Needless to say, one of the fundamental undercurrents of this perception was religion. Early modern travel narratives insisted on an association between a fatalistic attitude and Islam: they maintained that because their religion teaches them that their fate is predetermined, they believed they did not have to take any precautions, nor did they need to fear the plague. Notwithstanding the perceived differences of religion, a common assumption of the genre was that the *Turkish* mind was characterized by ignorance and superstition. It is not difficult to find depictions of the Muslim members of Ottoman society as ignorant, credulous, and incapable of understanding the concept of contagion. For example, Busbecq voiced contempt for what he believed was the result of their incapacity to comprehend the concept of contagion: "And so they handle the garments and linen in which plague-stricken persons have died, even though they are still wet with the contagion of their sweat; nay, they even wipe their faces with them."[86] Examples such as this abound in the genre. The particular stereotype that Muslims are incapable of rational thinking or comprehending "natural" phenomena was continuously nurtured and confirmed by various examples of the genre. In a similar vein, these travel narratives claimed that the *Turks* lacked an appreciation for antiquities and that they failed to understand the concept of history.[87] Hence, the denial of the existence of sciences in the Ottoman Empire is a commonly used topos of the genre. After careful

---

[85] Brentjes, *Travellers*, introduction and 1:447.

[86] Busbecq, *Turkish Letters*, 189.

[87] A. Wunder, "Western Travelers, Eastern Antiquities, and the Image of the Turk in Early Modern Europe," *Journal of Early Modern History* 7, nos. 1–2 (2003): 89–119.

scrutiny of numerous such narratives, Brentjes demonstrates that there is almost complete silence on the sciences in most accounts, and others, who did write about it, did so very briefly, especially in comparison to the Safavid case. In contrast, while the stereotypical accounts emphasized that Muslim Ottoman subjects had no interest in sciences, they exaggerated the role of Christian or Jewish immigrants or converts from Europe in the sciences. Brentjes contests this view by arguing that the demands of the humanist quest for knowledge, specimens, and manuscripts must have been facilitated by local networks of knowledge and patronage and the presence of sources. Thus, she suggests that the perceived difference in the state of the sciences between Europe and the Ottoman Empire came to play a central role in the self-identification of Europeans.[88] It may be helpful to think of the case of plague and the criticism for the lack of the concept of contagion among the *Turks* in this context.

Whatever the causes of this may have been, the trope of the *Turkish fatalism* ultimately succeeded. Perhaps the best example to illustrate this triumph is Daniel Defoe's famous novel *A Journal of the Plague Year*, published in 1722. Writing more than a half-century after Rycaut's *The Present State of the Ottoman Empire*, Defoe did not refrain from using the theme of predestination in his journalistic account of the 1665 Plague of London:

The Turks and Mahometans in Asia and in other Places... presuming upon their profess'd predestinating Notions, and of every Man's End being predetermin'd and unalterably before-hand decreed, they would go unconcern'd into infected Places, and converse with infected Persons, by which Means they died at the Rate of Ten or Fifteen Thousand a Week, whereas the Europeans or Christian Merchants, who kept themselves retired and reserv'd, generally escap'd the Contagion.[89]

Presumably, this would be not only familiar to an early-eighteenth-century English audience reading Defoe's work but also credible when used as part of an account of the Great Plague of London, which must have been still fresh in the communal memory of Londoners more than a half-century later. Here Defoe's use of the trope is not only indicative of its ultimate achievement over competing explanations, but at the same time, the alleged Muslim behavior is proven to be wrong, when contrasted with the attitudes of the *Europeans or Christian Merchants*. In other words, the *Turkish fatalism* is now defined as the alterity of Europeans' attitudes toward plague in view of its different effects on them. Defoe was an inadvertent forerunner of a new age.

It is well documented that plague was in decline in western and northern Europe starting in the late seventeenth and eighteenth centuries. Even though the process was gradual and not without major historical epidemics,

---

[88] Brentjes, *Travellers*, 1:437–40, 450–56.
[89] Daniel Defoe, *A Journal of the Plague Year: Authoritative Text, Backgrounds, Contexts, Criticism* (New York: W. W. Norton, 1992), 14.

such as the Great Plague of London in 1665, the Baltic plague of 1709–13,[90] or the Plague of Marseille in 1720–21, Europeans did not fail to observe that plague was diminishing. Knowing full well that plague continued in the eastern Mediterranean and Russian lands, they believed they had to keep strict regulations of quarantine and implement cordons sanitaires. Hence, the eighteenth century was a turning point in the European imagination about the changing locus of plague. The implications were twofold. On one hand, the European imagination came to dissociate itself from the plague, as this validated beliefs regarding the locus of plague outside of Europe. On the other, plague conveniently stopped being a major source of worry when the Ottomans were no longer an immediate military threat to Europe. Thus, plague now could be freely exoticized and associated with the *Turk* and the physical space they inhabited, as a convenient and dramatic way to emphasize the perceived differences. It was nevertheless the Enlightenment that irreversibly attached the plague to the image of the *Turk* while standardizing the trope of *Turkish fatalism*.

The great *Encyclopédie* of Diderot and D'Alembert, which was composed in the 1750s to 1770s, brought a theoretical framework and scientific precision to this trope. For example, the entry on "Peste" (Plague), composed by Louis de Jaucourt, said,

All the plagues that have appeared in Europe have been transmitted through the communication of the Saracens, Arabs, Moors or Turks with us, and *none of our plagues had any other source* ... The plague ... is conserved among them [the Turks] by way of their bizarre way of thinking about predestination: convinced that they cannot escape the orders of their God, they do not take any precautions to prevent the progress of the plague and to secure themselves from it, in this manner they communicate it to their neighbors.[91]

The entry on "Turquie" (Turkey), composed by the same Louis de Jaucourt, follows:

One of the scourges of Turkey which solely depends on the climate, is the plague, whose main seat is in Egypt. European states have devised admirable means to stop the progress of this ill; forming a line of troops around an infected country to prevent all communications; quarantining suspected vessels; perfuming clothes, papers, and

---

[90] Karl-Erik Frandsen, *The Last Plague in the Baltic Region, 1709–1713* (Copenhagen: Museum Tusculanum Press, 2010).

[91] Louis de Jaucourt, "Peste," in *Encyclopédie, ou dictionnaire raisonné des sciences, des arts et des métiers*, ed. Denis Diderot and Jean le Rond d'Alembert (Sociétés Typographiques, 1751–72), 12:452, emphasis mine: "toutes les pestes qui ont paru en Europe y ont été transmises par la communication des Sarrasins, des Arabes, des Maures, ou des Turcs avec nous, & toutes les pestes n'ont pas eu chez nous d'autre source ... La peste ... se conserve chez eux [les Turcs] par leur bizarre façon de penser sur la prédestination: persuadés qu'ils ne peuvent échapper à l'ordre du Très-haut sur leur sort, ils ne prennent aucune précaution pour empêcher les progrès de la peste & pour s'en garantir, ainsi ils la communiquent à leurs voisins."

letters that come form infected places. In this respect, the Turks have no policing; they watch the Christians flee the danger in the very same cities, which leaves them alone as the victims.[92]

Once it found its way into the *Encyclopédie*, this particular stereotype of the *fatalistic Turk* came to be consolidated, and thus became the common stock of Enlightenment learning, with lasting effects until the modern era.[93] As such, this vision was imagined to constitute a pivotal difference that made the "West" different from the "East," perhaps best articulated in artistic expression.[94]

A keen observer of Ottoman society, the Venetian *bailo* Bernardo was very perceptive in detecting the change of attitude toward flight from plagues. So was Rycaut in exposing the two camps of opinion (though equally dismissing them both for different reasons). Yet, the intellectual climate of the Republic of Letters in early modern Europe discarded these observations in favor of one that better suited the needs of Europe, which sought to assert a self-identity using the plague as a demarcation between Europe and what was east of it. This particular vision came to constitute a definition of the European healthscape, imagined as "plague-free," conveniently in contrast with the "plague-ridden" East. This legacy of early modern travel writers and their widely disseminated accounts shaped the vision of early modern Europeans as much as that of modern historians. The assumed differences between these societies vis-à-vis their response to plague still continue to be repeated in modern scholarship. As such, the fatalistic argument and the assertion of Muslim indifference do a great disservice to the student of plague in Ottoman history by not only obscuring the actual behavior of people of the past but cultivating essentialist binaries between Western-Christian and Eastern-Muslim constructs and imagining the Eastern-Muslim experience of plague as timeless, uniform, and thus not worthy of historical inquiry. Thus, perhaps, it is not at all a coincidence that

---

92 "Turquie," in ibid., 16:759: "Un des fléaux de la Turquie qui dépend uniquement du climat, est la peste, dont le siege principal est en Egypte. On a imaginé dans les états de l'Europe un moyen admirable pour arrêter les progrès du mal; on forme une ligne de troupes autour du pays infecté, pour empêcher toute communication; on fait faire une quarantaine aux vaisseaux suspects; on parfume les hardes, les papiers, les lettres qui viennent du lieu pestiferé. Les Turcs n'ont, à cet égard, aucune police; ils voient les Chrétiens dans la même ville échapper au danger, dont ils sont eux seuls la victime."

93 For a critical reading of disaster – for which plague worked as the ultimate example – in French Enlightenment thinking, see Daniel Gordon, "Confrontations with the Plague in Eighteenth-Century France," in Johns, *Dreadful Visitations*, 3–29.

94 E.g., see the contrast in the depiction of the "civilized" bodies and the sick, dying, and dehumanized bodies in an Oriental setting in Antoine-Jean Gros's 1804 painting *Bonaparte Visits the Plague Stricken in Jaffa* (*Bonaparte visitant les pestiférés de Jaffa*), commissioned by Napoleon himself. For an analysis of the painting, see, e.g., Christine M. Boeckl, *Images of Plague and Pestilence: Iconography and Iconology* (Kirksville, MO: Truman State University Press, 2000), 138–41.

the history of early modern Ottoman plagues has so far remained largely unexplored.

Conclusion

This chapter has offered a critical assessment of historical and historiographical factors that shaped Ottoman plague studies. First, it has presented the recent outburst of interest on the subject in Ottomanist scholarship over the last decade, in conjunction with the rise of historiographical trends such as environmental history and the history of animals. Then, it traced the development of studies on the history of Ottoman plagues from their origin in the early Turkish republic. It has been shown here that these studies were spearheaded by physicians who worked in public health campaigns to eradicate epidemic diseases and improve the overall health of the young nation-state. Setting the tone of scholarship, this tradition has largely ignored the history of epidemic diseases before the modern era.

The chapter has highlighted the reasons for the absence of studies devoted to the history of pre-1700 Ottoman plagues, such as the problem of presentist conceptions of past plagues, flaws in historical reasoning, and the absence of plague in early Ottoman chronicles. It has been argued that plague became a topos in Ottoman chronicles in the late sixteenth century, in conjunction with the rise of an urban context, by which the full effects of epidemics became more visible; the articulation of a certain meaning of plague; and the larger changes in the conception and writing of history.

The chapter has surveyed the development of misconceptions about the history of Ottoman plagues in the non-Ottomanist literature. Early modern Europeans saw the Ottomans as fatalistic in facing the plague, not taking any precautions to protect themselves from it, and thus as the ultimate plague exporters to Europe. These misconceptions circulated widely in Europe and even found their way into the work of contemporary scholarship, which utilized these sources. The scholarship that has developed since the 1970s has revolved around epidemiological binaries between Christian-Europe and Muslim-Ottoman with respect to both epidemiological experiences and responses to them.

With a view to outlining how this epidemiological orientalism was constructed, the chapter traces the genealogy of the trope of the *fatalistic Turk* in the early modern European travel literature. Using a selection of travel accounts penned in the early modern era, it highlights how stereotypes about the Ottomans' responses to plague were constructed, modified, and circulated. With a close reading of the intellectual climate of early modern Europe, it has demonstrated how accounts contrary to the stereotypical thinking were discarded at the expense of ideas that better served the needs of European society. Moreover, it has been suggested here that the trope of the *fatalistic Turk* went beyond the genre of travel writing and came to figure as an important difference, one that helped differentiate the "West" from the "East." As such, plague and responses to it contributed to the articulation of a European self-identity and healthscape, imagined to be separated from the sickly and "plague-ridden" East. Such epidemiological imaginaries were powerful tools in reducing the Ottoman experience of plague to a series of ahistorical fables and thus have largely obstructed it from becoming historicized.

3

The Black Death and Its Aftermath (1347–1453)

Perhaps few other subjects of historical inquiry inspire as much curiosity and fascination as the infamous Black Death of the fourteenth century, which continues to attract the attention of scholars and the broader public alike. A great number of studies have explored the history of this pandemic across the Afro-Eurasian zone, predominantly focusing on Europe. To this day, there exists a growing number of works devoted to this subject, contributing to an immense body of scholarship. The volume and breadth of this scholarship notwithstanding, the Black Death has been (and continues to be) a most controversial subject, especially around hotly debated issues like the nature of the disease, its origins and spread, its short- and long-term consequences, and the like. Above all, great attention was devoted to establishing the biological identity of the pathogen that caused the pandemic, so much so that it divided the field of scholarship into two camps over the last decades: those who believed it was caused by *Yersinia pestis* and their skeptics. More recently, new scientific tools and technologies have afforded the scholarly community novel methods for determining the identity of the pathogen. Especially molecular archaeology and genomics have contributed invaluable insights to resolve this controversy. Where we stand today, there is consensus in the international scholarly community that the Black Death was a pandemic of plague caused by *Y. pestis*.[1]

These controversies continue to shape current ways of thinking about the history of plague in the scholarship. In what follows, some of these controversies are revisited, primarily for the purpose of studying their implications for reconstructing the history of plague in the Ottoman context. In other

---

[1] For the consensus, see Green, "Editor's Introduction to *Pandemic Disease in the Medieval World*"; Lester K. Little, "Plague Historians in Lab Coats," *Past and Present* 213, no. 1 (2011): 267–90; James L. Bolton, "Looking for *Yersinia pestis*: Scientists, Historians, and the Black Death," in *Society in an Age of Plague* (*The Fifteenth Century, XII*), ed. Clark and Rawcliffe, 15–38 (Woodbridge, UK: Boydell Press, 2013). Also see Chapter 1.

words, the goal here is not to review the historiography of the Black Death per se, but to highlight how that body of scholarship has shaped avenues of thinking about the history of the disease in the Ottoman context. As we shall see, some of those avenues, by dwelling on models drawn from other historical contexts, have obstructed or obscured the study of plague in the Ottoman context. For this purpose, I first revisit the (now moribund) controversy over the pathogen of the Black Death (was it *Y. pestis* or not?) and then review the controversy over the origins of the pandemic (was it of proximate, i.e., Ottoman, origin or distant, i.e., East Asian, origin?). Following this, I trace the initial spread of the Black Death to our immediate area of attention (core areas that the Ottomans would come to rule). Then, I narrow down our geographic focus to Anatolia during the Black Death, trace the places that were affected, and identify the possible trajectories of disease spread. Narrowing the focus even further, I zoom in on the small Ottoman polity in northwest Anatolia at the time of the Black Death and explore to what extent its population was affected. In particular, I examine the factors that may have affected their exposure to the disease and investigate the possible links between the Black Death and early Ottoman expansion. To do so, I revisit some controversies about whether they were spared by the Black Death and about the relationship between nomadism and plague. Only after addressing these controversial issues will I move on to reconstruct a narrative of plagues in the area in the first post–Black Death century and analyze them with respect to their basic epidemiological features.

Controversy over the Pathogen: *Yersinia pestis* or Not?

In the last decades of the twentieth century, a revisionist literature started to develop, questioning the biological identity of the disease that caused the Black Death. Since the 1970s, scholars have raised doubts regarding the symptoms, transmission, and speed of propagation of plague outbreaks because what they saw in historical records was incompatible with what the biology of the disease seemingly required. At the time, the scientific knowledge of plague was largely drawn from a body of scholarship that developed in the context of the Third Pandemic. Following the discovery of the pathogen in 1894, scientists continued to make observations in South and East Asia (in India and China, in particular), which resulted in a vast body of scientific literature. Throughout the twentieth century, it was this body of knowledge that informed plague historians and, in due course, perplexed them. The discrepancy between what historians found in the sources that described the European experience of the Black Death and what the plague science of the time set down was simply too large to be dismissed easily.

First, there was the problem that the symptoms of the disease observed by the twentieth-century scientists did not quite match what historians saw in their sources for the late medieval plagues. Second, the role of rodent

hosts and vectors posed another challenge for historians of Europe, especially those who were working on northern European countries with colder
climates. It was puzzling to see no mention of rats in the historical sources.
Third, the speed and patterns of propagation of the pandemic also raised
doubts. A rat- and flea-borne disease would move slowly, in a recognizable
pattern, such as from house to house and from neighborhood to neighborhood, whereas an epidemic that spread from person to person, such as via
airborne transmission, would be fast and in random directions. Bubonic
plague, as described in that scientific literature, was supposed to be carried
by rats and thus to move slowly. However, the descriptions in the historical sources about the swift spread of the disease were in stark contrast
with this. And finally, the virulence of the disease and the high mortality
it caused as discussed in the historical sources were incompatible with the
scientific knowledge. Bubonic plague, the biology of the time dictated, was
not very virulent and did not cause high levels of mortality. So, how were
the historians to make sense of these discrepancies?

This led some to deny altogether that the Black Death was an epidemic of
plague caused by *Y. pestis*. The first among these was the British bacteriologist J. F. D. Shrewsbury, who, in his authoritative monograph *A History
of Bubonic Plague in the British Isles* (1970), marginalized the significance
of plague as a demographic factor.[2] While not rejecting the role of bubonic
plague altogether, Shrewsbury's work set the stage for others, who, in the
following decades, would take a more acutely skeptical stand. Following
this, the British zoologist Graham Twigg published his *The Black Death:
A Biological Reappraisal* (1984), in which he firmly rejected the possibility
of accepting *Y. pestis* as the causative agent of the Black Death.[3] Then,
in 1995, Koenraad Bleukx contested the possibility of plague as the cause
of the Black Death drawing from the English experience.[4] The next year,

---

[2] John Findlay Drew Shrewsbury, *A History of Bubonic Plague in the British Isles* (Cambridge:
    Cambridge University Press, 1970). In a review published in 1971, Christopher Morris
    critically evaluated the merits and shortcomings of this work, especially drawing attention to
    how Shrewsbury misinterpreted the evidence to downplay the importance of bubonic plague.
    See Morris, "The Plague in Britain," *The Historical Journal* 14, no. 1 (1971): 205–15.

[3] Graham Twigg, *The Black Death: A Biological Reappraisal* (London: Batsford Academic and
    Educational, 1984). Even though the beginning of this controversy is generally attributed
    to the work of Twigg in 1984, Benedictow rightly argues that it can be traced back to the
    1970s, especially to the work of Shrewsbury. It is clear that Twigg has been much influenced
    by Shrewsbury's ideas, with frequent references to the latter's work. See Ole J. Benedictow,
    *What Disease Was Plague? On the Controversy over the Microbiological Identity of Plague
    Epidemics of the Past* (Leiden: Brill, 2010), 16.

[4] Koenraad Bleukx, "Was the Black Death (1348–1349) a Real Plague Epidemic? England as a
    Case Study," in *Serta Devota in Memoriam Guillelmi Lourdaux, 2: Cultura Medievalis*, ed.
    Werner Verbeke, Marcel Haverals, Rafaël De Keyser, and Jean Goossens, 65–113 (Leuven:
    Leuven University Press, 1995).

Gunnar Karlsson denied the possibility of rat-borne plague on grounds that rats were absent in the fifteenth-century epidemics in Iceland.[5] This was followed by the collaborative work of demographer Susan Scott and zoologist Christopher J. Duncan (2001, and again 2004), which denied the possibility of a bacterium altogether, owing to the fast spread of the Black Death.[6] The most adamant voice of the skeptic camp, however, was offered by historian Samuel K. Cohn in his *The Black Death Transformed* (2002), which polarized the scene even further. Cohn categorically refused the possibility of considering rat-based plague caused by *Y. pestis* as the disease responsible for the Black Death.[7]

As much as they agreed in their rejection of *Y. pestis*, the skeptics failed to concur in identifying the disease involved. For example, whereas Twigg made a case for anthrax, Scott and Duncan argued for an Ebola-like virus. Rejecting the possibility of plague, Bleukx considered other disease possibilities but ultimately stayed agnostic. As for Cohn, he took it so far as to reject all explanations of plague to the extent of claiming that it was anything but *Y. pestis*–caused plague. What these scholars had in common was their insistence on the discrepancy between the historical sources (mostly on the Black Death as experienced in Britain or in other northern European contexts) and the scientific knowledge of plague as experienced in South Asia during the Third Pandemic – a body of knowledge that they seem to have taken outside of its ecological and colonial context.[8]

Taken as a whole, the work of the skeptics fostered reticence, a climate of reluctance in the scholarship to identify a past disease using modern microbiological knowledge.[9] The lingering effect on the scholarship continued until molecular archeology and genetics authoritatively demonstrated that

---

[5] Gunnar Karlsson, "Plague without Rats: The Case of Fifteenth-Century Iceland," *Journal of Medieval History* 22, no. 3 (1996): 263–84.

[6] Susan Scott and Christopher J. Duncan, *Biology of Plagues: Evidence from Historical Populations* (Cambridge: Cambridge University Press, 2001). Three years later, the authors have published a more popular version: Scott and Duncan, *Return of the Black Death: The World's Greatest Serial Killer* (Chichester, UK: John Wiley, 2004).

[7] Samuel K. Cohn, *The Black Death Transformed: Disease and Culture in Early Renaissance Europe* (London: Arnold/Oxford University Press, 2002). Also see Cohn, "The Black Death: End of a Paradigm," *The American Historical Review* 107, no. 3 (2002): 703–38.

[8] A corrective has recently been offered by Katherine Royer, "The Blind Men and the Elephant: Imperial Medicine, Medieval Historians, and the Role of Rats in the Historiography of Plague," in *Medicine and Colonialism: Historical Perspectives in India and South Africa*, ed. Poonam Bala, 99–110 (London: Pickering and Chatto, 2014).

[9] There were critical voices, however. See, e.g., John Theilmann and Frances Cate, "A Plague of Plagues: The Problem of Plague Diagnosis in Medieval England," *Journal of Interdisciplinary History* 37, no. 3 (2007): 371–93. Some effort has been made to offer a dialogue between these various voices. See, e.g., Nutton, *Pestilential Complexities*. For a revisiting of the differing and often controversial scholarly opinions on the subject, which are critically assessed as "alternative theories," see Benedictow, *What Disease Was Plague?*

the Black Death was a pandemic of plague caused by *Y. pestis*.[10] The effects of this controversy on the study of Ottoman plagues were rather indirect. While a general sense of reticence governed the field,[11] the lack of molecular archeological findings further aggravated the chasm between the new science of plague and the Ottoman sources.[12]

Controversy over the Origins of the "Oriental Plague": Proximate or Distant?

With the Third Pandemic, the focus of scholarly attention shifted from the Ottoman plague ports of the Near East to the European colonies in South and East Asia. This shift also surfaced in discussions about plague's area of origin. Throughout the twentieth century, there was an increasing belief in the international scholarly community that the origin of the Third Pandemic might also have been the origin of earlier plagues, in particular, the Black Death. Even though the German medical historian J. F. C. Hecker had suggested in his *Der Schwarze Tod im vierzehnten Jahrhundert* (1832) that the Black Death originated in China, it was the research that was produced during the Third Pandemic, backed up by the germ theory, that made an impact on the international scholarly community. In particular, the work of the Chinese epidemiologist Wu Lien-Teh and the reports of the Indian Plague Commission have been influential in shaping ideas of plague's area of origin in the twentieth century.[13]

From the 1970s onward, just as the identity of the disease that caused the Black Death was under the spotlight, the question of its area of origin was also revisited. In 1973, the French historian Emmanuel Le Roy Ladurie published an influential article in which he introduced the concept of "the unification of the globe by disease." In his search for understanding larger structural changes in history, Le Roy Ladurie proposed that a "microbial unity" characterized the world from the fourteenth to the seventeenth century as a conceptual tool to approach the Black Death and its recurrent waves.[14] In this, he was inspired by population studies of the 1960s that analyzed the consequences of the encounter of the populations of the New World, free from the diseases of the Old World – a phenomenon that came

---

[10] It is interesting to see a manifestation of this skepticism as late as 2013. See, e.g., Phyllis Pobst, "Should We Teach That the Cause of the Black Death Was Bubonic Plague?," *History Compass* 11, no. 10 (2013): 808–20.

[11] See, e.g., Sam White, "Rethinking Disease in Ottoman History"; White, *Climate of Rebellion*, 85–87.

[12] Varlık, "New Science and Old Sources."

[13] J. F. C. Hecker, *The Epidemics of the Middle Ages*, trans. B. G. Babington (London: Trübner, 1859), 17–19; Wu Lien-Teh, "Original Home of Plague."

[14] Le Roy Ladurie, "Un concept."

to be known as the *Columbian Exchange*.[15] Likening the consequences of the introduction of new diseases into the American continent to those of the Black Death, Le Roy Ladurie proposed the concept of microbial unity to refer to what he saw was an intensification in the circulation of disease. Accepting the origins of the Black Death as the Crimean port of Caffa (now Feodosia) and possibly its Asian hinterland, he also acknowledged the biological consequences of the Pax Mongolica – a network of caravan routes that united Asia under the Mongols. The intellectual climate of historical scholarship was ripe for overarching structures.

The American historian William McNeill published his influential *Plagues and Peoples* (1976), in which he combined the existing evidence on the Black Death with that drawn from Chinese history of epidemics. The result was a powerful hypothesis to explain how epidemics spread across continents. McNeill held that the expansion and strengthening of overland caravan trade routes of Eurasia under the Mongol Empire, starting from the thirteenth century, put the wild rodents of the steppe into contact with carriers of plague. Hence, he argued, a plague epidemic that originated in China in the 1330s spread westward along the Silk Road over the next decade and a half, until it reached the Black Sea region, whence it was distributed to the Mediterranean basin.[16] In doing so, McNeill, like Le Roy Ladurie and Alfred Crosby, not only emphasized the agency of disease in history but also opened up the field to global inquiries.

McNeill's hypothesis quickly came to be accepted in the scholarship and remained the conventional view about the origins and spread of the Black Death for more than three decades. Its vision inspired a number of works to adopt a broader geographic scope in studying the plague experiences of non-European regions.[17] Most prominently, Michael W. Dols's *The Black Death in the Middle East* appeared in 1977, sharing some of McNeill's ideas

---

[15] In a series of works, Woodrow Borah and Sherburne Cook explored the drastic effects of disease brought by the Spanish conquerors on the population of Mexico. They calculated the population of central Mexico on the eve of the conquest as 25.2 million, 19 million of which is calculated to have died within the following three decades. Within less than a century, the population had fallen to fewer than 2 million. See Borah and Cook, *The Population of Central Mexico in 1548* (Berkeley: University of California Press, 1960); Borah and Cook, *The Aboriginal Population of Central Mexico on the Eve of the Spanish Conquest* (Berkeley: University of California Press, 1963); Cook and Borah, *The Indian Population of Central Mexico, 1531–1610* (Berkeley: University of California Press, 1963). For a concise summary of methodology and figures, see Borah and Cook, "Conquest and Population: A Demographic Approach to Mexican History," *Proceedings of the American Philosophical Society* 113, no. 2 (1969): 177–83. For coining the term "the Columbian Exchange," see Alfred W. Crosby, *The Columbian Exchange: Biological and Cultural Consequences of 1492* (Westport, CT: Greenwood Press, 1972).

[16] McNeill, *Plagues and Peoples*, esp. Chapter 4 and appendix.

[17] E.g., we see the beginning of publications on the history of the Black Death in Russia. For these, see Uli Schamiloglu, "Preliminary Remarks on the Role of Disease in the History of the Golden Horde," *Central Asian Survey* 12, no. 4 (1993): 447–57, note 30. Just before

about the Asian origins of the pandemic and its westward spread across the continent.[18]

This particular hypothesis was most sternly criticized by John Norris in a 1977 article. He wrote, "The Black Death did not originate in China, India or 'Central Asia' as has been supposed, and was not 'brought' westward by the Mongols or anyone else." Analyzing epidemiological evidence from China, India, and Central Asia, Norris dismissed all as origins of the epidemic. He convincingly demonstrated how a tradition of scholarship misinterpreted others' work, reflecting general prejudices that were largely shaped by observations drawn from the Third Pandemic. Instead, he proposed that "it was probably moved northward over the course of centuries, by means of transmission among the wild rodent colonies, from Kurdistan and Iraq to Southern Russia."[19] The controversy continued between Norris and Dols, and in some way made it clear that the geographic origins of the pandemic could not be established by means of historical sources alone.[20]

To shed further light on the question, Uli Schamiloglu published an article in 1993 that focused on the disease experience of the Golden Horde. While not dismissing the westward spread model adopted by McNeill and Dols, Schamiloglu also took into consideration a northward spread of the disease from the Golden Horde to the Russian territory.[21] In 2004, Ole J. Benedictow published a comprehensive volume, *The Black Death, 1346–1353: The Complete History*, in which he explored the questions of origins and spread at length.[22] Benedictow argued that neither China nor India seem to have been affected by the Black Death of the mid-fourteenth century; they did not experience major outbreaks of plague until the seventeenth century. He surveyed known plague foci across the Afro-Eurasian zone to determine which one may have triggered the pandemic. With this in view, he adopted the *principle of proximate origin*, which he defined as "the plague focus closest to the area from where the Black Death was shipped to Europe, i.e., Kaffa in the Crimea," which is "narrowly and unambiguously associated with the area of the plague focus that stretches from the north-western shores of the Caspian Sea into southern Russia."[23] He supports this by descriptions

---

McNeill, Lawrence N. Langer published a piece on the Black Death in Russia. Langer, "The Black Death in Russia: Its Effects upon Urban Labor," *Russian History* 2, no. 1 (1975): 53–67.

[18] Dols, *Black Death*.

[19] J. Norris, "East or West? The Geographic Origin of the Black Death," *Bulletin of the History of Medicine* 51, no. 1 (1977): 1–24, quotations on 1.

[20] Dols, "Geographical Origin of the Black Death," *Bulletin of the History of Medicine* 52, no. 1 (1978): 112–13; Norris, "Response," *Bulletin of the History of Medicine* 52, no. 1 (1978): 114–20.

[21] Schamiloglu, "Preliminary Remarks."

[22] Benedictow, *Black Death, 1346–1353*; see Chapter 5 for origins, Part II for spread.

[23] Ibid., quotations on 50 and 51, respectively.

in historical sources regarding the geographic origins of the outbreak and thus arrives at the conclusion that the Black Death spread westward from this area of origin toward Caffa in the Crimea, but not from more distant locations such as China or India.

Benedictow's claim about the absence of the Black Death in China and India was further elaborated. In an article published in 2011, George D. Sussman addressed the question whether the Black Death was in India and China. Sussman argued that the Black Death occurred neither in India nor in China. Instead, he suggested that the first identifiable descriptions of plague in these regions can be dated to the seventeenth century.[24] Soon after this, Paul D. Buell published an article titled "Qubilai and the Rats," in which he adamantly denied that the Black Death was in China. Treating the idea of the Chinese origins of the Black Death as a myth, Buell examined why China was spared from the pandemic, despite its proximity to Central Asia and the significance of a nomad connection. Buell argued that both political and economic policies seeking new maritime connections and the differences in disease environments inhibited the arrival of the Black Death there.[25] The controversy over origins does not seem to be settled yet. Most recent historical interpretations of genetics research seem to trace the Black Death back to its east Asian origins.[26]

The Initial Spread of the Black Death

Leaving aside the rather dark journey of plague to Caffa, we are much better informed about the spread of the infection across the Mediterranean world. When it did, the news of where the disease came from spread along with it. The contemporaries of the Black Death – whether they were in Italian cities, in Constantinople, or in Aleppo – heard the circulating rumors about where

[24] On the basis of a number of sources, George D. Sussman demonstrates how the European scientific vision of the plague's origins shifted toward China and the Indian subcontinent, irreversibly, as a result of the Third Pandemic. See Sussman, "Was the Black Death in India and China?," *Bulletin of the History of Medicine* 85, no. 3 (2011): 319–55. For a discussion of descriptions of bubonic plague in the autobiography of seventeenth-century Mughal emperor Jahangir (r. 1605–27), see B. M. Ansari, "An Account of Bubonic Plague in Seventeenth Century India in an Autobiography of a Mughal Emperor," *The Journal of Infection* 29, no. 3 (1994): 351–52.

[25] Paul D. Buell, "Qubilai and the Rats." Buell also speculated that the geographic origin of Justinianic plague may have been the same as that of the Second Pandemic. He wrote, "Does the presence of this biovar possibly indicate that the Justinian plague too had a Central Asian origin? Possibly it came from the same reservoir associated with the second pandemic, the only difference being that we simply lack the historical information present in the 14th century." See 131. Later research demonstrated authoritatively that the origin of all three pandemics can be traced to the Qinghai-Tibet Plateau. See Chapter 1.

[26] Robert Hymes, "Epilogue: A Hypothesis on the East Asian Beginnings of the *Yersinia pestis* Polytomy," *The Medieval Globe* 1 (2014): 285–308.

the disease had come from. Some of these rumors found their way into the chronicles of that era. For example, Gabriele de' Mussis (d. 1356), a lawyer from Piacenza, wrote in his *Historia de Morbo*,

Among those who escaped from Caffa by boat were a few sailors who had been infected with the poisonous disease. Some boats were bound for Genoa, others went to Venice and to other Christian areas. When the sailors reached these places and mixed with the people there, it was as if they had brought evil spirits with them: every city, every settlement, every place was poisoned by the contagious pestilence, and their inhabitants, both men and women, died suddenly.[27]

This version of the story that the sailors brought home the disease from the Genoese colony of Caffa is well known. According to it, in the year 1346, a mysterious illness started causing great mortality in the lands of the Golden Horde. When it broke out in the Mongol army besieging the fortress of Caffa, the Mongols started catapulting the corpses over the walls. This was how, it was reported, the Genoese colony contracted the disease, which some brought back home on their flight.[28] Another story of origins comes from Ibn al-Wardi (d. 1349), an eyewitness to plague in Aleppo, who wrote on the basis of what he heard from Muslim merchants returning from Crimea. According to his account, even though the disease had started in the more distant lands of Asia, it was witnessed in the lands of the Uzbeks in the months of October and November 1346, before it moved to Crimea and Byzantium.[29] Similar stories of origin must have also been circulating in Byzantine Constantinople, as testified by the chronicles of the time. More than a decade after the disease's first arrival to Constantinople, historian Nicephorus Gregoras (d. 1360) wrote,

A serious and pestilential disease invaded humanity. Starting from Scythia and Maeotis and the mouth of the Tanais, just as spring began, it lasted for that whole year, passing through and destroying, to be exact, only the continental coast, towns as well as country areas, ours and those that are adjacent to ours, up to Gadera and the columns of Hercules.[30]

---

[27] Gabriele de' Mussis, "The Arrival of the Plague" [*Historia de Morbo*], in *The Black Death*, trans. and ed. Rosemary Horrox (Manchester: Manchester University Press, 1994), 14–26, quotation on 18–19.

[28] This is a very famous story, which has been accepted as an instance of premodern biological warfare. Benedictow offers a very insightful analysis for why this story must be a myth. Benedictow, *Black Death*, 51–53.

[29] Michael W. Dols, "Ibn al-Wardī's *Risālah al-Naba' 'an al-Waba'*: A Translation of a Major Source for the History of the Black Death in the Middle East," in *Near Eastern Numismatics, Iconography, Epigraphy and History, Studies in Honor of George C. Miles*, ed. Dickron K. Kouymjian (Beirut, 1974), 444; Dols, *Black Death*, 40. Dols believed that Ibn al-Wardī's reference to the origin of the disease in the "land of darkness" should be interpreted as inner Asia or Mongolia but not China.

[30] Christos S. Bartsocas, "Two Fourteenth Century Greek Descriptions of the 'Black Death,'" 394–400, quotation on 395; Aberth, *Black Death*, 15–16.

To be sure, there were other such stories about the origins of the pestilence that circulated in different circles and cities at the time. In most accounts, there was emphasis on the universal nature of the pestilence, the great mortality it caused, and its movement from place to place. Though fragmentary, these narratives afford a possible trajectory followed by the epidemic, if not a precise origin. Recent scholarship, however, cautions us about accepting these accounts of the origin, path, or scope of the epidemic uncritically, as they may be "the path of rumours rather than pestilence itself."[31]

Taken as a whole, what can be rather cautiously assumed on the basis of fragmentary accounts is that the infection spread, not along a single trajectory, but rather in multiple directions both on the sea and over land. In fact, the historical scholarship on the Black Death has meticulously endeavored to put these accounts into a spatial and temporal sequence. According to this narrative, the sea journey of the Black Death first carried it to Constantinople, to the Aegean and eastern Mediterranean port cities and islands, such as Alexandria and Cyprus, and to the western Mediterranean port cities. In the meantime, the infection seems to have also spread southward along the eastern shores of the Black Sea, into the Caucasus and the Anatolian peninsula, and further south into Syria.[32] Even though the maritime journey of the Black Death and its notorious stops at Mediterranean metropolises have been better documented, its overland spread, especially in inland areas and in the countryside, is more difficult to trace. There is a bias on the part of the sources that should be remembered while thinking of sketching the pandemic's itinerary. It is also important to remember that plague's spread to different areas necessitates paying attention to regional circumstances with respect to the disease's speed and direction of spread as well as the mortality it caused.[33]

Anatolia and Its Surroundings during the Black Death

It is not clear exactly when the Black Death first arrived at Anatolia or the Balkans. It seems most likely that Constantinople was among the first to be struck. Benedictow claims that plague broke out there in early July 1347.[34]

---

[31] Ann G. Carmichael, "Universal and Particular: The Language of Plague, 1348–1500," in Nutton, *Pestilential Complexities*, 17–52, 27. Carmichael notes that there were rumors circulating in central Italy about plague in distant places, the most famous of which was statistics on plague in Paris about a year before the disease actually reached the city.

[32] For the initial spread of the Black Death, see Benedictow, *Black Death*, 57–67; Biraben, *Les hommes et la peste*, 1:48–55, 71–85; Kōstēs, *Ston kairo tēs panōlēs*; Schamiloglu, "Black Death in Medieval Anatolia"; Dols, *Black Death*, 35–67.

[33] David C. Mengel, "A Plague on Bohemia? Mapping the Black Death," *Past and Present* 211, no. 1 (2011): 3–34.

[34] Benedictow believes that the infection should have been first imported to the city in the first half of May, owing to the time it takes for the epizootic to turn into an epidemic. See Benedictow, *Black Death*, 61.

Gradually increasing its force, the outbreak seems to have reached its climax in the Byzantine capital in November and December of the same year (Map 1).[35] Eyewitness accounts describe the destruction of the plague in most gruesome terms. According to the influential Byzantine statesman Demetrios Kydones (d. 1397/8), day by day the dead came to outnumber the living. Another eyewitness, the Byzantine emperor John VI Kantakouzenos (d. 1383), who lost his thirteen-year-old son Andronikos to the plague, wrote, "No words could express the nature of the disease."[36]

After Constantinople, the infection may have been carried further inland into its surrounding areas, especially by those who fled the city. This movement, however, is difficult to trace in the sources. What can be more easily discerned is the maritime spread of the disease along the Aegean ports and islands, probably in fall 1347.[37] Plague was recorded in Thessaloniki, the second city of the empire after Constantinople, which was already troubled by the revolts of the zealots and other crises. Even though we do not know enough about the effects of the plague on its population, when combined with the effects of other crises that befell the town, it must have been severe.[38] The infection then spread quickly to the Aegean islands of Limnos and Euboea, to Crete, and to Koroni and Methoni in the Peloponnese, still in 1347. The next year, plague is documented on the islands of Rhodes, Crete, and Cyprus and in the Peloponnese.[39]

Although the trajectory of the Black Death's spread leading toward the European ports of the Mediterranean is relatively better known, this was not the only line of epidemic propagation. Meanwhile, plague seems to have taken a foothold on the Black Sea coast of Anatolia. It was recorded in Trabzon in September 1347, where it lasted for seven months and caused great mortality. According to the testimony of the Florentine chronicler

---

[35] Ibid.; Stephane Barry and Norbert Gualde, "La peste noire dans l'Occident chrétien et musulman, 1347–1353," *Canadian Bulletin of Medical History/Bulletin canadien d'histoire de la médecine* 25, no. 2 (2008): 467.

[36] Barry and Gualde, "La peste noire," 467–68; Marie-Hélène Congourdeau, "La peste noire à Constantinople de 1348 à 1466," *Medicina nei secoli* 11, no. 2 (1999): 377–90, 379; Bartsocas, "Two Fourteenth Century Greek Descriptions of the 'Black Death,'" 395–96, quotation on 396.

[37] Benedictow, *Black Death*, 61. Benedictow argues that plague started spreading on both sides of the Aegean coastline in late summer 1347, and by autumn, it had covered the entire coastline.

[38] Joseph Nehama, *Salonique: La ville convoitée* (Tarascon, France: Cousins de Salonique, 2004), 103–5. Nehama mentions a famine and an epizootic (cattle plague) in the years preceding this in Thessaloniki. During the zealots' revolts in Thessaloniki, an epizootic (in 1342 or 1343) killed hundreds of beasts; the carcasses were piled up on the streets. Also see John W. Barker, "Late Byzantine Thessalonike: A Second City's Challenges and Responses," *Dumbarton Oaks Papers* 57 (2003): 5–33, 18.

[39] Kōstēs, *Ston kairo tēs panōlēs*, 317–18.

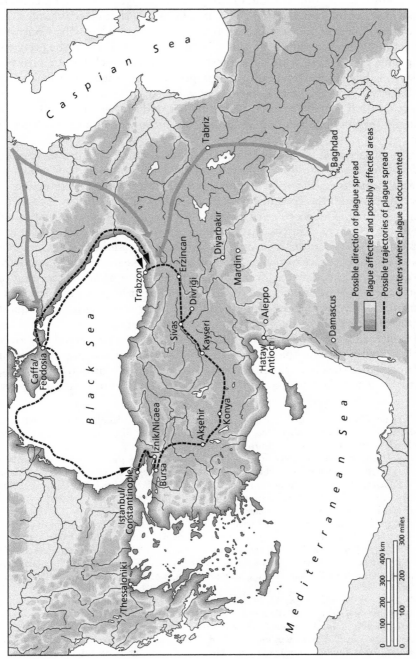

MAP 1. Anatolia and surroundings during the Black Death, circa 1346–49.

Possible direction of plague spread

Plague affected and possibly affected areas

Possible trajectories of plague spread

Centers where plague is documented

Giovanni Villani, "only one out of five persons survived."[40] It is not entirely clear how the infection arrived there. It seems likely that those who fled the infection along the eastern shores of the Black Sea or across the Caucasus brought the disease with them. There is further evidence about the presence of plague in Tabriz in 1346–47, as testified in the chronicles written for the Jalayirid dynasty.[41] Drawing from the presence of plague in Tabriz, and in Baghdad in 1347, Dols assumes a possible southward movement of the Black Death from the Caucasus to Azerbaijan, and further south to Baghdad and the Persian Gulf, but this seems difficult to confirm with the evidence at hand.[42]

The progression of the epidemic within the Anatolian peninsula is more difficult to trace. We do not know exactly what route the infection followed at this time, but it seems safe to assume that the initial direction of spread was from the coastline toward the interior, though not necessarily unidirectional. The presence of plague in Bursa in 1348 can be established from the Ottoman sources. As has been shown in the previous chapter, fifteenth-century Ottoman chroniclers Aşıkpaşazade and Neşri present evidence for the presence of plague. Both accounts make one isolated reference to plague, in association with the death of the Karesi prince. According to Aşıkpaşazade, the dominions of the Karesioğulları principality in northwestern Anatolia were integrated into the Ottoman territories with the conquest of the fortress of Bergama. Thereupon, Orhan (r. 1324–62) had the Friday sermon read and coins minted in his name as a sign of sovereignty over Karesi dominions. Aşıkpaşazade notes that the Karesi prince was brought to Bursa after the conquest of Bergama, where he lived for two more years, until he succumbed to plague.[43] The same piece of information, almost

---

[40] William Miller, *Trebizond, the Last Greek Empire* (Amsterdam: Hakkert, 1968), 53; Schamiloglu, "Black Death in Medieval Anatolia," 265; Dols, *Black Death*, 63; Benedictow, *Black Death*, 61; Kōstēs, *Ston kairo tēs panōlēs*, 317.

[41] The Jalayirids were a dynasty of Mongol origin that ruled in Iraq and northwestern Persia after the disintegration of the Ilkhanid power in the area in the 1330s. One of these chronicles, Abū Bakr al-Quṭbī al-Ahrī's *Ta'rīkh-i Shaikh Uwais*, has been already noted by Michael Dols. See Dols, *Black Death*, 45n32. Two other chronicles confirm the presence of plague in Tabriz and its surroundings in 747 H. (April 1346–47). See Zayn al-Dīn b. Ḥamd Allāh Muṣṭawfī Qazvīnī, *Zayl-i Tārīkh-i Guzīda*, ed. İraj Afshār (Tehran: Naqsh-i Jahān, 1372 [1993]), 41; Ḥāfiẓ Abrū, *Zayl-i Jāmi' al-Tavārīkh*, ed. Khānbābā Bayānī (Tehran: 'Ilmī, 1317 [1939]), 178. I am grateful to my colleague Pat Wing for bringing these sources to my attention. For further discussion of these chronicles, see Patrick Wing, "The Jalayirids and Dynastic State Formation in the Mongol Ilkhanate," PhD diss., University of Chicago, 2007.

[42] Dols, *Black Death*, 44–46, 62. Norris disagrees with Dols's argument about a possible southern movement of the disease. He points out that some of those outbreaks may be introduced from local enzootic foci. See Norris, "East or West?," 15.

[43] Aşık Paşazade, *Osmanoğulları'nın Tarihi*, ed. Kemal Yavuz and Yekta Saraç (Istanbul: Koç Kültür Sanat Tanıtım, 2003), 104, 372. Elizabeth Zachariadou noted this more than two decades ago: "Ashikpashazade reports that Karasi's son, who had been taken prisoner,

verbatim, appears in Neşri's chronicle.[44] Even though this is an isolated reference, it can be taken as evidence that plague was in Bursa. In both cases, the dating of the plague is problematic.[45] It is equally difficult to determine where the outbreak was introduced from and how long it lasted. Located on the northwestern tip of the Anatolian peninsula, Bursa presumably received the infection from Constantinople or its surroundings. However, it is difficult to trace the journey of the infection from Bursa toward the interior of Anatolia.

Another piece of evidence comes from Sivas, a town east of central Anatolia. The source for this is a chronology composed in Persian by a certain Zeynü'l-Müneccim bin Süleyman el-Konevi in July 1371. In this chronology, the entry for the year 748 H. (1347–48) reads, "Plague, pestilence, and death."[46] The source does not specify where the epidemic took place. If we were to assume that the author was in Sivas at the time, we may take this as some evidence about the plague's whereabouts. The source mentions the Hijri year 748, which corresponds to a time frame between April 1347 and March 1348. Given the fragmentary nature of the evidence, one possible suggestion is that the infection first arrived at Trabzon, on the Black Sea coast, where it was documented to last from fall 1347 to probably early spring 1348. From there, it may have been carried into its hinterland.

The land route between Trabzon and Tabriz was one of the most heavily used trade arteries on the eve of the Black Death.[47] This was the itinerary

---

died of plague two years after the conquest of his emirate: *iki yıl diri oldu; ahir yumrucak çıkardı; Allah rahmetine vardı.* He probably died during the Black Death of 1348." See Elizabeth A. Zachariadou, "The Emirate of Karasi and That of the Ottomans: Two Rival States," in *The Ottoman Emirate (1300–1389): Halcyon Days in Crete I: A Symposium Held in Rethymnon 11–13 January 1991* (Rethymnon: Crete University Press, 1993), 230. Curiously, the later Ottomanist scholarship did not seem to take notice of this important point.

44 Mehmed Neşri, *Kitab-ı Cihan-Nüma = Neşrî Tarihi* (Ankara: TTK, 1995), 1:166–67: "Rivâyet olunur ki, çünki Karasi vilâyeti Orhan Gazi'ye müsellem oldı, Karasi-oğlını dahi hisardan âmânla çıkarub, Bursa'ya gönderdiler. İki yıl diri olub, âhir tâ'undan vefat itdi."

45 The only event in the chronology offered is the annexation of the Karesi lands, which, according to historian Elizabeth Zachariadou, can be dated to 1345–46. See Zachariadou, "Emirate of Karasi," 230.

46 Osman Turan, *İstanbul'un Fethinden Önce Yazılmış Tarihî Takvimler* (Ankara: TTK, 2007), 71.

47 A. H. Lybyer, "The Ottoman Turks and the Routes of Oriental Trade," *The English Historical Review* 30, no. 120 (1915), 578. For the urban markets of Anatolia in the fourteenth century, see Kate Fleet, "The Turkish Economy, 1071–1453," in *The Cambridge History of Turkey, I: Byzantium to Turkey, 1071–1453*, ed. Kate Fleet, 227–65 (Cambridge: Cambridge University Press, 2009). For the trade networks connecting Tabriz to the Black Sea in the late medieval era, see Patrick Wing, "'Rich in Goods and Abounding in Wealth:' The Ilkhanid and Post-Ilkhanid Ruling Elite and the Politics of Commercial Life at Tabriz, 1250–1400," in *Politics, Patronage and the Transmission of Knowledge in 13th–15th Century Tabriz*, ed. Judith Pfeiffer, 301–20 (Leiden: Brill, 2014).

that the Castilian ambassador Ruy Gonzalez de Clavijo would follow some fifty years later, on his way to the court of Timur in Samarkand.[48] At Erzincan, this route intersected with Anatolia's principal caravan route, which connected urban centers like Sivas, Kayseri, Konya, Akşehir, İznik, İzmit, and Istanbul. Crisscrossing Anatolia, the caravan route also partly coincided with the pilgrimage route. Under the rule of the Seljuks, it was improved by the building of caravanserais and was fully functional in the fourteenth century.[49] On the eve of the Black Death, when Ibn Battuta traveled in Anatolia, he too traveled along this route.[50]

Given these overland connections, it may be assumed that plague moved from Trabzon to Erzincan, and then to Sivas, some time between late fall 1347 and early spring 1348, on the basis of el-Konevi's chronology. Another piece of evidence that supports this trajectory is the incidence of plague in Divriği (Tivrik) in September 1348, as documented in Armenian sources.[51] A town in eastern central Anatolia about one hundred miles southeast of Sivas, Divriği was not directly situated on a caravan route, as it was surrounded by mountains and was difficult to reach. This may be the reason why the infection arrived there slightly later.

Tracing the movement of plague toward east and southeast Anatolia is challenging. Even though the Mamluk sources offer some evidence for the presence of plague in Anatolia, it is difficult to establish a precise trajectory of spread. For example, Ibn al-Wardi notes the presence of plague in Byzantine lands, Cyprus, and the islands.[52] Al-Maqrizi's account is more detailed about the infection in Anatolia. He suggests that when the disease arrived at Antioch in 1348–49, people of the town fled north toward central Anatolia, carrying the disease with them to Karaman and Kayseri. Similarly, when plague hit Mardin and Diyarbakır, the local Kurdish population tried to save themselves by fleeing from this area. The presence of the disease on the mountains of Karaman and in Lesser Armenia is also noted in the Mamluk sources without necessarily a precise timeline.[53]

---

[48] Departing Trabzon, the embassy went though Maçka and the Zigana pass, before reaching Erzincan, from where they moved to Erzurum. For this segment of their journey, see Ruy González de Clavijo, *Narrative of the Embassy of Ruy Gonzalez de Clavijo to the Court of Timour at Samarcand, ad 1403–6* (London: Hakluyt Society, 1859), 61–79.

[49] Stefanos Yerasimos, *Les voyageurs dans l'empire ottoman, XIVe-XVIe siècles: bibliographie, itinéraires et inventaire des lieux habités* (Ankara: TTK, 1991), 62–64.

[50] Ibn Battuta, *Travels in Asia and Africa, 1325–1354*, trans. H. A. R. Gibb (London: Routledge, 1929).

[51] Avedis K. Sanjian, *Colophons of Armenian Manuscripts, 1301–1480: A Source for Middle Eastern History* (Cambridge, MA: Harvard University Press, 1969), 86; also cited in Dols, *Black Death*, 46.

[52] Dols, "Ibn al-Wardī's *Risālah al-Naba' 'an al-Waba'*," 448.

[53] Gaston Wiet, "La grande peste noire en Syrie et en Égypt," in *Études d'Orientalisme dédiées à la mémoire de Lévi-Provençal* 1 (Paris: Maisonneuve, 1962), 369–72; Schamiloglu, "Black Death in Medieval Anatolia," 10; Dols, *Black Death*, 62.

On the basis of this evidence, the widespread presence of plague in southeast Anatolia can be confirmed. However, it is still difficult to establish a clear temporal and spatial sequence. Although al-Maqrizi suggests that plague was brought to Antioch from Syria, there is no corroborating evidence to support this. Even though this is not entirely implausible, it is equally possible that it was introduced by way of sea.[54] The fact that the chronicler stresses that people fled toward central Anatolia makes it difficult to argue that it was brought there from central Anatolia. Despite the lack of precision regarding directionality, the presence of the disease in eastern and southeastern Anatolia is confirmed.

Shifting our attention back to central Anatolia can offer additional insights into the trajectories of plague's spread in the interiors of the peninsula. Al-Maqrizi's mention of the plague in Karaman and Kayseri is significant. As he suggests, these places may have received the infection from those who fled from Antioch. It seems more likely, however, that the infection was carried there along the caravan route. As an important stop between Sivas and Konya, Kayseri was located on the caravan route of prime importance. Equally significant in this context is the availability of anecdotal evidence about the presence of plague in Konya. The hagiography of Hacı Bektaş mentions Pir Ebi Sultan, one of the disciples of the mystic, who would have lived at the time of the Black Death.[55]

Another piece of evidence points out that the Black Death may have visited Akşehir, a town in southwestern Anatolia. Şeyyad Hamza, a fourteenth-century poet, composed an elegy to his children whom he lost to the plague. The poem (a *kaside* of fifty couplets) expresses his great pain in losing his loved ones. Not only does the poem openly mention the epidemic and describe the hitherto unheard-of mortality but it also states the year, that is, 749 H. (April 1348–March 1349). This is further corroborated by the tombstone of the poet's daughter Aslı Hatun (Asl[ı]Hatun binti Şeyyad Hamza) found in the town's cemetery, which also carries the same date.[56] It is not known where the poet lived; however, the tombstone of his daughter suggests that he was in Akşehir when plague broke out. If this indeed were the

---

54 Dols suggests a maritime introduction on the basis of Ibn Khatimah's account. See Dols, *Black Death*, 62.

55 For a more detailed discussion of the case of Pîr Ebi Sultan in the hagiography of Hacı Bektaş, see Chapter 7. Also see Hacı Bektaş Veli, *Manakıb-ı Hacı Bektâş-ı Velî "Vilâyetnâme"* (Istanbul: İnkılap Kitabevi, 1995), 86–87. The tomb of this mystic in Konya has become a shrine especially visited for healing powers against fevers. See İbrahim Hakkı Konyalı, *Konya Tarihi* (Konya: Enes Kitap Sarayı, 1997), 700–701.

56 This poem can be considered as the earliest known piece of poetry written in response to the Black Death in Turkish by an eyewitness. Metin Akar, "Şeyyad Hamza Hakkında Yeni Bilgiler," *Türklük Araştırmaları Dergisi* 2 (1987): 1–14; Orhan Tavukçu, "Şeyyâd Hamza'nın Bilinmeyen Bir Şiiri Münasebetiyle," *International Journal of Central Asian Studies* 10, no. 1 (2005): 181–95. For Aslı Hatun's tombstone, see Rıfkı Melûl Meriç, "Şeyyad Hamza'nın Kızına Ait Mezartaşı," *Taşpınar Mecmuası* 28 (1935): 60–63.

case, plague may have reached this town, which was located along the same caravan route that crisscrossed Anatolia. Several decades later, Bertrandon de la Broquière, the pilgrim-spy sent by the Duke of Burgundy, would pass through Akşehir on his way back from the Holy Lands. Traveling to Constantinople with a returning pilgrim's caravan, he recounts stopping over at Akşehir, a little town at the foot of a high mountain, three days' distance from Konya.[57]

One additional piece of evidence comes from the hagiography of the fourteenth-century Anatolian mystic Abdal Musa. According to the testimony of this source, Genceli, a town in western Anatolia, was hit by a great disaster, which forced its population to flee. Even though Abdal Musa's hagiography does not specify what disaster it was, this could be supplemented by evidence from the hagiography of his disciple, Kaygusuz Abdal, which makes specific references to Abdal Musa's power over plague.[58] If this was indeed a reference to plague, this piece of evidence corroborates geographically, other sources of information about the spread of the Black Death in Anatolia along the main caravan route.[59]

Despite the fragmentary nature of evidence, it should be possible to offer some general observations about the spread of the Black Death in Anatolia. First, it seems plausible to assume a faster spread over maritime routes and a relatively slower spread over land routes. Second, the infection may have been introduced from different points along the Anatolian coast, such as Constantinople or Trabzon, whence it spread to the interior. The inland dissemination of the infection from these points onward can be assumed to have followed overland and perhaps river routes. It may be assumed that plague circulated via multiple channels within Anatolia at this time. Third, what appear to be piecemeal and disjointed pieces of evidence become meaningful when Anatolia's historical routes are considered. It seems plausible that the Black Death moved along the main caravan route, either from Trabzon to Sivas, and then to Kayseri, Konya, Akşehir, and Bursa, or less likely in the opposite direction. The fact that the Trabzon and Divriği outbreaks were earlier than the Akşehir incidence suggests that the infection moved from east to west along this trajectory. It is also possible to trace some offshoots

[57] Bertrandon de la Brocquière, *The Voyage D'Outremer* (New York: P. Lang, 1988), 77.

[58] For a more detailed discussion of the hagiographies of Abdal Musa and Kaygusuz Abdal, see Chapter 7. Also see Abdurrahman Güzel, ed., *Abdal Mûsâ Velâyetnâmesi* (Ankara: TTK, 1999); *Kaygusuz Abdal (Alâeddin Gaybî) Menâkıbnamesi* (Ankara: TTK, 1999).

[59] I have not been able to locate the town of Genceli. According to Abdurrahman Güzel, the editor of the hagiographies, this was an ancient site about three hours away from Antalya, yet he does not specify exactly where. Following the biography of the mystic, it should be possible to assume a location between Bursa and Antalya in western Anatolia. One possible location is the Genceli village in Dinar, Afyonkarahisar, about one hundred miles southwest of Akşehir, which was on the main route and was shown to be affected by plague.

of the infection from this main artery toward relatively isolated locations (e.g., Divriği, Genceli, and some towns in southeast Anatolia), which suggests that the disease diffused from centers along the main trajectory toward areas of lesser circulation. Fourth, and most important, the Black Death was by no means limited to the coastal areas or sea-level port cities. As has been demonstrated here using the fragmentary evidence available, plague was seen deep in the interior of Anatolia, well into highland locations that were difficult to access. Given the topographic and climatic diversity of Anatolia, plague manifested in a wide ecological spectrum. One of the microecologies was the area claimed by the Ottoman polity, which at the time of the Black Death was limited to a rather small area in northwestern Anatolia.

The Black Death and the Ottomans: Revisiting Controversies

When the initial wave of the outbreak hit Anatolia, the Ottoman polity was a small principality on the southern outskirts of the Byzantine Empire. As one of the Turkoman principalities that emerged in Anatolia at the turn of the fourteenth century, the Ottomans started to wage war on the Byzantine frontier. Under the leadership of Orhan – son of Osman (d. 1324), the eponymous founder of the dynasty – the Ottomans managed to capture important Byzantine strongholds, such as Bursa (1326), İznik (1331), and İzmit (1337). On the eve of the Black Death, they had incorporated the neighboring principality of Karesi, which allowed them access to the Dardanelles. Hence, Ottoman territory extended over a fairly large area south and east of the Marmara Sea by mid-century. Especially after the annexation of the Karesi emirate's landholdings, the Ottomans came into direct contact with the Byzantines, whereupon the Dardanelles and the Bosphorus straits came to separate their territory.

Given the proximity of Ottoman and Byzantine areas in the mid-fourteenth century, it seems almost impossible to assume that plague did not circulate between them. As we have seen, the initial wave of the Black Death seems to have found its way to Bursa, and perhaps to other locations controlled by the Ottomans at this early point of their history. As the Ottoman expansion across the Dardanelles followed soon afterward, their dominions became even closer than before. Evidently, the successive waves that affected the neighboring Byzantine areas also spread to the Ottoman side. Even though we are not always in a position to establish precise trajectories and areas of influence of these outbreaks, the circulation of epidemics between the Byzantine and Ottoman areas in the first post–Black Death century is almost certain.

There was a palpable correlation between plague and the Ottoman expansion, both temporally and spatially: the two expanded almost concurrently. The Ottomans' most fervent expansion in the Balkans and Anatolia took place while plague was periodically visiting those areas. What was the nature of the relationship between the Ottoman growth and the plague, especially in the first post–Black Death century? Such a relationship was proposed in the scholarship quite early on. Writing about Ottoman history in the early twentieth century, Herbert Adams Gibbons saw plague as one of the factors that facilitated the early Ottoman expansion. He commented, "Between 1348 and 1431, nine great plagues are recorded. These dates coincide with the most aggressive period of Ottoman conquest." According to Gibbons, the initial outbreak of the Black Death and its successive waves had a heavy toll on the Greek-Christian urban populations of the Balkans and Anatolia. In the wake of the plague, these areas were not in a position to form a strong opposition to the Ottoman advancement. Hence, Gibbons concluded, "Orkhan . . . was aided by the 'black death.'"[60] A decade later, historian Lynn Thorndike built on the observation of Gibbons and proposed that one of the consequences of the Black Death was the rapid Ottoman expansion. He wrote, "The Black Death in the fourteenth [century] [i]n part . . . may have been responsible for the expansion of the Ottoman Turks and the final decline of civilization in the Balkan peninsula and Asia Minor."[61] Even though these arguments were not thoroughly pursued in the scholarship, they left behind a residual imaginary of the early Ottoman society as having been mostly free from plague in its early centuries.

Despite its problematic implications, the argument that the Black Death may have facilitated the Ottoman expansion proved to be resilient, especially coupled with the absence of narrative accounts of early Ottoman plagues. Toward the end of the century, we still hear the same argument, albeit in a different form. For example, historian Metin Kunt argued that the Black Death was one of the factors that contributed to the ease of early Ottoman conquests. He suggested that the Turkoman emirates of Anatolia were not as much affected by the Black Death as were the populations of the Byzantine Empire, Europe, and the Middle East. He explained this difference by the lack of immunity to plague among the latter groups of people – something the Turkomans of Anatolia possessed, owing to their Central Asian origin. Kunt reasoned that because the origin of the plague was also Central Asia, the people of Central Asian descent would have the immunity to protect them from it.[62] At the time he advanced this hypothesis about two decades ago, plague's Central Asian origins were widely accepted. But there did

---

[60] Herbert Adams Gibbons, *The Foundation of the Ottoman Empire; a History of the Osmanlis up to the Death of Bayezid I (1300–1403)* (New York: Century, 1916), 95–96.

[61] Thorndike, "Blight of Pestilence," 456.

[62] Metin Kunt, "State and Sultan up to the Age of Süleyman: Frontier Principality to World Empire," in *Süleyman the Magnificent and His Age: The Ottoman Empire in the Early Modern World*, ed. Metin Kunt and Christine Woodhead (London: Longman, 1995), 11.

not seem to be any scientific basis for such facile explanations of genetic immunity acquired from ancestral area of origin, and today we know that this assumption cannot be supported by scientific evidence.[63]

The question whether early Ottoman expansion was facilitated by the Black Death had to address historical factors. With this in view, it was Uli Schamiloglu's pioneering article that revisited the question. Schamiloglu acknowledges the widespread mortality in mid-fourteenth-century Anatolia owing to the Black Death, and unlike Kunt, he believes that other Turkish principalities in the area were also devastated by it. This, Schamiloglu explained, was caused by two reasons: first, the principalities that were located directly on coastal areas suffered more heavily from the epidemic, and second, the Ottomans seem to have suffered less than their rivals because they were largely nomadic. He clarifies, "Epidemic disease does not spread as easily among nomadic populations, and this has been offered as an explanation of why nomadic populations became relatively stronger in the medieval Arabian Peninsula or following the collapse of the Golden Horde. For this same reason the Ottoman nomadic population could have remained largely unaffected by the plague while Byzantium and the other Turkish principalities suffered from depopulation and instability. As a result the Ottomans would have suddenly gained in relative size and strength."[64]

Most recently, J. R. McNeill reiterated the same argument that "the lightning success of the Ottomans from 1347 onwards" was partly owed to plague's devastating effects on their rivals. Like Schamiloglu, McNeill also held that the Ottomans were relatively spared from the devastating effects of the Black Death and its recurrent waves because they had neither port cities nor a predominately urban society. McNeill argues that the pastoral nomadism of the Ottomans must have spared them from the devastating demographic losses experienced in the southeast Balkans and northwest Anatolia.[65]

Despite their different emphases, there seem to be three elements common to these arguments: (1) that the Ottomans successfully rose to power; (2) that there is solid evidence to show the devastating effects of the plague

---

[63] A recent study proved this wrong by demonstrating that the evolutionary changes caused by plague in the immunity system of populations did not result from their ancestral area of origin but from exposure to the infection. See Hafid Laayouni et al., "Convergent Evolution in European and Rroma Populations Reveals Pressure Exerted by Plague on Toll-like Receptors," *PNAS* 111, no. 7 (2014): 2668–73. For questions of immunity, see Stephen R. Ell, "Immunity as a Factor in the Epidemiology of Medieval Plague," *Review of Infectious Diseases* 6, no. 6 (1984): 866–79; Fabian Crespo and Matthew B. Lawrenz, "Heterogeneous Immunological Landscapes and Medieval Plague: An Invitation to a New Dialogue between Historians and Immunologists," *The Medieval Globe* 1 (2014): 229–57.

[64] Schamiloglu, "Black Death in Medieval Anatolia," 271.

[65] J. R. McNeill, "The Eccentricity of the Middle East and North Africa's Environmental History," in Mikhail, *Water on Sand*, 27–50, esp. 40–41.

on the Byzantines and other parts of Anatolia; and (3) that there is a dearth
of (comparable) evidence on Ottoman plagues, at least for the first century
following the Black Death. The first two premises are well supported by historical evidence, and there is no need to discuss them any further.[66] However,
the third deserves more careful consideration. As discussed in Chapter 2, the
absence of evidence cannot be taken as evidence for absence. It is critical
to understand the meaning of plague for early Ottoman society and their
attitudes toward it to historicize that silence. Besides, it is no secret that we
do not have a wealth of written sources for the first century of Ottoman
history. In other words, there is a general dearth of Ottoman sources to
shed light on this early phase of their history, not least on the question of
the presence or absence of plague in their realm. Under the circumstances,
one wonders whether the silence about plague has any exceptional meaning
or should be considered as being just another dark aspect of early Ottoman
history, one of its "black holes."[67] Nonetheless, it is simply not true that
the Ottoman sources are completely silent about plague. As we have seen,
there are scattered references to plagues in the sources that have not been
hitherto brought together systematically. In the absence of a general framework with which to read early Ottoman plagues, those scattered references
can be easily overlooked.

Regardless, the question whether (and to what extent) the Ottomans were
affected by the Black Death remains to be addressed. It is true that we lack
detailed evidence to establish the degree of devastation plague caused in
early Ottoman society. We equally lack evidence to establish with precision

[66] For a discussion of Byzantine population loss as a result of the Black Death, see Klaus-Peter
Matschke, "Research Problems Concerning the Transition to Tourkokratia: The Byzantinist
Standpoint," in *The Ottomans and the Balkans: A Discussion of Historiography*, ed. Fikret
Adanır and Suraiya Faroqhi, 79–113 (Leiden: Brill, 2002), esp. 82–83. In addition to the
better-reported demographic decline in the large urban centers, such as in Constantinople,
the rural Byzantine population is also shown to have suffered great losses, at least by half.
For a study of the rural population of eastern Macedonia, see Jacques Lefort, "Population
and Landscape in Eastern Macedonia during the Middle Ages: The Example of Radolibos,"
in *Continuity and Change in Late Byzantine and Early Ottoman Society*, ed. Anthony Bryer
and Heath W. Lowry, 11–21 (Birmingham: University of Birmingham Centre for Byzantine
Studies, 1986); Jacques Lefort, "Rural Economy and Social Relations in the Countryside,"
Dumbarton Oaks Papers 47 (1993): 101–13. For a discussion of the fourteenth-century
population of Anatolia, see Elizabeth Zachariadou, "Notes sur la population de l'Asie
mineure turque au XIVè siècle," *Byzantinische Forschungen* 12 (1987): 221–31.

[67] Since Colin Imber's 1993 article, the metaphor of the "black hole" has been associated
with early Ottoman history. See Imber, "The Legend of Osman Gazi," in Zachariadou,
The Ottoman Emirate, 67–73; Colin Heywood, "Filling the Back Hole: The Emergence of
the Bithynian Atamanates," in *The Great Ottoman Turkish Civilisation*, ed. Kemal Çiçek,
Ercüment Kuran, Nejat Göyünç, and İlber Ortaylı (Ankara: Yeni Türkiye Yayınevi, 2000),
1:107–15. Also see Eugenia Kermeli and Oktay Özel, eds., *The Ottoman Empire: Myths,
Realities and "Black Holes": Contributions in Honour of Colin Imber* (Istanbul: Isis Press,
2006).

how the other parts of Anatolia were affected. Hence, we do not know whether they were *more* or *less* affected than the Ottomans. What we do know instead, on the basis of limited information, is that the coastal areas appear to have been affected first, before plague found its way toward inner areas. Was that why it has been suggested that Anatolia littoral was more heavily affected by plague than the interior? Perhaps. But it should also be remembered that this might be an artifact of the sources. Precisely because of their maritime communications with other port cities, the news of their being visited by plague would circulate more easily than news of visitations in inner areas of Anatolia. Hence, it is important not to lose sight of the distinction between *what is reported* and *what happened*.

Moreover, there is not enough evidence to suggest that the coastal areas were more heavily affected. Comparable cases can be found in the way the Black Death spread elsewhere, especially in areas that have been better scrutinized in the scholarship. For example, a range of inland locations in continental Europe has been recorded to experience the plague, yet until recently, historians of plague have not problematized the etiological and epidemiological disparities between the outbreaks of plague experienced in port cities and those in the hinterland. Even the better-studied cases of European cities during the Black Death do not suggest that such distinctions were clearly identified.[68] At the same time, one may need to reconsider how inland the Ottomans were at the time of the Black Death or during the first century that followed it. By 1347, after the annexation of Karesi lands, the Ottoman dominions reached the eastern and southern shores of the Marmara Sea up to (or at least close to) the Bosphorus and the Dardanelles, which were very densely populated areas at the time.[69] In the subsequent era, they acquired possession of several port cities on the Black Sea, the Aegean, and the Mediterranean. It can even be argued that Ottoman expansion over the first post–Black Death century increased its degree of exposure to new infections. Arguably, because the Ottomans were extended over an ever-growing realm, they were, as a result, in greater contact with possible incoming or persisting infections. Presumably, as they expanded further in the Balkans, they came into contact with places where plague epidemics recurred periodically.

---

[68] See Carmichael, "Plague Persistence in Western Europe"; Neil Cummins, Morgan Kelly, and Cormac O'Grada, "Living Standards and Plague in London, 1560–1665," SSRN Scholarly Paper (Rochester, NY: Social Science Research Network, July 3, 2013), http://papers.ssrn .com/abstract=2289094.

[69] According to the Byzantine historian Pachymeres, Bithynia was a prosperous and densely populated area in the late thirteenth century. See Lefort, "Rural Economy and Social Relations," 105n27. On the basis of the eyewitness testimonies from the first half of the fourteenth century (e.g., al-Umari and Ibn Battuta), Zachariadou concludes that this area was prosperous and well populated on the eve of the Black Death. See Zachariadou, "Notes sur la population."

Be that as it may, we know full well that plague was not limited to coastal areas or to port cities. In fact, it may be interesting to note that most of the evidence about the Black Death in Anatolia comes, not from the coastline, but from the interior. There is even evidence for plague's occurrence in places away from the main highways and at high altitude. For example, both Sivas and Divriği have altitudes of more than four thousand feet (1,285 and 1,250 meters, respectively). Similarly, both Akşehir and Kayseri were established on the foot of a mountain range, at an altitude of about thirty-five hundred feet (1,050 meters). It may be the case that this is simply a coincidence, but taken as a whole, it suggests at least that the disease was not limited to the sea-level Anatolia littoral – quite the contrary. Recent research from Madagascar, where plague is still enzootic, offers clues to understanding why altitude matters for maintaining the infection. The highlands of the island (above eight hundred meters) offered the ecological circumstances where plague was sustained in the rodent and flea population.[70] With this in view, historian Ann Carmichael recently argued that the European Alps likely served as an ecological zone for plague maintenance.[71] In this context, it should be possible to consider that the mountain ranges of Anatolia and the Balkans comprised ecologically favorable niches for sustaining plague.[72]

It has also been suggested that other Anatolian principalities were more affected by plague than the Ottomans because they were "closely connected to port cities."[73] Nevertheless, there is no convincing evidence that the Ottomans were less connected to port cities than were others. On the contrary, there is evidence that the fourteenth-century Anatolia was a closely connected network in which a range of mobilities and exchange took place. Tracing the trajectories of plague that went in and out of Ottoman domains can offer some understanding of how they were related to the larger world around them. Sources of the time suggest a certain degree of connectedness. For example, on the eve of the Black Death, Ibn Battuta traveled in and out of the Ottoman domains with ease.[74] Johann Schiltberger mentions that the Ottomans had access to the eastern shores of the Bosphorus at the turn of the fifteenth century, and he crossed it to get to Constantinople or Pera.[75] Similarly, Bertrandon de la Broquière in the early 1430s commented on the

---

[70] Amy J. Vogler et al., "Phylogeography and Molecular Epidemiology of *Yersinia pestis* in Madagascar," *PLoS Neglected Tropical Diseases* 5, no. 9 (2011): e1319; Voahangy Andrianaivoarimanana et al., "Understanding the Persistence of Plague Foci in Madagascar," *PLoS Neglected Tropical Diseases* 7, no. 11 (2013): e2382.

[71] Carmichael, "Plague Persistence in Western Europe."

[72] I have argued this elsewhere with particular reference to the type of rodent and flea species and other animals that could have played a role in maintaining the infection in the wilderness. See my "New Science and Old Sources."

[73] See, e.g., J.R. McNeill, "Eccentricity," 40.

[74] Ibn Battuta, *Travels in Asia and Africa*.

[75] Johann Schiltberger, *The Bondage and Travels of Johann Schiltberger* (New York: Burt Franklin, 1879), 79. For exchanges between the Byzantine and Ottoman courts at this time,

lively trade in Bursa on his travel to Pera with a group of Genoese merchants and on the Venetian, Catalan, Genoese, and Florentine merchants who lived in Edirne.[76]

It may help to remember that the cities of Anatolia formed a tightly knit network of international trade in the fourteenth century. Several urban centers along the caravan routes were linked, as evidenced in a network of caravanserais across the region. For example, Anatolian cities on the Black Sea coast were linked to Syria and Egypt via overland caravan routes.[77] A great many cities of Anatolia were instrumental in grain, cloth, and slave trade.[78] These trading networks were connected to larger networks that involved the Mediterranean, the Black Sea, and its Asian hinterland. In fact, it was this increased level of integration between interregional networks in the first half of the fourteenth century that enabled the distribution of the disease.[79] In the words of historian Cemal Kafadar:

> In this world of dizzying physical mobility – crisscrossed by overlapping networks of nomads and seminomads, raiders, volunteers on their way to join military adventures, slaves of various backgrounds, wandering dervishes, monks and churchmen trying to keep in touch with their flock, displaced peasants and townspeople seeking refuge, disquieted souls seeking cure and consolation at sacred sites, Muslim schoolmen seeking patronage, and the inevitable risk-driven merchants of late medieval Eurasia – it is not at all surprising that information traveled. So did lore and ideas, fashions and codes, of course.[80]

We may perhaps add plague to the list; this would have been the Anatolia that encountered the Black Death in the mid-fourteenth century.

Yet there was something that moved even faster than the plague: news! News of plague always moved faster than the infection itself, owing to the incubation period needed for the epidemic to take place.[81] Hence, it is

---

see Nevra Necipoğlu, "Circulation of People between the Byzantine and Ottoman Courts," in *The Byzantine Court: Source of Power and Culture; Papers from the Second International Sevgi Gönül Byzantine Studies Symposium, Istanbul 21–23 June 2010*, ed. Ayla Ödekan, Engin Akyürek, and Nevra Necipoğlu (Istanbul: Koç University Press, 2013), 105–8.

76   Bertrandon de la Brocquière, *Voyage D'Outremer*, 83–88, 108.

77   Yaşar Yücel, *Çoban-oğulları Candar-oğulları Beylikleri: XIII-XV. Yüzyıllar Kuzey-Batı Anadolu Tarihi* (Ankara: TTK, 1980), 137–38.

78   Kate Fleet, *European and Islamic Trade in the Early Ottoman State: The Merchants of Genoa and Turkey* (Cambridge: Cambridge University Press, 1999); Fleet, "Ottoman Grain Exports from Western Anatolia at the End of the Fourteenth Century," *JESHO* 40, no. 3 (1997): 283–93; Fleet, "Turkish Economy."

79   Abu-Lughod, *Before European Hegemony*, 124.

80   Cemal Kafadar, *Between Two Worlds: The Construction of the Ottoman State* (Berkeley: University of California Press, 1995), 61.

81   Based on the reports of the Indian Plague Research Commission, Benedictow calculates the time between the rodent epizootic and human epidemic as about twenty-four days. See Benedictow, *Black Death*, 18.

possible that Ottoman urban populations fled their settlements upon hearing news of plague. By the same token, it is also possible that not only Orhan and his court but the entire Ottoman elite fled to infection-free areas upon hearing news of disease.[82] If so, can this be the reason why there is nothing written about those years in the Ottoman chronicles? For instance, Aşıkpaşazade skips over the years when the Black Death visited Ottoman areas. So does Neşri. Perhaps Orhan was following what common wisdom of nomadic and semi-nomadic lifestyle would have prescribed about leaving low-lying urban areas for highland pastures, a principle that his successors would also follow to avoid epidemics. This, however, is mere speculation and cannot be established in the absence of evidence. Nevertheless, it may be possible to make inferences about epidemics when Ottoman sultans were documented to have moved to "the mountains." For instance, Oruç often noted such occasions when the sultan moved to highland retreats (*yayla*) without necessarily mentioning an outbreak.[83] As we shall see in the next chapters, tracing those dates may provide some evidence about outbreaks, especially if supported by other sources.

Regardless, if we were to believe that the Black Death affected the Ottomans less than others, we still need to explain how they differed from others who surrounded them and reflect on what social and economic practices may have spared them. At this point, we may need to revisit the proposition that Ottoman society was less affected by the Black Death because they were mostly nomadic. According to this argument, nomadic societies are not as badly affected by epidemic diseases as urban societies, and because the Ottomans were largely nomadic at that stage, they would have been mostly unaffected by the Black Death. The merits of the argument in offering insights about why the Ottomans might have been less affected by plague notwithstanding, it is necessary to comment briefly on the widespread presence of nomadism in late medieval Anatolia.

Following the Battle of Manzikert in 1071, large numbers of nomadic Turkoman groups started penetrating Anatolia, which spread pastoral nomadism virtually overnight across the peninsula. Hence, at the turn of the fourteenth century, the presence of such groups in the area where the Ottomans were to rule was no exception. In this area, large groups of pastoral nomads alternated between summer pastures (*yaylak*) in higher altitudes and winter pastures (*kışlak*) in the lowlands and valleys. As we are often reminded, pastoral nomadic groups were also involved in agriculture

---

[82] In fact, Ibn Battuta suggested that Orhan was always on the move. See Ross E. Dunn, *The Adventures of Ibn Battuta, a Muslim Traveler of the Fourteenth Century* (Berkeley: University of California Press, 1986), 152.

[83] E.g., Oruç notes that Murad stayed in a plateau near Edirne in the years 830 H. (1426–27), 832 H. (1428–29), 834 H. (1430–31), 835 H. (1431–32), and 838 H. (1434–35), though this cannot be taken as direct evidence for the presence of outbreaks in every one of those years, in the absence of corroborating evidence. See Oruç, *Tarih*.

and other economic activities (e.g., manufacturing, trade) and for that purpose were in touch with settled societies. Though it may be so, it is still difficult to determine to what extent the Ottomans were nomadic (or rather more nomadic than others in Anatolia) at the time of the Black Death. In the absence of clear evidence about the number of nomads, semi-nomads, and town dwellers, it is difficult to single out the Ottomans as being *more* nomadic than others. To a large extent, the Anatolian principalities had nomadic or semi-nomadic groups in their populations, in addition to those who lived in towns. If for anything, there is evidence that the Ottomans were going through a process of sedentarization, by which they were becoming *less* nomadic on the eve of the Black Death.[84] In the preceding decades, urban centers, such as Bursa, İznik, and İzmit, had been integrated into Ottoman domains.[85] For example, a visitor in the early 1330s, Ibn Battuta, found Bursa to be a lively commercial center.[86]

Moreover, the relationship between nomadism and plague seems to be more complicated than suggested. It is true that epidemics thrive in urban settings where people live in close proximity to each other; epidemiological studies have shown this with great authority. Nevertheless, there is also evidence for the spread of epidemics outside of urban centers, to the countryside, and to areas where nomads had extensive contacts.[87] The assumption that nomadic groups were relatively immune to plagues is mostly borrowed from studies of nomads of the desert and those of Central Asia.[88] Yet, instead of accepting this as a blanket statement, it may be necessary to consider the type of nomadism in Anatolia itself at the time of the Black Death and reflect on practices that affected their exposure to infection.[89] After all, one may expect to see differences between the sheep-herding Turkomans of Anatolia and the camel-herding Bedouins of the Arabian Peninsula and North Africa

---

[84] Rudi Paul Lindner, *Nomads and Ottomans in Medieval Anatolia* (Bloomington: Research for Inner Asian Studies, Indiana University, 1983), 29–32; Feridun Emecen, "Batı Anadolu'da Yörükler," in *İlk Osmanlılar ve Batı Anadolu Beylikler Dünyası*, 175–85 (Istanbul: Kitabevi, 2001).

[85] This trend seems to have continued in the subsequent era. Over the course of the fifteenth and sixteenth centuries, nomadic population seems to have decreased in proportion to sedentary population. For example, the nomads were only 15 percent of the Anatolian population in 1520. Halil İnalcık, *An Economic and Social History of the Ottoman Empire, 1300–1914* (New York: Cambridge University Press, 1994), 34. Also see Reşat Kasaba, *A Moveable Empire: Ottoman Nomads, Migrants, and Refugees* (Seattle: University of Washington Press, 2009).

[86] Ibn Battuta, *Travels in Asia and Africa*, 136.

[87] Dols, *Black Death*, 154–69; Lawrence I. Conrad, "The Plague in the Early Medieval Near East," PhD diss., Princeton University, 1981, 465–69; Stuart J. Borsch, *The Black Death in Egypt and England: A Comparative Study* (Austin: University of Texas Press, 2009), 24–54.

[88] McNeill, *Plagues and Peoples*; Conrad, "Plague in the Early Medieval Near East," 465–69.

[89] Pastoral nomadism needs to be better understood. For a recent call to research in this field of inquiry, see Edmund Burke, "Pastoralism and the Mediterranean Environment," *IJMES* 42, no. 4 (2010): 663–65.

in how they interacted with their disease environments. In the way of offering an explanation, it was once suggested that fleas found the smell of goats and horses repulsive and did not approach them. Building on this, Leila Erder held that this might have spared the goat-herding nomads of Anatolia from bubonic plague.[90] Braudel also noted that the nomads of Anatolia associated summer pastures in highlands with better health and that they rushed to leave their "flea-ridden" winter pastures as soon as spring came.[91] In addition, it is also held that nomads protected themselves from epidemics by leaving behind the dead and the dying.[92] A piece of evidence to substantiate this practice comes from an anecdote recorded in a sixteenth-century hagiography, in which an Anatolian nomad (*yürük*) is shunned by a mystic for having left a plague victim behind. To no avail, the nomad tried to prove their custom right by claiming that it was their *ancient practice*.[93]

That these possible methods that may have favored the nomads notwithstanding, recent research suggests quite a different picture, in which the nomads are also at risk of infection. Moreover, they may help spread infection by bridging areas where plague is enzootic (or sylvatic) to places where it can become epidemic. For example, evidence from nomads in modern North Africa shows their risk of contracting the infection and of propagating it.[94] These studies highlight the exposure of nomads to plague owing to their contact with rodents and their ectoparasites. By the same token, the role of nomadic peoples in transmitting plague has also been brought into focus in historical studies of plague. For example, the recent work of Paul Buell draws attention to the relationship between Central Asian steppe nomads and the plague, both in the Second and the Third pandemics, and possibly in the First as well.[95] Finally, recent research from Madagascar also reveals new insights about the transmission of enzootic plague from highlands to lowlands that may have implications for understanding the involvement of nomads in the process. As mentioned earlier, plague is sustained in the

90   Erder claims that Biraben suggested this, but I have not been able to access the cited work. See Leila Erder, "The Measurement of Preindustrial Population Changes: The Ottoman Empire from the 15th to the 17th Century," *Middle Eastern Studies* 11, no. 3 (1975): 293n30. Yet, Solomon Schweigger noted that the horses were disturbed by fleas in sixteenth-century Istanbul. See Schweigger, *Sultanlar Kentine Yolculuk*, 58.

91   Fernand Braudel, *The Mediterranean and the Mediterranean World in the Age of Philip II*, vol. 1 (Berkeley: University of California Press, 1995), 97.

92   Erder mentions this practice but does not present examples. See Erder, "Measurement of Preindustrial Population Changes," 293.

93   İbn Isa-yı Saruhanî, *Akhisarlı Şeyh Îsâ Menâkıbnâmesi (XVI. yüzyıl)*, ed. Sezai Küçük and Ramazan Muslu (Sakarya: Aşiyan Yayınları, 2003), 96–97, 109.

94   Idir Bitam et al., "New Rural Focus of Plague, Algeria," *Emerging Infectious Diseases* 16, no. 10 (2010): 1639–40; Kmar Ben Néfissa and Anne Marie Moulin, "La peste nord-africaine et la théorie de Charles Nicolle sur les maladies infectieuses," *Gesnerus-Swiss Journal of the History of Medicine and Sciences* 67, no. 1 (2010): 30–56.

95   Buell, "Qubilai and the Rats," 130–32.

highlands of the island because of the abundance of flea vectors (*Xenopsylla cheopis* and *Synopsyllus fonquerniei*).[96] If plague finds a favorable environment to preserve itself from one season to the next in the highlands, the infection can be carried either by animals or humans (or their ectoparasites) to the lowlands, where commensal rodents can sustain the infection.

Drawing from this model, it is possible to reconsider the role of pastoral nomads bridging the disease ecologies of Ottoman highlands and lowlands, especially in view of their seasonal movements and their closer involvement with animals. Nomads interacted with settled societies in various ways. For example, they supplied raw materials for the textile and leather industries, such as wool, dyes, and hides. They also produced carpets, rugs, and other textile items. They supplied transportation animals, such as donkeys, horses, and camels. They participated in harvests in western Anatolia as migrant workers and also served in various military undertakings of the Ottoman state.[97] All of these activities brought the nomads into contact with settled populations of towns and cities. Such economic interactions most likely took place in the outskirts of Ottoman towns, where businesses such as tanneries, soap factories, and slaughterhouses were located and low-income families and day laborers resided.[98] These businesses attracted a great number of commensal rodents, exposed laborers to potentially infected materials, and thus functioned as possible gateways of infection leading to urban outbreaks.[99] All of these links could amplify the exchange of infection between the highlands and the lowlands, as facilitated by the mediation of nomads.

Nevertheless, the connection between epidemics and nomads still remains undertheorized in historical studies. More research is needed on the environmental and climatic contexts of the fourteenth-century Anatolia in which the Ottomans lived and interacted with others. Given the available evidence, what can rather cautiously be concluded is that when plagues were introduced from outside, such as was the case in the mid-fourteenth century, nomadic communities as well as those who left towns early could escape the disease. But when plague started to gain a foothold in an area, either sustained by commensal urban rodents or the wild rodents of the countryside,

---

[96] Vogler et al., "Phylogeography and Molecular Epidemiology."

[97] About the various ways nomads were integrated into the Ottoman economy, see Kasaba, *A Moveable Empire*, 31–35.

[98] Yaron Ayalon, "When Nomads Meet Urbanites: The Outskirts of Ottoman Cities as a Venue for the Spread of Epidemic Diseases," in *Plagues in Nomadic Contexts: Historical Impact, Medical Responses, and Cultural Adaptations in Ancient to Mediaeval Eurasia*, ed. Kurt Franz et al. Leiden: Brill, forthcoming.

[99] It is generally held that some professionals in premodern cities were at higher risk of infection. Among these were butchers, bakers, millers, and artisans of cloth and paper, by virtue of their handling meat, grains, and textiles, all instrumental media in the dissemination of plague. See Audoin-Rouzeau, *Les chemins de la peste*, 233–38.

nomads were as much at risk of infection as others – if not more so, because of their potential contacts with plague-hosting animals and arthropod vectors. In other words, for incoming plagues arriving from the sea, nomads may have been relatively secure, but they were at risk for outbreaks from local enzootic origins. In the Ottoman case, this may suggest an increased incidence of the infection among nomadic groups only after plague established enzootic foci in the post–Black Death era.

A Narrative of Recurrent Waves of the Black Death (1347–1453)

The onslaught of the Black Death was a brutal but brisk episode in the Ottoman world and beyond. This first wave lasted from a few months to as much as a year in different places. Here, as in other areas, plague soon receded, leaving behind decimated populations. But the worst was yet to be seen in the repeated waves that would follow. After this initial outbreak, plague was to return periodically to this region for several centuries. What follows is a survey of the recurrent outbreaks of the Black Death until the pivotal point of the Ottoman conquest of Constantinople in 1453.

Plague came and went in waves. Yet the outbreaks did not necessarily follow a recognizable pattern of circulation, spread, and recurrence, at least during this first post–Black Death century. Successive waves of plague returned to places already visited by the Black Death and to those that were left untouched. All in all, both Anatolia and the Balkans were exposed to the infection, like other parts of the Afro-Eurasian world. This exposure does not allow us to make certain grand claims. For example, what the evidence does not allow us to assume is that this area immediately turned into a hotbed of plague, exporting the infection to Europe.

The successive waves of plague did not affect all places at the same time, which sometimes allows tracing the movement of the infection. The patterns of circulation are easier to outline when spread via maritime contacts; overland propagation is more difficult to trace. Byzantine sources adopted a system of counting waves of plagues: they chronicled ten successive waves.[100] A similar system of counting can be found in the chronicles of the Morea.[101] Despite its obvious methodological problems (the Byzantine-centric nature of evidence, limited applicability to larger areas, etc.), this plague count is a helpful tool that is followed loosely here.

---

[100] Peter Schreiner, *Die byzantinischen Kleinchroniken 2. Teil: Historischer Kommentar* (Vienna: Verlag der Österreichischen Akademie der Wissenschaften, 1977), 271–72, 290–92, 308, 311, 324, 337, 344, 361–62.

[101] "The Great Deaths: The First Death happened in 1347; The Second Death in 1362; The Third Death in 1373; The Fourth Death in 1381; The Fifth Death in 1390; The Sixth Death in 1396; The Seventh Death in 1409; The Eighth Death in 1417; The Ninth Death in 1423; The Tenth Death in 1440," according to Diana Gilliland Wright. See http://surprisedbytime .blogspot.com/search/label/Black%20Death.

In the case of Constantinople, the second wave of the plague came in 1361, about fourteen years after the initial outbreak. Even though the infection was present in other Mediterranean ports at the time (e.g., Alexandria in 1357–58 and 1361, Venice in 1359–61, Genoa in 1360–61, and Ragusa/Dubrovnik in 1361), it is difficult to determine the exact route of transmission to Constantinople. The next year, while still in the Byzantine capital, plague is also documented in Trabzon, Crete, Cyprus, Limnos, and the Peloponnese. There is also evidence for a large-scale epidemic in Anatolia in 1362–63, as suggested by the aforementioned chronology of el-Konevi.[102] Notarial accounts from Cyprus offer some information about the course of the epidemic in the island. It seems that plague took hold in Cyprus in summer 1362 and continued into the fall of that year, probably peaking in spring of the next.[103] In 1363, sources recorded the infection also in Constantinople, Edirne,[104] and Trabzon, as well as in the Peloponnese. In 1364, plague is still in the Byzantine capital in October and November, and in Crete, where it lasted until the following year.[105] In 1368, the disease was in Ioannina in Epirus, which is documented to have suffered terribly from the outbreak, leaving thousands of victims behind.[106] This second wave of plague lasted about four to five years in this area, and even longer in other parts of the Mediterranean world.[107]

A third wave of plague arrived in 1372. This time the infection started in Thessaloniki and Constantinople in the first year, being quickly carried to areas that had maritime contacts with these cities. In the following years, plague was recorded in Epirus, in the Peloponnese, and in Crete.[108] Especially Epirus seems to have suffered terribly in 1374, with combined effects of plague and warfare. Crete was under the influence of the epidemic until 1376. This wave of the plague reached even well-isolated communities, such as the monastic community of Mount Athos, as suggested by documents that indicated the presence of the infection there in the year 1378.[109]

---

[102] Turan, *Tarihî Takvimler*, 73: "764 te umumî ölüm, vebâ ve taun."

[103] Aysu Dincer, "Disease in a Sunny Climate: Effects of the Plague on Family and Wealth in Cyprus in the 1360s," in *Economic and Biological Interactions in Pre-industrial Europe, from the 13th to the 18th Century* (Florence: Firenze University Press, 2010), 534.

[104] This may have been Edirne's first plague under Ottoman control, after its conquest. For the date of the conquest, see İnalcık, "Edirne'nin Fethi (1361)," in *Edirne: Edirne'nin 600. Fetih Yıldönümü Armağan Kitabı* (Ankara: TTK, 1993), 137–59.

[105] Köstēs, *Ston kairo tēs panōlēs*, 318. Biraben shows plague was in Constantinople every year between 1363 and 1366. Biraben, *Les hommes et la peste*, 1:440.

[106] Costas Tsiamis et al., "Epidemic Waves of the Black Death in the Byzantine Empire (1347–1453 AD)," *Le Infezioni in Medicina: Rivista Periodica Di Eziologia, Epidemiologia, Diagnostica, Clinica e Terapia Delle Patologie Infettive* 19, no. 3 (2011): 195.

[107] Biraben, *Les hommes et la peste*, 1:378, 389, 394, 430, 440.

[108] Köstēs, *Ston kairo tēs panōlēs*, 319.

[109] Tsiamis et al., "Epidemic Waves of the Black Death," 195.

A fourth wave of plague appeared in Constantinople at the turn of the decade, possibly introduced by the Genoese fleet.[110] This is also evidenced by the presence of plague on Anatolia's Black Sea coast, perhaps distributed from infected ports as a result of contacts with Genoese ships. For example, plague seems to have affected the area close to the port of Samsun – a Genoese port – in the year 1380. The evidence for this comes from a mausoleum built in a village on the mouth of the Kızılırmak River, about five miles north of modern-day Bafra in Samsun. This mausoleum was built in March 1381 by a certain Emirza bin Hüseyin Bey, a local leader of the İsfendiyarids.[111] The inscription at the entrance of the mausoleum clearly indicates that there was a plague epidemic in 1380, during which the aforementioned ruler lost his children one after another.[112] The mausoleum included tombstones of six individuals, five of whom were Emirza Bey's children (four daughters and one son). All died in the months of October and November 1380.[113] This wave of the plague continued throughout the 1380s, with sporadic outbreaks in the ports of the Peloponnese and in Athens, before it returned to Constantinople again in 1386.[114] The Byzantine statesman Demetrios Kydones wrote in his letters about the state of the city during this outbreak and commented that the capital seemed to be cut off from the rest of the world.[115] In the meantime, plague remained active in Crete until the end of the decade.

A fifth wave arrived in the 1390s, perhaps from Venice and Ragusa, which were also infected.[116] Plague probably traveled eastward via the Peloponnese before arriving at Constantinople in 1391. It is possible that the contagion also reached northern Anatolia in the fall of that year, as suggested in the letters of Manuel II Palaiologos, who joined the Ottoman campaign in that year. Manuel mentions in his letters that sickness was affecting the soldiers, alongside scarcity of supplies and cold weather, but does not give much

---

[110]   Ibid.

[111]   For the İsfendiyarids (İsfendiyaroğulları), see J. H. Mordtmann, "Isfendiyār Oghlu," *EI²*.

[112]   Zeki M. Oral, "Durağan ve Bafra'da İki Türbe," *Belleten* 20, no. 79 (1956): 385–410; Günhan H. Danışman, "Emirza Bey Türbesi, Bafra," *Anadolu Araştırmaları* 10 (1986): 543–46.

[113]   M. Sami Bayraktar, "Bafra ve Çarşamba'da Beylikler Döneminden Kalan Tarihi Yapılar," *Uluslararası Sosyal Araştırmalar Dergisi* 6, no. 25 (2013): 120, inscription on 118. This may be one of the earliest known family mausoleums from fourteenth-century Anatolia with clear indication to plague. Unfortunately, the mausoleum was pillaged; the graves and tombstones were destroyed in March 2012.

[114]   Kōstēs, *Ston kairo tēs panōlēs*, 319–20. Dols noted an outbreak of plague in Eygpt in 781 H. (1379–80), which reached Syria the next year and continued until 783 H. (1381–82), but it is not clear whether these were related to the outbreak in northwest Anatolia. See Dols, *Black Death*, 307.

[115]   Tsiamis et al., "Epidemic Waves of the Black Death," 195–96; Congourdeau, "La peste noire," 380.

[116]   Biraben, *Les hommes et la peste*, 1:395, 440.

information on the nature of the disease.[117] In the following years, plague was in Cyprus and Crete, and it reappeared in Constantinople in 1398. At the close of the fourteenth century, the disease was on the southern shores of the Peloponnese, especially in Methoni and Koroni.[118]

In the beginning of the fifteenth century, new outbreaks of plague affected this area. An outbreak was recorded in Koroni in 1400, which also affected the island of Corfu the next year. In the following years, sporadic cases were recorded in the nearby ports and islands.[119] Ruy Gonzalez de Clavijo's account mentions an outbreak in the year 1403. During his journey toward Constantinople, because of high winds, his ship had to anchor close to the island of Tenedos (Bozcaada), opposite the coast of northwest Anatolia, before entering the Dardanelles. On October 14, they heard news of plague from a vessel coming from Gallipoli, specifically, that "a great pestilence raged at Gallipoli."[120] Even though Gallipoli would have been under Ottoman control at that time, we do not seem to find reference to this outbreak in the Ottoman sources.

What appears to be the next wave started in 1408. Plague was in Crete that year. The next year, it spread to Cyprus and to Constantinople, where it lasted through 1410. Byzantine chronicles described these outbreaks as exceptionally vehement, taking as many as ten thousand lives in Constantinople alone.[121] In the years 1410 and 1411, the epidemic is also documented to be in the Peloponnese (Koroni and Methoni) and in Corfu, Cyprus, and Crete.[122] It was especially punishing on the island of Corfu in 1410, killing, among others, the much-needed archers, as understood from the island's appeal to the Venetian Senate requesting replacements.[123] There is evidence for the circulation of the infection in the Ionian Sea in the middle years of the decade, with a recurrent eruption in Corfu in 1413 and in the nearby island of Cephalonia in 1416.

Plague returned to Constantinople in 1417 in a severe episode. On account of the raging epidemic, Venetian ships avoided unloading their

---

[117] Manuel II Palaeologus, *The Letters*, ed. and trans. George T. Dennis (Washington, DC: Dumbarton Oaks Center for Byzantine Studies, 1977), 45–46. Dennis commented that this outbreak may be the same as the one raging the capital in the same year (62n1). This is also mentioned in Elizabeth A. Zachariadou, "Manuel II Palaeologos on the Strife between Bāyezīd I and Ḳāḍī Burhān Al-Dīn Aḥmad," *Bulletin of the School of Oriental and African Studies* 43, no. 3 (1980): 475.

[118] Kōstēs, *Ston kairo tēs panōlēs*, 320.

[119] Ibid., 333.

[120] Ruy González de Clavijo, *Embassy of Ruy Gonzalez de Clavijo*, 26.

[121] Congourdeau, "La peste noire," 380; Nevra Necipoğlu, *Byzantium between the Ottomans and the Latins: Politics and Society in the Late Empire* (Cambridge: Cambridge University Press, 2009), 186–87.

[122] Kōstēs, *Ston kairo tēs panōlēs*, 333–4.

[123] Tsiamis et al., "Epidemic Waves of the Black Death," 196.

cargo in its ports.[124] Byzantine historian Doukas wrote, "Large numbers of the populace succumbed to the bubonic plague...the dreaded disease continued to consume and destroy bodies, neither respecting nor sparing any age." The victims included Russian princess Anna, the fourteen-year-old bride of Manuel's eldest son, the future emperor John VIII Palaiologos. Doukas writes that Anna's death of plague in August 1417 was greatly mourned in the capital.[125] More interesting was the death of Yusuf, the youngest son of Bayezid I (r. 1389–1402), from plague in the Byzantine capital, where he was brought after his father's defeat by Timur in 1402.[126] Doukas writes that Yusuf converted to Christianity and was baptized under the name Demetrios before he succumbed to plague.[127] The fifteenth-century Ottoman historian Kemal's account confirms Yusuf's death from plague, but there is no reference to his conversion. Kemal also mentions Ahmed and Mahmud, other sons of Bayezid who died from plague, which may suggest the spread of the epidemic into the Ottoman areas as well.[128] There is also evidence that plague was carried to the Black Sea shores. The Byzantine historian George Sphrantzes's sister died during this outbreak along with her daughter and husband, Gregory Palaiologos Mamonas, in a Black Sea town in winter 1416–17.[129]

Over the following few years, plague is documented in Crete, Cyprus, Peloponnese, and Epirus. It returned to the Byzantine capital in 1420, where it remained until the next year. When the Ottoman army laid siege to Constantinople in 1422, the already reduced population of the city was in a state of panic.[130] Thessaloniki was also affected in 1422 and 1423, during the critical years when the city was brought under Venetian rule while under siege by the Ottoman army. In 1426, plague seems to have moved southward,

---

[124]   Congourdeau, "La peste noire," 380.

[125]   Doukas, *Decline and Fall of Byzantium to the Ottoman Turks* (Detroit, MI: Wayne State University Press, 1975), quotation on 112, 288n119. For Anna's tomb, see Alexander van Millingen et al., *Byzantine Churches in Constantinople; Their History and Architecture* (London: Macmillan, 1912), 128.

[126]   Dimitris J. Kastritsis, *The Sons of Bayezid: Empire Building and Representation in the Ottoman Civil War of 1402–1413* (Leiden: Brill, 2007), 41.

[127]   Doukas, *Decline and Fall*, 112, 288n120, n122. He was buried at the monastery of Studion. For his tomb, see van Millingen et al., *Byzantine Churches in Constantinople*, 47–48. Congourdeau also mentions Yusuf's baptism and claims that he died during the outbreak of 1409–10, based on Sphrantzes's account. See Congourdeau, "La peste noire," 380. Yusuf's case has also been noted in Lowry, "Pushing the Stone Uphill," 100–102. Yet, Lowry suggests that this went unnoted by the Ottoman chroniclers.

[128]   See Kemal, *Selâtîn-Nâme (1299–1490)* (Ankara: TTK, 2001), 135: "Ki sultânuñ beş oğlı olmışıdı / Hudâ emrine üçi varmışıdı / Biri Ahmed biri Mahmûd Yusuf Han / Ta'ûndan gitdi bunlar bilgil iy can / Ki dördüncüsi durur Mustafâ Han / Beşinci[si]niñ ismidür Murâd Han."

[129]   William Miller, "The Historians Doukas and Phrantzes," *The Journal of Hellenic Studies* 46, Part 1 (1926): 66; Necipoğlu, *Byzantium between the Ottomans and the Latins*, 246.

[130]   Ibid., 187–88.

as it was recorded in Chalcis (Negropont).[131] It was also in other Venetian colonies and in Venice itself throughout the decade.[132]

The next outbreak in 1429–30 is better documented. Mamluk sources suggest that the epidemic spread to Egypt from Syria.[133] Ottoman sources mention the presence of plague in Bursa. According to a historical calendar of the fifteenth century: "and in this year a terrible pestilence [*ölet*] and epidemic [*vebâ*] befell the city of Bursa, which caused many people to perish."[134] Following this statement, the entry lists the death of a number of Ottoman elites from Bursa.[135] Meanwhile, Constantinople was visited again by the infection after a decade. Plague was documented there in 1431, in 1435, and again in 1438.[136] In 1431, the infection was recorded in Ragusa and in the Peloponnese, yet it is difficult to suggest a precise direction of spread given the paucity of evidence. Plague erupted again in the Byzantine capital in 1435, in the midst of ongoing negotiations with the papacy to hold a council for the union of the churches. Among those who died in Constantinople was the papal envoy Simon Fréron, who had come there to prepare the council. His colleague, John of Ragusa, fled to the countryside to escape the plague. Meanwhile, Venice banned its ships from approaching the western shores of the Black Sea, which suggests the presence of the infection in that area as well. The eastern shores of the Black Sea were not spared; plague is documented in Trabzon in the same year.[137]

This outbreak is also mentioned in the chronicle of Oruç, who dates it to 838 H. (August 1434–July 1435). Oruç wrote, "A great pestilence broke out that caused terrible deaths in Rum-ili, to such an extent that the

---

[131] Kōstēs, *Ston kairo tēs panōlēs*, 334–35; Tsiamis et al., "Epidemic Waves of the Black Death," 196.

[132] Biraben, *Les hommes et la peste*, 1:395.

[133] Dols, *Black Death*, 205.

[134] The earlier source for this is a historical calendar, written around 1445 and presented to Murad II. See Turan, *Tarihi Takvimler*, 25: "ve Bursa şehrinde begayet ölüt ve vebâ düşelden ve çok halk-ı 'âlem helâk olub Murad han karındaşları ve Emîr Süleyman beg oğlı Orhan beg ve Emîr Seyyid ve İbrahim Paşa ve Çorak beg ve Vezir Hacı 'İvaz Paşa ve Şeyh Fahreddin Efendi oğılları ve Mevlânâ Şemseddin 'ulemâ-i Sultan Fenâri oğlı vefatlarından berü." Here Turan read the word as *ölüt*, but it seems more likely to be *ölet*, which translates as "pestilence." Another source that mentions it is an anonymous calendar written in 1452–53 and presented to Mehmed II. See Atsız, "Fatih Sultan Mehmed'e Sunulmuş Tarihi bir Takvim," *İstanbul Enstitüsü Dergisi* 3 (1957): 17–23.

[135] It is not indicated whether those people died as a result of the epidemic. It is possible that simply because their deaths were listed right after that record for the outbreak, it could be interpreted that they died of plague. This is a rather lengthy entry with a long list of events, which complicates dating the outbreak. The fact that the Ottoman conquest of Thessaloniki is mentioned within the same entry suggests that this could be 1430 or the year before.

[136] Kōstēs, *Ston kairo tēs panōlēs*, 335–36.

[137] Ibid., 335; Tsiamis et al., "Epidemic Waves of the Black Death," 196; Congourdeau, "La peste noire," 380–81; Necipoğlu, *Byzantium between the Ottomans and the Latins*, 195.

entire population of this area was almost wiped out. The whole world came to ruins." During this time, our chronicler noted, Murad II (r. 1421–51) stayed in a countryside retreat near Edirne, perhaps to avoid the plague.[138] It appears that the disease lingered for a few more years in the Balkans. Doukas noted that Murad's troops suffered heavy losses from "pestilential disease" during a six-month-long siege of Belgrade in spring and summer 1436.[139]

It seems that plague had spread to a very large area. Traveling in the Mediterranean around this time, the Spanish traveler Pero Tafur encountered plague on several occasions. For example, while he was on his way to the Holy Land, probably in 1436, he received news of a plague in Paphos, a coastal city on the southwest of Cyprus, from which he had to take refuge in a village on a nearby mountain.[140] On his return to Constantinople, in the early months of 1438, Pero Tafur records that ships had to wait for two months on the Bosphorus before entering the city because it was feared that they would bring the plague with them. Tafur commented,

Orders having been issued that no ships coming from the Black Sea were to enter the harbour, either at Constantinople or Pera, because it was feared that they would bring the plague with them, they built a shelter two leagues from Constantinople where the ships could discharge their cargo, and where they had to remain for sixty days unless they were prepared to put to sea again. Certainly the foreign nations bring much sickness with them, and I myself saw in that lodging men dead of plague.[141]

Following this prolonged episode, sporadic outbreaks were noted in the 1440s, scattered over the Peloponnese, in Chios, and in the other islands of the area, as well as in the environs of Constantinople.[142] For example, there is evidence for an outbreak in Negropont toward the end of the decade, where it was said to have decimated two-thirds of the city's population over two years. It was also noted in the Morea, Thrace, Peloponnese, and Corfu at that time.[143]

---

138 *Oruç, Tarih*, 59 [facsimile 40b]: "Vebâ-yı ekber o[l]dı, Rûm-ili'nde halk şol kadar kırıldı ki, az kalup dükeniyazdı, âlem harâba vardı tamâm hicretün sene 838." For Murad's countryside retreat (*Keşürlik yaylası*, a plateau northeast of Edirne), see 59n344.

139 Doukas, *Decline and Fall*, 178. Oruç dates this siege slightly later, to 843 H. (June 1439–40).

140 Tafur, *Travels and Adventures*, 68. Also, plague was in Anatolia, Bursa, Aleppo, and Damascus in 1437. See Biraben, *Les hommes et la peste*, 1:431.

141 Tafur, *Travels and Adventures*, 138. Tafur was familiar with such measures adopted elsewhere in the Mediterranean. For example, he makes it clear he was very impressed with Venice. Also he praises the strict policies of the Duke of Milan in the following way: "No one can enter the city unless first, on entering the Duke's dominions, he obtains a certificate which establishes that he comes from a healthy country, uncontaminated by plague. This regulation is most rigidly enforced, and they say that it is now sixty years since there has been an outbreak of plague in any part of the country" (180).

142 Kōstēs, *Ston kairo tēs panōlēs*, 336.

143 Ibid.; Tsiamis et al., "Epidemic Waves of the Black Death," 197.

TABLE 1. *Frequency of Plagues in the Mediterranean World Following the Black Death*

Area	Time Frame	Average Frequency
Byzantine Constantinople, the Aegean, and Balkans littoral	1347–1453	10.6
France	1347–1536	11.0–12.0
Egypt	1347–1517	8.0–9.0
Syria	1347–1517	9.5

Source: Data are from Michael Dols, "The Second Plague Pandemic and Its Recurrences in the Middle East: 1347–1894," *JESHO* 22, no. 2 (1979): 162–189; Dols, *The Black Death in the Middle East* (Princeton, NJ: Princeton University Press, 1977); Jean-Noël Biraben, *Les hommes et la peste en France et dans les pays européens et méditerranéens* (Paris: Mouton, 1975).

An Analysis of Recurrent Waves of the Black Death (1347–1453)

After having presented a narrative sketch of the Black Death within a century of its outbreak, it may be helpful to make some general observations about the emerging patterns of spread and periodicity of outbreaks. Following the method adopted by the sources, it is possible to identify ten major waves of plague, separated by interepidemic phases of inactivity, a pattern compatible with modern knowledge of plague epidemiology. Most of the recorded cases come from Byzantine sources, complemented at times by Mamluk and Ottoman sources as well as eyewitness testimonies of travelers. We hear more about the cases of plague in the Byzantine capital as well as other port cities and islands of the Aegean and the Mediterranean. On the basis of this Byzantine-centric evidence, the maritime circulation of the disease in the Mediterranean, Aegean, and Black Sea can be identified with confidence. Yet, as we have seen in the case of the Black Death and in some outbreaks of its recurrent waves, the circulation of the disease was not limited to the sea; it was also distributed overland. With this in view, considering plague as "waves" is more intuitive for a conception of plague as something that is introduced from the sea, affecting different coastal cities in a spatial and temporal succession. Overland spread did not necessarily follow a predictable pattern.

In the main, it may be possible to estimate the overall frequency of plagues in this 106-year period as 10.6 years. Not all places experienced epidemics at the same rate. Some places, such as Constantinople and Peloponnese, had more frequent exposures, whereas others, such as Crete, Cyprus, and the Ionian islands, had fewer exposures. Taken as a whole, this figure is comparable to the frequency of outbreaks in other parts of the Mediterranean world in the post–Black Death centuries (Table 1). For example, it is similar to the frequency of epidemics in France but less frequent than those in Egypt and Syria.[144]

Over all, the data at hand are too fragmentary to determine the precise patterns of spread for the epidemics of this era. As stated earlier, maritime propagation of the disease is much more visible than spread via overland connections, which seems to be an artifact of the sources. However, ports were close to each other in the Mediterranean Sea, and the type of coastal navigation practiced made the spread of such infections easier. In this case, the rats (and their fleas) on ships would mostly account for transportation by maritime trade.

In this particular part of the Mediterranean world, one of the main trajectories was the connection between the ports of Italian city-states (e.g., Venice, Genoa) and Constantinople, with frequent stops along the way in places such as Corfu, Methoni, Koroni, and Limnos. Alternatively, a trajectory connecting Italian trading colonies (e.g., Crete, Rhodes, Cyprus) also holds true for plague itineraries. It may also be observed that there is no strict temporal correspondence or synchrony between the epidemics observed in Constantinople and other Aegean ports and islands and those in Egypt and Syria in this period – which may suggest that the exchanges with those areas were not as active and direct as those in Venetian and Genoese colonies in the area. At this stage, it appears that plague was circulating within a rather limited network of exchange, though this was to change after 1453, as shown in the next chapters of this book.

If we rather focus on Anatolia itself for the Black Death and its recurrent waves of plague over the first century, the movement of the disease does not seem to present an easily recognizable pattern. As we have seen, the infection was likely diffused from the coast to the interior, following major caravan routes. The direction of spread seems to be primarily from east to west but was perhaps accompanied by movements in different directions. Yet, this east to west spread did not seem to lead to a continuous chain of contagion that found itself outside Anatolia. It spread into its interiors, diffusing further into less accessible areas. On the whole, the peninsula seems to be a recipient of the infection in this era but not necessarily a distributor of it.

Conclusion

This chapter has presented a general overview of the history and historiography of the Black Death. It has highlighted major issues of contention, including the controversy over the identity of the pathogen (*Y. pestis* or not) and the origins of the pandemic (whether proximate or distant). It emphasized how the body of scientific knowledge drawn from South and East Asia

---

[144] Biraben, *Les hommes et la peste*, 1:121; Dols, "Second Plague Pandemic," 168–69.

during the Third Pandemic both informed and obscured historical analyses of the Black Death. It discussed how the discrepancies between the historical sources and the body of plague science especially revolved around issues such as symptoms, rats, speed and patterns of propagation, and mortality rates. In doing so, it has reviewed the revisionist literature of the Black Death (produced by plague skeptics) since the 1970s, with an emphasis on contested issues and the development of overarching theoretical frameworks.

The chapter traced the spread of the Black Death, first around, then inside, the Anatolian peninsula and, to a lesser extent, the Balkans. Drawing from a number of secondary and primary sources (including those that have been hitherto unexplored by historians of plague), it established the presence of plague, not only on Anatolia littoral (e.g., in Trabzon, Constantinople), but also in its interior (e.g., Sivas, Konya, Akşehir). The spread of the disease in Anatolia followed the major trade routes; it moved from the coast to the interior and most likely from east to west.

The chapter has also revisited some earlier suggestions about the link between plague and early Ottoman expansion. While not denying such a connection, it suggests that the nature of this link deserves to be more closely investigated. For that purpose, it has offered a critical review of hypotheses that saw early Ottoman expansion as resulting from the Black Death. It also evaluated the degree of connectedness in Anatolia at the time of the Black Death, the state of the nomads, and how they could be related to plague. Instead of accepting that the rise of the Ottomans was owed to the Black Death, it is argued here that their rise occurred in spite of it. If anything, it maintains that it was plague that resulted from Ottoman expansion.

Following this, the chapter surveyed the state of the plague from the Black Death to the Ottoman conquest of Constantinople (1347–1453). Both a narrative and an analysis of the outbreaks over the first post–Black Death century have been presented. In this era, plague outbreaks recurred periodically with an average frequency of 10.6 years. The survey has shown that the duration, persistence, and mortality of those outbreaks varied from place to place and over time. The most prominent pattern was the maritime spread of the infection, as facilitated by the Byzantine Empire's connections with the Venetians and the Genoese. Overall, both patterns of spread and frequency were compatible with modern plague epidemiology (appearing in waves, patchiness, phases of epidemic activity vs. latency) and with the frequency of outbreaks recorded in other parts of the Mediterranean world. As shown in the next chapters, this activity began to diverge from the plague experience of the western Mediterranean over the next century.

PART II

PLAGUE OF EMPIRE

4

The First Phase (1453–1517)

Plague Comes from the West

La peste nous vient de l'Asie, & depuis deux mille ans toutes les pestes qui ont
paru en Europe y ont été transmises par la communication des Sarrasins, des
Arabes, des Maures, ou des Turcs avec nous, & toutes les pestes n'ont pas eu
chez nous d'autre source.[1]

As we saw in the last chapter, by 1453 the Ottoman lands both in Anatolia
and the Balkans had been repeatedly visited by waves of plague for more than
a century. Here it is argued that the Ottoman conquest of Constantinople
in 1453 marks an important turning point in the Ottoman experience of
plague. Over the course of the next century and a half, both the trajectories
of plague's dissemination and the frequency of its recurrence were to change
significantly, so much so that the disease would turn into a constant presence
in the Ottoman healthscape – a presence that unremittingly persisted almost
as long as the empire itself. In this sense, perhaps it would not be wrong to
consider the Ottoman experience of plague as shaped by the workings of an
empire and to call it a *plague of empire* (Figure 1).

These changes, I argue, can be best understood in the framework of
Ottoman expansion in the long sixteenth century (1453–1600) and its
broader political, social, economic, and ecological ramifications. Here the
outbreaks of this era are studied both spatially and temporally with a view
to reconstructing a historical narrative of plague and establishing its links
to more general changes in Ottoman history. The chapter explores the connection between plague and the Ottoman expansion, especially with respect
to the role of conquest, urbanization, and networks of disease exchange.
More specifically, we pursue how the growth of Ottoman rule may have
stimulated an increased level of communication, interaction, and mobility
between individual domains that were brought together by conquest and

---

[1] Louis de Jaucourt, "Peste," in Diderot and d'Alembert, *Encyclopédie*, 12:452.

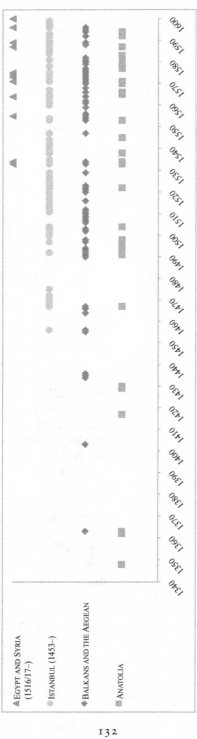

FIGURE 1. Outbreaks of plague in Ottoman-controlled areas (1347–1600).

by the formation of administrative, military, and commercial networks of a centralizing empire (Map 2).

The outbreaks of plague of the long sixteenth century show significant differences with respect to their scope, spread, and frequency of recurrence. First, the intervals between the occurrences of individual outbreaks gradually diminished. Second, the regions touched by outbreaks steadily expanded to cover a broader area. And last, the patterns of epidemic spread both within and outside the Ottoman lands changed. With that in view, it might be helpful to identify the distinct phases of plague activity in this era so as to offer a more nuanced vision.

The long sixteenth century is predominantly characterized by rapid territorial expansion in Ottoman history, though it is possible to detect significant turning points in this process, upon which a periodization of plagues can be based. However, this might seem to imply an underlying assumption that conquest was the sole factor triggering the expansion of plague. This assumption could leave us with a portrayal of Ottoman power as active in respect of conquest but passive in respect of other factors. Both in conjunction with conquest and independent of it, processes of trade, urban growth, and increased communication and mobility both within and outside Ottoman realms are also crucial factors for understanding plague periodization. In particular, the plague outbreaks that affected various regions under Ottoman rule in the long sixteenth century are presented here in three distinct phases: the *First Phase* (1453–1517), the *Second Phase* (1517–70), and the *Third Phase* (1570–1600).

The First Phase (1453–1517)

This First Phase is delimited by two important Ottoman conquests. The beginning date 1453 is the Ottoman conquest of Constantinople – a turning point in Ottoman history. It not only signifies the end of the Byzantine Empire but also underscores a new beginning in Ottoman ideological assertions and definitions of identity as heirs to universal sovereignty. More important, it has direct bearings to the history of plague. As a city with a notorious history of plagues, Constantinople added a new dimension to the Ottoman repertoire of plague experience. The city was located in the midst of trade routes connecting the Black Sea and its Eurasian hinterland to the Mediterranean world and consequently had always been under a greater risk of infection. The adding of Constantinople to the Ottoman dominions brought a new impetus to various forms of mobility, resulting in severe outbreaks soon after the conquest. These outbreaks continued more or less in the same manner until the end of the First Phase in 1517, when the Ottomans incorporated Mamluk territory, which not only integrated new trajectories of contamination but also introduced new elements to Ottoman disease ecologies.

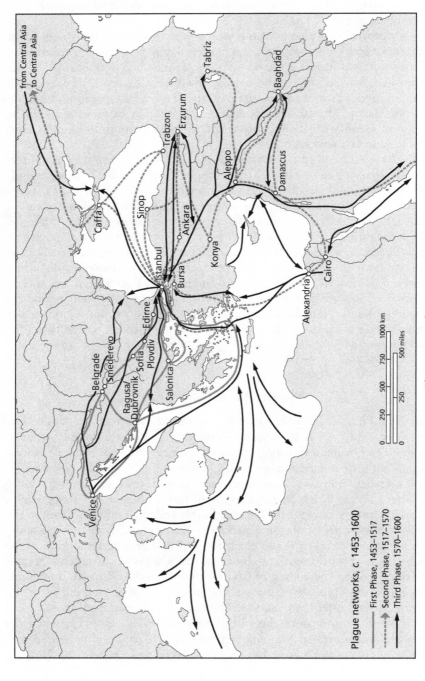

Plague networks, c. 1453–1600

First Phase, 1453–1517
Second Phase, 1517–1570
Third Phase, 1570–1600

from Central Asia
to Central Asia

Caffa

Trabzon
Erzurum
Tabriz

Sinop

Ankara

Baghdad

Istanbul

Bursa

Konya

Aleppo

Damascus

Belgrade
Smederevo

Edirne

Sofia
Plovdiv

Ragusa/
Dubrovnik

Salonica

Alexandria

Cairo

Venice

0   250   500   750   1000 km

0   250   500 miles

MAP 2. Plague networks, 1453–1600.

What is critical here is that the years 1453 and 1517 are not simply markers of conquest; more important, the sixty-four years between them witnessed the formation of a new plague trajectory – a rather limited span of circulation along an east-west axis in the eastern Mediterranean. During this period, plague's movements were facilitated by myriad forms of mobility, including warfare, trade, travel, and migration. The full effect of plague manifested in the newly budding Ottoman urban centers. The long sixteenth century witnessed the rise and development of new urban clusters throughout the Ottoman realm. Such areas, where people lived in close proximity, provided the best environment for the local and regional spread of the disease.

Mobilities that facilitated the dissemination of the infection, on one hand, and urbanization that aggravated its effects, on the other, were intertwined. Following 1453, urban industries developed owing to refinements of trade and increased resources stemming from conquests, which contributed to the establishment of welfare institutions in urban areas, such as mosques, schools, and hospices. Such institutions transformed smaller Ottoman towns into flourishing urban centers, which in turn acted as magnets attracting further immigration from their hinterlands. In other words, contradictory as it may seem, urban populations were increasing even as plague was taking a significant toll.[2] Plague might have served as a temporary check to rising urban populations but did not necessarily determine their long-term decrease. Urban populations can barely be isolated from their rural hinterlands, especially in times of crisis. As elsewhere in the early modern era, the population of Ottoman towns was sustained with a constant influx of immigration from rural areas. Every time plague hit an urban center and killed a certain proportion of its population, there would be an increased demand for labor and therefore renewed incentive to emigrate to the city once the plague receded. Recurring outbreaks served merely as a momentary obstruction of population growth and oddly even offered urban centers the prospect of

---

[2] For population growth in the Ottoman Empire in the sixteenth century, the classic hypothesis is framed in M. A. Cook, *Population Pressure in Rural Anatolia 1450–1600* (London: Oxford University Press, 1972). Leila Erder challenged this vision on grounds that the increase in the number of "hane" given in fiscal registers does not necessarily translate into an increase in population, which does not match with other historical developments of the century. Instead, she suggested that adopting a changing multiplier of "hane" may well lead to the conclusion of a decrease in population. See Erder, "Measurement of Preindustrial Population Changes." In association with theories of population growth in the sixteenth century, some scholars have tried to explain population growth by the assumed absence of plague in that era. See, e.g., Panzac, "Wabā'," *EI²*; Dols, "Second Plague Pandemic," 176. Also see İnalcık, *An Economic and Social History of the Ottoman Empire*; Jennings, "Urban Population in Anatolia in the Sixteenth Century"; Panzac, "La population de l'empire ottoman et de ses marges du XVe au XIXe siècle: bibliographie (1941–1980) et bilan provisoire," *Revue de l'Occident Musulman et de la Méditerranée* 31, no. 1 (1981): 119–37; Panzac, "Population," in Ágoston and Masters, *Encyclopedia of the Ottoman Empire*, 467–69.

increasing their population through immigration and thus revitalizing their economy. As discussed in greater detail in the following pages, the cases of Bursa, Edirne, and Istanbul illustrate this complex dynamic between urban demographics and plague outbreaks in the First Phase (Map 3).

Although plague seems to have broken out in many areas sporadically, it came and went in waves. On the basis of scarce, brief, and scattered references in the sources, it is possible to identify three waves of plague activity: the first from 1466 to 1476; the second from 1491 to 1504; and a recurrent episode between 1511 and 1514.

The First Wave (1466–1476)

In summer 1467, a great plague broke out in Istanbul. This was an extremely violent outbreak that caused terrible suffering heretofore unknown, as described by the Greek historian Kritovoulos of Imbros in his history written for Sultan Mehmed II:

It [plague] was also introduced into the great City of Constantinople, and I hardly need to say what incredible suffering it wrought there, utterly unheard-of and unbearable. More than six hundred deaths a day occurred, a multitude greater than men could bury, for there were not men enough. For some, fearing the plague, fled and never came back.... They abandoned the sick uncared-for and the dead unburied.... The City was emptied of its inhabitants, both citizens and foreigners. It had the appearance of a town devoid of all human beings, some of them dead or dying of the disease, others, as I have said, leaving their homes and fleeing, while still others shut themselves into their homes as if condemned to die. And there was great hopelessness and unbearable grief, wailing and lamentation everywhere. Despair and hopelessness dominated the spirits of all.[3]

Such were the gloomy words of Kritovoulos, whose account gives the impression that the city had never experienced such a serious outbreak before. Yet, this was neither the first outbreak Istanbul had seen, nor was it the last. The city had not only notoriously suffered the Plague of Justinian of the mid-sixth century and its recurrent waves until the mid-eighth but also the Black Death, when the plague returned in 1347 in a devastating epidemic, followed by recurrences throughout the rest of the fourteenth century and into the next.[4] This may have been the first major outbreak the new owners of the city saw, which was perhaps why its effects were felt and

---

[3] Kritovoulos, *History of Mehmed the Conqueror*, 220–21.

[4] During the first half of the fifteenth century, Byzantine Constantinople witnessed an outbreak in almost every decade. For example, the outbreak of 1406–7 affected the whole Black Sea region. See Georg Sticker, *Abhandlungen aus der Seuchengeschichte und Seuchenlehre* (Giessen: Töpelmann, 1908), 1:82. Biraben does not mention any outbreaks for the city after 1396, until the Ottoman conquest. See Biraben, *Les hommes et la peste*, 1:440–41. A list of plague outbreaks affecting Byzantine Constantinople can be traced in Schreiner, *Die byzantinischen Kleinchroniken*. Also see Chapter 3.

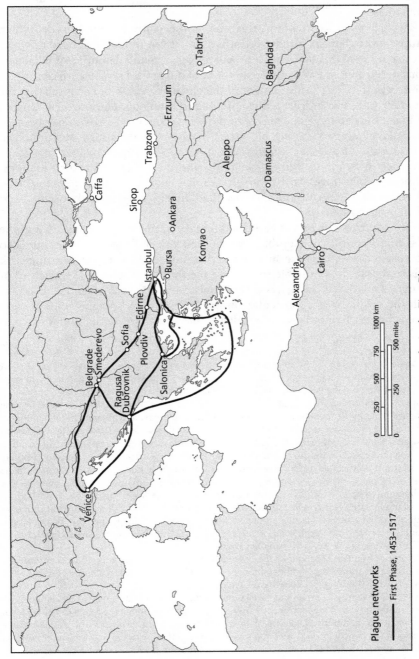

MAP 3. Plague networks in the First Phase, 1453–1517.

Plague networks

—— First Phase, 1453–1517

described in such a dramatic tone by Kritovoulos, who might have been an eyewitness.[5]

According to Kritovoulos, this was an especially violent episode, which caused more than six hundred deaths a day. Even though it is hard to verify the accuracy of this figure with other sources, it is still definitive of what was considered a most severe outbreak for Istanbul in the late fifteenth century. If we accept this figure as the height of the outbreak, it can be surmised that the city may have lost at least a third, if not half, of its population.[6] It is hard to estimate the demographic profile of those affected, but Kritovoulos observed that plague spread among all ages.[7] This outbreak is also mentioned in the account of another Byzantine historian, Sphrantzes, who refers to its presence in Istanbul, Edirne, Gallipoli, and their immediate surroundings. Although Sphrantzes fails to give a detailed account, as Kritovoulos does, he writes that tens of thousands perished during this outbreak, on the basis of what he had heard.[8]

This outbreak deserves closer examination, not only because it was the first major outbreak Istanbul experienced under Ottoman rule, but also because it shows the nascent characteristics of the First Phase. Starting with this outbreak, it is possible to observe the formation of a new trajectory of plague spread. To understand this new trajectory, it is essential to establish the origin of this particular outbreak. Where did plague come from?[9] According to Kritovoulos, a pestilence hit all of Macedonia and Thrace in

---

[5] Between the conquest and the outbreak of 1467, Istanbul was hit by a short outbreak of plague in summer 1456. The plague that broke out in the Balkans in 1455 seems to have reached Istanbul the next year. See Lowry, "Pushing the Stone Uphill," 103.

[6] It is very hard to make estimates about the total number of deaths caused. If we accept the figure given by Kritovoulos, i.e., six hundred deaths per day, and assume that the outbreak lasted with the same intensity for one month, this will give us a toll of eighteen thousand deaths. Since the outbreak lasted until the early autumn as well, a total of fifteen thousand to twenty thousand deaths can be estimated. However, the population of the city is not precisely known. It is estimated as fifty thousand at the time of the conquest in 1453. A census made after the plague in 1477 shows a population of between sixty thousand and one hundred thousand people, which is suggested to be closer to the lower figure. See Halil İnalcık, "Istanbul," *EI*[2]; Kafesçioğlu, *Constantinopolis/Istanbul*, 178–79. A mortality ratio of one-third can be accepted for this outbreak. Also cf. Lowry's estimate between fifty thousand and seventy-five thousand, which seems too high. Lowry, "Pushing the Stone Uphill," 123.

[7] Kritovoulos, *History of Mehmed the Conqueror*, 220.

[8] George Sphrantzes, *The Fall of the Byzantine Empire: A Chronicle by George Sphrantzes, 1401–1477*, trans. Marios Philippides (Amherst: University of Massachusetts Press, 1980), 89; Lowry, "Pushing the Stone Uphill," 107.

[9] The fact that plague broke out in Istanbul in the middle of the summer can be taken as an indication that it was introduced from outside, if the accounts are reliable. The seasonal character of recurrent plagues is in stark contrast with this onset. When plague became enzootic to the commensal rodent population of Istanbul or to the wild rodent population in its immediate hinterland, it started earlier in the spring, when favorable tempeature supported it.

the middle of summer 1467. He does not know from where the disease first came up to Thrace, but he notes that it spread to all of the cities in that region, both inland and coastal.[10] In reality, the outbreak affected a much wider region than Kritovoulos had known. Though continuously present in many European cities over the previous century, a new wave of pestilence was introduced in the early 1460s. By 1463, plague was in various parts of France, Spain, Italy, and Central Europe. Rome, Florence, Bologna, and Venice were all suffering from this pestilence in 1463, which spread to Naples the next year.[11] In the following years, plague spread to an even larger area, including England, Hungary, northern Europe, and the southeast Balkans.[12] This wave of pestilence seems to have spread to Ottoman areas from the port cities of the Mediterranean, most probably from Venice, which was suffering from plague in 1464.[13]

How was Venice connected to Istanbul to make it possible for plague to spread in the 1460s? There were two main arteries that connected Venice to Istanbul in the late fifteenth century: a maritime route and an overland route. The standard maritime route leading east traversed the Adriatic and reached southern Peloponnese and then Crete. From there, it either went north to the Aegean, through Athens and Chios to the Dardanelles and Istanbul, or continued east through Cyprus toward Jerusalem. Being the main route eastward, this trajectory was used, not only by official envoys sent to Istanbul, but also by pilgrims traveling to Jerusalem. The maritime route could at times be disadvantageous; it was longer and subject to the dangers of the sea. Thus the overland route was often preferred in the late fifteenth century for being safer and faster.[14] The overland route that connected the Adriatic to Istanbul offered two alternative itineraries: a northern branch and a southern branch. The northern branch started from Ragusa and crossed through Albania, Macedonia, and Bulgaria to reach Edirne and Istanbul. Being a major caravan route, this was the most important artery connecting Ragusa to Istanbul.[15] In addition to being a trade route, it was frequently used by French and Venetian imperial envoys as well as by pilgrims until the

---

[10] Kritovoulos, *History of Mehmed the Conqueror*, 219.

[11] Pasquale Lopez, *Napoli e la peste 1464–1530: politica, istituzioni, problemi sanitari* (Napoli: Jovene, 1989), 21.

[12] Biraben, *Les hommes et la peste*, 1:366.

[13] Ibid., 1:396. The presence of plague in Venice in 1464 is also confirmed by Sticker, *Abhandlungen*, 1:85.

[14] Yerasimos, *Les voyageurs*, 25–31. For a typical itinerary followed from Venice to Istanbul in the late fifteenth century, see Eve Borsook, "The Travels of Bernardo Michelozzi and Bonsignore Bonsignori in the Levant (1497–98)," *Journal of the Warburg and Courtauld Institutes* 36 (1973): 146.

[15] Among the goods that were transported over this caravan route were items manufactured in Ragusa, such as glass, cloth, soap, and wax, as well as goods imported from Italy for the Balkan markets. See Franz Babinger and C. E. Bosworth, "Raghusa," *EI²*.

mid-sixteenth century. The southern route, alternatively, connected Ragusa and Istanbul through Thessaloniki and southern Thrace.[16]

It is most likely that plague traveled along the overland routes in the Balkans to reach Ottoman areas. Once the infection was introduced to Ragusa on the Adriatic coast in 1464,[17] it seems to have followed the northern branch toward Thrace, infecting along the way destinations in Bosnia and Herzegovina in 1464 and in Macedonia in 1466. Its presence in Thessaly might be indicative of its spread through the southern branch simultaneously. Moving along one or more of these routes, plague reached the Ottoman dominions in the Balkans in 1466.[18]

At this time Mehmed II was on a military expedition in Albania. The army had set forth in early 1466 and reached there in June.[19] When Mehmed's army was prepared to go back to Istanbul, probably late in summer 1466, they received news of a terrible plague in the Balkans, upon which they changed their itinerary. Looking for an area free from the pestilence, they moved northeast toward Bulgaria. Ottoman chronicler Oruç recorded that the sultan and the army stayed in Philippopolis before returning to Istanbul.[20] This piece of information is confirmed by the report of a Milanese ambassador to Venice (dated October 9, 1466) that mentioned that the sultan was still in the mountains with his army for fear of plague, planning to spend the winter in Sofia without returning to Edirne or Istanbul, and that he established himself on a mountaintop, and that no visitor was permitted to approach his encampment closer than a distance of one day's journey.[21] According to Oruç, the sultan and the army returned from Philippopolis to Istanbul after spending a few days in Edirne before the end of 1466.[22]

The outbreak of 1466 seems to have affected certain areas of Ottoman dominions in the Balkans, but there is no clear evidence for its exact duration and effects. The next year, however, when plague reached Edirne and Istanbul in summer 1467, its devastating effects are much better documented.[23] According to Kritovoulos, plague spread from Edirne and Istanbul to Gallipoli, then crossed the Dardanelles and affected the southern shores

---

[16] Yerasimos, *Les voyageurs*, 31–41.

[17] Most probably plague spread to Ragusa from Venice, which was infected the same year. See Biraben, *Les hommes et la peste*, 1:441.

[18] Ibid.

[19] Although Tursun Bey claims that Mehmed left Edirne for the Albanian campaign in spring 1466, Babinger documents that the army was in Philippopolis around late February and early March 1466. See Babinger, *Mehmet the Conqueror*, 251; Tursun Bey, *Târîh-i Ebü'l-feth*, ed. Mertol Tulum (Istanbul: Baha Matbaası, 1977), 140.

[20] Oruç, *Tarih*, 119.

[21] The Venetian report is cited in Babinger, *Mehmet the Conqueror*, 253–54.

[22] Oruç, *Tarih*, 119.

[23] Unlike Biraben, who dates the outbreak to 1466, Sticker dates it to 1467. See Sticker, *Abhandlungen*, 1:85.

of the Marmara sea, and moved inland to Bursa and further east of it, spreading to areas as far east as western-central Anatolia in the same year.[24] Although we are fairly well informed about the effects of this outbreak in Istanbul, its presence and effects in other Ottoman regions remain largely unknown.

Ottoman chronicles of the fifteenth and sixteenth centuries, though they are generally silent about the occurrences of plague, can reveal some important clues about plague outbreaks, especially when those coincided with military campaigns and the movements of the sultan and the court. In this particular case, while Istanbul and a substantial part of Ottoman lands were struck, Mehmed was away on military expedition. After he had returned from the first Albanian campaign in late fall 1466, the sultan spent the winter in Istanbul and then set out for a second campaign to Albania in early spring 1467.[25] Toward mid-summer 1467, he withdrew from Albania only to find out that plague was wreaking havoc in the entirety of Thrace and Macedonia and in the cities he was planning to travel through, as well as in Istanbul. He proceeded northeast with his army to plague-free areas of northwestern Bulgaria. Upon finding out that the region between Nikopolis and Vidin, on the southern bank of the Danube, was untouched by the plague, he spent the entire autumn 1467 with his army there. Informed by messengers that came nearly every day, he eventually found out that Istanbul was free from plague and returned to the city.[26] This account is also confirmed by the chronicle of Neşri, and later by that of Hoca Saadeddin (probably using the former as his source). Hoca Saadeddin reports that Mehmed's army heard news of an outbreak in Thrace, returning from Albania. He notes that the sultan did not enter cities but preferred to go to the countryside and spend his time in the vineyards and the gardens on the Black Sea coast until winter came. When the outbreak ceased and the disease was cleared, he left Rusokastro (Rus Kasrı) and Aytos (Aydos) near the Black Sea coast of Bulgaria and returned to Istanbul.[27] Whereas Kritovoulos, Neşri, and later Hoca Saadeddin all date the sultan's return to Istanbul to the beginning of winter 1467, Babinger suggests that he might have spent the entire winter in the Balkan mountains, because the news of his return to Istanbul seemed to have reached Venice toward March 1468.[28]

---

[24] Kritovoulos, *History of Mehmed the Conqueror*, 220. Biraben also confirms the presence of plague in Bursa and Anatolia in *Les hommes et la peste*, 1:441. Sticker confirms the Edirne and Gallipoli outbreaks. See Sticker, *Abhandlungen*, 1:85.

[25] Kritovoulos, *History of Mehmed the Conqueror*, 218. Oruç mentions the second campaign without giving the exact timing of the year in 1467; see Oruç, *Tarih*, 119.

[26] Kritovoulos, *History of Mehmed the Conqueror*, 222.

[27] Saadettin, *Tacü't-tevarih*, 3:93–94. Note that the areas for the army's retreat are different from those offered by Kritovoulos. See Kritovoulos, *History of Mehmed the Conqueror*, 222.

[28] Babinger, *Mehmet the Conqueror*, 263.

The reconstruction of the accounts of these two outbreaks in two consecutive years, that is, 1466 and 1467, sketchy as they are in the sources, poses a great deal of confusion, especially because they are further complicated by the similarity of the narratives of the two Albanian campaigns. To establish the exact chronology of these two outbreaks, it is important to pay close attention to the similarities of their accounts. Among the fifteenth-century Ottoman chroniclers, Oruç is the only one who accurately refers to the outbreak of 1466. After mentioning that Mehmed spent the winter in Philippopolis returning from his first Albanian campaign, he notes that there occurred a great plague that year. The sultan, according to him, returned from Philippopolis to Edirne, where he stayed a few days before returning to Istanbul. But he is completely silent about the second outbreak of 1467.[29] Interestingly enough, the accounts of Neşri and later that of Hoca Saadeddin mention only the second outbreak, during the Albanian campaign of 1467, but fail to mention that of the previous year, while Aşıkpaşazade and Tursun Bey fail to mention the plague altogether on either occasion.[30] Tursun Bey, for example, writes that the "glorious sultan" returned to Edirne after the Albanian campaign, without mentioning the plague.[31] The same is true for Kritovoulos and Sprantzes, who left fairly lengthy descriptions of the second outbreak, without even mentioning the first.

The confusion that surfaces in the primary sources seems to have obstructed a correct chronology of these outbreaks in the modern scholarship as well. For example, Babinger mistakes Kritovoulos's account of the second outbreak for the first one and dates it to 1466 instead of 1467. When he writes about Mehmed's delaying his return to Istanbul because of the 1466 outbreak, he uses Kritovoulos's account that described the 1467 outbreak. However, there is no indication in the sources that the 1466 outbreak reached Istanbul. Had it been so, neither Kritovolous nor Sphranztes would insist emphatically on their observation that no such terrible outbreak had occurred for some years, if at all.[32] As for Lowry, he establishes the date of the second outbreak correctly as 1467 on the basis of Kritovoulos and Sphrantzes but fails to note the first outbreak. Without the prior knowledge of two different outbreaks, he misinterprets the valuable piece of information offered by Oruç regarding the first outbreak and dates it to 1467, to make it compatible with the accounts of Kritovoulos and Sphrantzes.[33]

[29] Oruç, *Tarih*, 119–20.
[30] Mehmet Neşrî, *Neşrî Tarihi*, ed. M. A. Köymen (Ankara, 1984), 2:174–75.
[31] Tursun Bey, *Tarih-i Ebu'l-feth*, 142.
[32] Kritovolous described the disastrous effects of this outbreak as "utterly un-heard of." See Kritovoulos, *History of Mehmed the Conqueror*, 220. Sphrantzes wrote, "No outbreak of such intensity occurred for many years." See Sphrantzes, *Fall of the Byzantine Empire*, 89.
[33] Lowry, "Pushing the Stone Uphill," 106.

Notwithstanding the confusion in chronology, the outbreaks of 1466 and 1467 mark the beginning of a decadelong wave of plague that would appear year after year in Ottoman cities. In fact, as soon as plague died out in 1467, a new one broke out in Istanbul in summer 1468. Mehmed returned from campaigning in Anatolia and arrived at Istanbul in late November 1468, this time despite the ongoing plague. However, the outbreak was once again serious enough to prompt him to vacate the city and return to the mountains during the winter. The epidemic seems to have continued through winter 1468 into the early months of 1469. The loss of population caused by this outbreak must have been equally severe, especially in Istanbul. The Florentine colony in Pera was very severely hit, causing the death of many people from leading merchant families and prompting many others to flee.[34] The next year (1470), plague was in Istanbul again, this time serious enough to interfere with trade, as mentioned in a Genoese report.[35] In 1471, the infection should be still lingering in the city, possibly the reason behind Mehmed's departure for the countryside.[36] During summer 1472, the epidemic was in Istanbul, whereupon the sultan left with his court but came back on August 25, despite the ongoing plague.[37] In the same year, Venice was affected by the plague more severely than in previous years.[38] Hungary, Serbia, and Rumeli were all visited by plague at this time.[39] In summer 1474, the Ottoman army was on another expedition in Albania. Plague broke out in the army camps when they laid siege to Scutari. When the janissaries began to perish en masse, the siege was lifted without capturing the city.[40] In May 1475, plague was seen in Istanbul once again, peaking later that summer. This was when the war captives from the newly conquered Caffa were brought in ships. After the conquest in June 1475, a great number of young girls and boys (reported to be anywhere between fifteen hundred and five thousand) were taken as war captives and brought to Istanbul on August 3. The ships were not allowed to be unloaded on account of the ongoing epidemic in the city.[41] This was also the outbreak that prompted Mehmed to leave once again. The sultan had his court moved

---

34 Babinger, *Mehmet the Conqueror*, 273–77.

35 Lowry, "Pushing the Stone Uphill," 124–25.

36 Babinger argues that Mehmed spent the spring in Istanbul but left on November 30, 1471, for Vize (southeast of Kırklareli), possibly to flee an outbreak in Istanbul and to "enjoy the pure air of Istranca mountains." See Babinger, *Mehmet the Conqueror*, 299.

37 Ibid., 309.

38 Benedetto Dei, *La cronica dall'anno 1400 all'anno 1500* (Florence: F. Papafava, 1984), 169.

39 Biraben, *Les hommes et la peste*, 1:441.

40 Benedetto Dei, *La cronica*, 171.

41 The Italians and Armenians on board were allowed to stay first in Üsküdar before they were taken to their newly assigned homes and quarters when plague died out. See Babinger, *Mehmet the Conqueror*, 345.

to the mountains, where they spent more than three months in seclusion on a hill between Edirne and Kırklareli, starting in June or July. In the beginning of the autumn, they moved further west to Philippopolis, and then to Sofia, where they stayed during the month of October. The sultan and the whole court were still waiting for the plague to die out in the winter, spending time in Vize.[42] The movement of the sultan and the court is also confirmed by Oruç, who writes that Mehmed spent some time in Çöke that year, without specifying the exact timing and without mentioning the outbreak. However, the lack of reference to the return of the sultan to Edirne or Istanbul before the next campaign season might be an indication that he stayed there until early spring 1476, which might suggest the end of this outbreak.[43] Indeed, plague seems to have gradually died out in the Ottoman lands after this, though it persisted in Italian cities in 1476 and in the years that followed.[44]

This was how the first wave of the First Phase affected the Ottomans over a decade (between 1466 and 1476). Studying this first wave reveals some interesting findings concerning the patterns of plague's propagation. First, plagues in this wave seem to have been introduced to Ottoman cities from the west, mainly through overland routes in the Balkans. The epidemic that affected the Italian cities in the early 1460s seems to have moved east toward the Adriatic, affecting Bosnia, Herzegovina, and Bulgaria along the way, before reaching Edirne and Istanbul. This particular propagation of plague and most characteristically its eastward movement is contradictory to what has been observed for later eras. The scholarship conventionally accepts a trajectory of plagues moving from east to west, that is, from Ottoman cities to European cities – at least in the eighteenth and nineteenth centuries.[45] Such an assumed directionality of epidemic spread may obscure the possible trajectories of the earlier eras. As demonstrated, the outbreaks in this first wave seem to have moved from west to east.

Second, plagues of this first wave seem not to have diffused too much into the Anatolian peninsula, spreading somewhat into its western-central regions. There is no evidence for its presence in eastern Anatolia or for its spread further east or south of it. Why? Perhaps this lack of evidence originates from a bias in the sources. The account of Kritovoulos, for example, though reliable for plague spread in core Ottoman areas, does not mention what happened further east. At the same time, it is important to remember that late-fifteenth-century Ottoman holdings in Anatolia were relatively sizeable but did not envelop the entire peninsula, which would only take place in the sixteenth century.

---

[42] Ibid., 342–46.

[43] Oruç gives the year as 880 H./1475–76. Çöke, a hill located thirty kilometers northeast of Edirne, was a retreat for the Ottoman sultans. See Oruç, *Tarih*, 57n325.

[44] Benedetto Dei, *La cronica*, 100–103, 153.

[45] For a detailed dicussion of this view in the historiography, see Chapter 2.

The Second Wave (1491–1504)

Following the first wave, there is no evidence for a new outbreak in Ottoman areas for about fifteen years. Although plague was present in several western Mediterranean ports around this time, it does not seem to have been communicated to Ottoman lands.[46] Nor was it present in the eastern Mediterranean regions in this interim period.[47] Why this interlude? Although warfare seems to have continued in several places in the Balkans and Anatolia between 1476 and 1491, there does not seem to be a new outbreak. Is it possible that a new wave of outbreaks was triggered by the Ottoman-Mamluk War (1485–91) that preceded it? Was this interlude needed for the rodent population to exceed a certain threshold and sustain a new epizootic? For reasons that are not entirely clear, plague reappears in Ottoman and eastern Mediterranean regions in 1491 – this time to continue intermittently for about fourteen years.

For reconstructing the historical narrative of plagues in this second wave, Ottoman chronicles supply some basic information, which can be complemented with non-Ottoman sources. As in the first wave, establishing the origin and initial spread of the outbreak is essential. According to Ottoman historians, this wave of plague also came from Thrace. Hoca Saadeddin indicates that the outbreak began in Thrace in 1491.[48] His account seems to suggest an eastward movement of the plague following overland routes. In conjunction with overland spread, it is also possible to conceive a maritime contagion for this outbreak. The fact that the disease was seen in Rhodes the same year might be indicative of a simultaneous maritime propagation.[49] When the plague first broke out, according to Hoca Saadeddin, Sultan Bayezid II (r. 1481–1512) left Istanbul for Edirne. However, upon hearing news of the epidemic, he did not stay in one place but visited different places before Edirne and, after staying there for a week, returned to Istanbul.[50] As was the case in the first wave outlined earlier, the accounts of chroniclers do not always coincide. The chronology of events given by Hoca Saadeddin later in the century differs from that offered by Oruç, a contemporary of events. The latter dates the outbreak, not to 1491, but to the year after. These conflicting accounts pose some difficulty for reconstructing the chronology of events. According to Oruç, Bayezid spent 1491 entirely in Istanbul and departed for Edirne in April 1492.[51] The account given by Hoca Saadeddin

---

[46] Plague was in Venice every year from 1477 to 1485 and in 1490; in Naples in 1478 and 1481; in Ragusa in 1481–3; and in other western Mediterranean port cities in southern France and Spain. See Biraben, *Les hommes et la peste*, 1: 380–81, 390, 396–97, 441–42.

[47] No plague outbreak is mentioned in Egypt and the Syria-Palestine region between 1477 and 1491. See Dols, "Second Plague Pandemic," 168–69.

[48] Saadettin, *Tacü't-tevarih*, 3:269–70.

[49] Plague was in Rhodes in 1491. See Biraben, *Les hommes et la peste*, 1:442.

[50] Saadettin, *Tacü't-tevarih*, 3:269–70.

[51] Oruç, *Tarih*, 146–48.

TABLE 2. *Loss of Business Owing to Plague, Reported by Shops Selling Fermented Millet Beer in Bursa (1491)*

Name	Current	Past	Loss (%)
Bozahane-i Balıkpazarı	65	80	19
Bozahane-i Gallepazarı	40	50	20
Bozahane-i Odalar	25	31	19
Bozahane-i Sedbaşı	40	50	20
Bozahane-i Pınarbaşı	16	25	36
Bozahane-i Cedid	30	40	25
Bozahane-i Tahte'l-kalʿa	25	42	40

Source: Bursa Şeriye Sicilleri, A 8/8, 221a (4 Zilhicce 896/October 8, 1491) as published in Yılmaz and Yılmaz, ed., *Osmanlılarda Sağlık* 2: 26–7, doc. 16.

on the movements of Bayezid is similar to what Oruç narrates for summer 1490.[52] Is it possible that the outbreak took place in summer 1490 and that Hoca Saadeddin, writing some time later, was slightly mistaken about the date?

Notwithstanding the ambiguity of the narrative sources, archival evidence confirms the presence of plague in the year 1491, at least in Bursa. According to a document from the court of Bursa, a certain Yusuf bin Mustafa from a nearby village went to the court to register the death of Süleyman, a novice janissary boy (*acemi yeniçeri*), from plague.[53] Another document from October 1491 refers to plague's effect on the businesses selling fermented millet beer (*boza*) in Bursa (Table 2). It appears that these shops suffered a considerable loss in their business when people stopped going there on account of the raging plague. Granted that they could demonstrate their circumstances, these businesses were partially subsidized for their losses due to plague.[54] Even though this document was issued in October, the businesses would have been exposed to the distressing effects of the plague for some time, before the matter was brought to the attention of the court. Other cases of deaths from plague continued later that autumn, through spring and summer 1492. The deaths of several other novice janissary boys from plague were registered at the court in Bursa.[55]

[52] According to Oruç, Bayezid left Istanbul for Edirne in July 1490 and spent the summer in different places before returning briefly to Edirne and to Istanbul in December 1490, but he does not mention an outbreak. Ibid., 146–47.

[53] Bursa Şeriye Sicilleri, A 8/8, 44a/1, 2 Cemaziyelevvel 896/March 13, 1491 [cited in OS 2:26, doc.14]. The death of Süleyman was registered on March 13, 1491, but we do not know exactly when he died, presumably shortly before this date.

[54] Bursa Şeriye Sicilleri, A 8/8, 221a, 4 Zilhicce 896/October 8, 1491 [cited in OS 2:26–7, doc.16].

[55] E.g., for the death of Kasım of plague in the village of Armut, see Bursa Şeriye Sicilleri, A 8/8, 262b, 18 Muharrem 897/November 21, 1491 [cited in OS 2:27, doc.18]; for the

Ottoman chronicles seem to agree on the outbreak of 1492. According to Hoca Saadeddin, plague broke out in summer 1492, which he mentions on the occasion of the army's stay in Edirne for the entire summer, on account of the plague raging in Istanbul until the winter.[56] Oruç, conversely, writes that the sultan left Edirne for a campaign to Belgrade in May 1492. After several months of campaigning in the Balkans, the army returned to Edirne in the early days of September 1492.[57] Unlike Hoca Saadeddin, Oruç mentions this outbreak independently of the army's movements. According to the latter, a great plague devastated Anatolia, the Balkans, and the Mamluk lands in 1492. On the basis of hearsay, Oruç reports some mortality figures pertaining to the Mamluk case.[58] According to Oruç, plague was still around in 1493 and possibly in early 1494; he commented that people suffered everywhere, including in Europe.[59] Hoca Saadeddin recorded that plague, accompanied by famine, excessive rainfall, and flooding, affected especially Anatolia for three successive years starting in 1495.[60] Oruç also mentioned the plague in Istanbul and Edirne, most probably in 1497.[61] In 1498, plague was still in Anatolia, Syria, and Egypt.[62]

The presence of plague in Istanbul in 1497 is also testified by Venetian sources. It appears that reports about the plague raging in the city since the early days of that year started to reach Venice in early spring. A letter dated January 12 recorded that plague killed three hundred a day in the capital.[63]

---

death of Hamza of plague in the village of Balıklı, see Bursa Şeriye Sicilleri, A 8/8, 268b/1, 2 Safer 897/December 5, 1491 [cited in *OS* 2:28, doc.20]; for the death of İlyas in the same Balıklı village, see Bursa Şeriye Sicilleri, A 8/8, 268b/2, 2 Safer 897/December 5, 1491 [cited in *OS* 2:28, doc.21]; for the death of Ali, İskender, and Nasuh of plague in the village of Serme, see Bursa Şeriye Sicilleri, A 8/8, 342b/1, 7 Cemaziyelevvel 897/March 7, 1492 [cited in *OS* 2:28, doc.22]; for the death of Ali of plague in the village of Katırlı, see Bursa Şeriye Sicilleri, A 8/8, 342b/2, 7 Cemaziyelevvel 897/March 7, 1492 [cited in *OS* 2:28, doc.23]; for the death of Nasuh in the village of Yenice, see Bursa Şeriye Sicilleri, A 8/8, 342b/3, 7 Cemaziyelevvel 897/March 7, 1492 [cited in *OS* 2:28, doc.24]; for the death of Hamza, see Bursa Şeriye Sicilleri, A 8/8, 409a, 12 Ramazan 897/July 7, 1492 [cited in *OS* 2:28–9, doc.25]; for the death of Hızır in the village of Armut, see Bursa Şeriye Sicilleri, A 8/8, 250b, 897/1492 [cited in *OS* 2:29, doc.27].

56 Saadettin, *Tacü't-tevarih*, 3:275–76.
57 Oruç, *Tarih*, 148–53.
58 Ibid., 153: Mamluk authorities recorded the deaths of twenty-seven thousand people in every five days, twenty thousand in every thirteen days, and thirty thousand in every seventeen days during the month of May, June, and July of 1492, respectively. Oruç then writes that in thirty-three days, there were 605,000 deaths in Cairo alone, which seems to be a grossly exaggerated figure. Cf. Dols, *Black Death*, 313.
59 Oruç, *Tarih*, 154, 163–65.
60 Saadettin, *Tacü't-tevarih*, 3:347.
61 Oruç, *Tarih*, 171. In 1497, plague was also reported in Anatolia, Albania, and Macedonia, along with Thessaloniki, Sofia, Novi Brdu, and Drac. See Biraben, *Les hommes et la peste*, 1:442.
62 According to Dols, plague was in Syria and Egypt in 1497–98. Dols, *Black Death*, 313.
63 *Sanudo*, 1:552.

Another letter of January 20 confirms the severity of the outbreak.[64] The outbreak seems to have lasted into the summer, as suggested by further reports. A letter dated June 25 records that plague was still severe in the capital.[65]

The widespread plague in western Anatolia around this time is confirmed by Florentine sources. The account of Bernardo Michelozzi and Bonsignore Bonsignori, two Florentine gentlemen traveling to the Levant in 1497–98, testifies to the presence of plague in western Anatolia in spring 1498. While traveling from Istanbul to Rhodes through Bursa and coastal Aegean cities, Michelozzi and Bonsignori had to change their plans to tour the ancient sites upon receiving news of plague in the region. Instead, they took refuge on the island of Chios on the Aegean, where they stayed for about a month (until mid-June), probably waiting for plague to abate. In mid-summer 1498, an outbreak was ravaging the island of Cyprus, most probably the plague. Plague was also recorded in Cairo and Alexandria at this time.[66]

Plague was once again raging in the capital in fall 1500, according to Venetian sources. This time, news of plague in Istanbul came from the testimony of two fugitive slaves, who also reported that the sultan (i.e., Bayezid II) was in Edirne at the time.[67] Soon after this, further reports of the sultan's stay in Edirne and the continued presence of plague in the capital reached Venice.[68] On the basis of these accounts, it appears that plague lasted in the capital from fall 1500 into the early winter of the next year. Yet plague does not seem to have receded any time soon after that. In summer 1501, plague was still in the Ottoman capital. According to the reports that found their way into Venetian sources in fall 1501, Bayezid had returned to the capital in the midst of plague.[69] An eyewitness to plague in Istanbul in summer 1501 was Florentine merchant Giovanni di Francesco Maringhi. According to his testimony, plague lasted until mid-winter 1502, taking a great many lives. He reports that the death toll in Istanbul alone was more than twenty-five thousand by the end of October 1501 and that this was one of the worst of the multiple outbreaks he had witnessed in the city since 1497.[70] High mortality in the capital is also confirmed by reports that reached Venice, according to which it is stated that seven hundred or more died every day.[71]

---

[64] Ibid.

[65] Ibid., 756.

[66] Borsook, "Travels of Bernardo Michelozzi and Bonsignore Bonsignori," 168, 172–73.

[67] *Sanudo*, 3:1073.

[68] Ibid., 3:1216, 1347, 1394.

[69] Ibid., 4:161.

[70] Heath Lowry, *Ottoman Bursa in Travel Accounts* (Bloomington: Indiana University Ottoman and Modern Turkish Studies Publications, 2003), 71–72; Lowry, "Pushing the Stone Uphill," 125–26.

[71] *Sanudo*, 4:179–80.

Evidence from Ottoman archival sources indicates the presence of plague in the Shirvan plains in Azerbaijan in June 1501. The document reports that Safavid groups were stationed on the eastern banks of the Kura River and that the Aqquyunlus were safeguarding the passageways and roads. Although this region did not come under Ottoman control until much later in the sixteenth century, this is an indication that the Ottomans were watching this area very closely at this critical time.[72]

News of plague in Istanbul in the year 1502 continued to arrive at Venice, however intermittently. Some reports suggested that mortality was even greater than that of the previous year, having reached eight hundred a day in mid-March.[73] In May, there were rumors in the city that the sultan had died because no one was allowed to enter the court on account of the plague.[74] Plague was still reported to affect the capital in late summer.[75] It was also reported that the infection was in Gallipoli[76] and in Macedonia. A report dated June 30, 1502, noted that plague was in Skopje and its environs in January and disappeared in February. When it returned in mid-March, it broke out in Skopje, affecting many in the area. Plague seems to have lasted in and around the town until fall of that year.[77] The disease was reported to have continued in the capital and elsewhere into the next year. Venetian sources attest to relatively lower mortality figures for 1503 (two hundred a day in Istanbul, and higher in Edirne).[78] Perhaps this was an indication that this epidemic wave was gradually coming to an end. Regardless, plague was ravaging the Aegean islands and port cities,[79] while it was still in Istanbul in 1504.[80] Ottoman sources give evidence of its presence in Bursa and its surrounding villages in May 1504. A number of novice janissary boys died from plague, which was registered at court in the presence of witnesses.[81]

---

[72] İlhan Şahin ed., *II. Bâyezid dönemine ait 906/1501 tarihli ahkâm defteri* (Istanbul: Türk Dünyası Araştırmaları Vakfı, 1994), 125.

[73] *Sanudo*, 4:242.

[74] Ibid., 4:267.

[75] Ibid., 4:390.

[76] Ibid., 4:480.

[77] "Citizens of Dubrovnik in Skopje report that the plague in Macedonia is exterminating Bulgarians and Turks equally," dated June 30, 1502. *Diversa notarie* 81, nos. 138–39 (from Dubrovnik State Archives). See http://www.promacedonia.org/en/ban/ma2.html.

[78] *Sanudo*, 4:805.

[79] Biraben, *Les hommes et la peste*, 1:442.

[80] *Sanudo*, 5:874, 914, 968, 1063, 6:10.

[81] For the death of Hamza in the village of Hamamlıkızık, see Bursa Şeriye Sicilleri, A 19/19, 122b/1, 16 Zilkade 909/May 1, 1504 [cited in *OS* 2:33, doc.41]; for the death of Ahmed in Kite, see Bursa Şeriye Sicilleri, A 19/19, 122b/2, 17 Zilkade 909/May 2, 1504 [cited in *OS* 2:33-4, doc.42]; for the deaths of Hasan and İskender in the village of Hacı Ivaz Paşa Kızığı, see Bursa Şeriye Sicilleri, A 19/19, 122b/3, 17 Zilkade 909/May 2, 1504 [cited in *OS* 2:34, doc.43]; for the death of Süleyman in the village of Hacı Ivaz Paşa Kızığı, see Bursa Şeriye Sicilleri, A 19/19, 122b/4, 17 Zilkade 909/May 2, 1504 [cited in *OS* 2:34, doc.44]; for the death of Ali in the village of Hacı Ivaz Paşa Kızığı, see Bursa Şeriye Sicilleri, A 19/19,

TABLE 3. *Plague Mortality in Istanbul,*
May 16–18, 1513

Date	Plague
10 Rebiülevvel 919/May 16, 1513	?
11 Rebiülevvel 919/May 17, 1513	?
12 Rebiülevvel 919/May 18, 1513	?
Total (in three days)	57

Source: Topkapı Palace Museum Archives, E. 6155.

The Recurrent Episode (1511–1514)

Sources do not seem to record the return of plague to core Ottoman areas until 1511. This may be a new wave of epidemic activity, but the presence of the disease in the Ottoman vassal states of Wallachia (between 1506 and 1511) and Moldavia (in 1512)[82] complicates the picture. This makes it difficult to determine whether this outbreak was a new wave or a recurrent episode of the second wave. Because of its dissimilarities to the previous two waves, it may be safer to assume that this was a recurrent episode. Wallachia and the Black Sea area may have been the origin for this episode, as no other areas seem to be infected around this time. Although plague was in Venice in 1510, it might be hard to link the origin of this outbreak to it, in the absence of evidence of plague in either Ragusa or in the ports of the Aegean.

In 1511, following a massively destructive earthquake in 1509, plague was once again in Istanbul.[83] Venetian dispatches from the capital note the presence of plague in fall 1512. According to this, there was an outbreak in the capital in October and November, whereupon it was said that three hundred died per day. It was also reported that the Venetian *bailo* and merchants left the city for the countryside on account of plague.[84] It is difficult to determine whether the outbreak continued over the winter months or receded, but it was again noted in spring of the following year. Ottoman archival documents testify to plague mortality in Istanbul in May 1513[85] (Tables 3 and 4). Venetian sources confirm its sustained presence into summer 1513. This time, the reports emphasized the severity of the outbreak,

123a/1, 17 Zilkade 909/May 2, 1504 [cited in OS 2:34, doc.45]; for the death of Hüseyin in the village of Hacı Ivaz Paşa Kızığı, see Bursa Şeriye Sicilleri, A 19/19, 123a/2, 17 Zilkade 909/May 2, 1504 [cited in OS 2:34, doc.46]; for the death of Ali in the village of Gölpınar, see Bursa Şeriye Sicilleri, A 19/19, 123a/3, 17 Zilkade 909/May 2, 1504 [cited in OS 2:34, doc.47].

82 Biraben, *Les hommes et la peste*, 1:442.
83 Ibid.; Süheyl Ünver, "Türkiyede Veba (Taun) Tarihçesi Üzerine," 72; İnalcık, "Istanbul."
84 *Sanudo*, 15:392, 410.
85 TSMA E.2544, E.6155. For a detailed discussion of the significance of these documents, see Chapter 8.

TABLE 4. *Mortality Report of Plague and Nonplague Deaths in Istanbul,
May 23–25, 1513*

Date	Plague	Nonplague	Total
17 Rebiülevvel 919/May 23, 1513	9	4	13
18 Rebiülevvel 919/May 24, 1513	14	8	22
19 Rebiülevvel 919/May 25, 1513	9	2	11
Total (in three days)	32	14	46

Source: Topkapı Palace Museum Archives, E. 2544, E. 6155.

noting a daily mortality of 250 to 300 in late July and early August.[86]
Presumably, the outbreak started to recede later in August, as reports suggest that mortality declined noticeably.[87] It was still in the capital in early September, and it was said that a total of sixty thousand died that year of plague.[88] This, however, seems to be an exaggerated figure; a more realistic estimate would be fifteen thousand to twenty thousand.

Around this time, plague was also in Syria (1511–14) and Egypt (1513–14), producing exceptionally high levels of mortality.[89] Prince Ahmed, son of Bayezid, lost two sons to plague in Cairo during this outbreak.[90] A sermon delivered by Rabbi Yosef ben Meir Garson in 1514 in Damascus reflects the deeply felt pain in the Jewish community on account of high mortality caused by plague.[91] News of plague in Aleppo in summer 1514 soon reached Venice, along with news of the Ottoman victory over Shah Ismail.[92] Even though Venetian sources noted that plague started anew in Istanbul in fall 1514, no further mention of it is made.[93]

An Analysis of the Outbreaks in the First Phase

An analysis of outbreaks in this phase with respect to length, area of origin, and trajectories of spread reveals their similarities and differences. First, with respect to length of duration, while the first and the second waves lasted intermittently over a decade or longer, the last episode was relatively short. The gaps in the outbreaks may be more indicative of lacunae in the sources than a real absence of epidemic activity; it is quite possible there

---

[86] *Sanudo*, 16:587–88; 17:35, 37, 79.

[87] Ibid., 17:110.

[88] Ibid., 17:159–60, 266.

[89] Dols, *Black Death*, 314; Dols, "Second Plague Pandemic," 168–69; Ünver, "Türkiyede Veba."

[90] Çağatay Uluçay, "Yavuz Sultan Selim Nasıl Padişah Oldu?" *Tarih Dergisi* 10 (1954): 138–39n46.

[91] Minna Rozen, *A History of the Jewish Community in Istanbul: The Formative Years, 1453–1566* (Leiden: Brill, 2002), 103.

[92] *Sanudo*, 19:64.

[93] Ibid., 19:326.

were outbreaks that went unrecorded. Second, a comparison with respect to the area of origin stresses similarities between the first and the second waves. In both instances, plague seems to have arrived to Ottoman lands from the west. In the first wave, plague very likely came from the overland caravan routes linking the Adriatic to Istanbul (most probably the northern branch). In the second wave, it most likely arrived through either the overland routes in the Balkans or via maritime links. The recurrent episode of the second wave implicates an alternative area of origin in the Black Sea basin, which may indicate the emergence of new patterns of plague activity.

On the basis of the available evidence, it is possible to surmise that in the First Phase, plague moved along an east-west axis in the Mediterranean. This trajectory of contamination seems to represent the main channel of interaction and mobility in the region. For example, the tightly knit trade networks operated by Ragusan merchants along the Balkan caravan routes were especially important for grain trade, as Ragusa monopolized international trade in the Balkans for the most part between 1490 and 1590.[94] It should be possible to trace the movement of plague and the grain trade along this trajectory.

Third, the spread of plague, once introduced to Ottoman regions, is quite informative. Whereas, in the first wave, there is no indication of the spread of plague deep into the Anatolian peninsula, there are explicit references to its devastating presence there during the second wave. Moreover, Anatolia might have served as a conduit for the overland transmission of plague to and/or from Syria and Egypt during the second wave. This might be indicative of an emergent network of plague between Anatolia and Syria and Egypt in the late fifteenth century, perhaps triggered by warfare between the Ottomans and the Mamluks between 1485 and 1491. Eventually, it is worth noting that accounts of plague were discretely interleaved with narratives of warfare, conquest, and various forms of human mobility. Perhaps it should not come as a surprise that the outbreaks of the first wave largely coincided with the Ottoman-Venetian War (1463-79).

What is perhaps not so obvious, but equally important, is the link between the propagation of plagues and the rise of trade networks, and even more significantly, the rise of Ottoman urban centers whose prominence at this time is beyond dispute: Bursa, Edirne, and Istanbul. Not only was each city on a major pathway for the movement of plague but also each underwent a process of urbanization, or, in truth, reurbanization, that was ingrained in the dynamics of urban plague mortality.

---

[94] Traian Stoianovich, "Pour un modèle du commerce du Levant: economie concurrentielle et economie de bazar 1500–1800," in *Istanbul à la jonction des cultures balkaniques, méditerranéennes, slaves et orientales, aux XVIe-XIXe siècles* (Bucharest: Association internationale d'études du Sud-Est européen, 1977), 191; Zdenko Zlatar, *Dubrovnik's Merchants and Capital in the Ottoman Empire (1520–1620): A Quantitative Study* (Istanbul: Isis Press, 2011).

Bursa, Edirne, and Istanbul: Urbanization and Plague

The process of urbanization, however slow in the beginning, took a definitive character in the sixteenth century, when several villages in Anatolia grew into new towns and undistinguished cities developed into thriving metropolises.[95] It is argued here that the urbanization of Ottoman towns in this era cannot be studied in isolation from plague and the heavy mortality it caused. As the first major urban center of the Ottoman polity, Bursa is vital for early Ottoman urban history. But what is most significant for the purposes of this study is its rise as an urban transit center for trade in the fourteenth and fifteenth centuries, which illustrates the complex relationship of conquest, urbanization, and trade to plague outbreaks.

Not much is known about the early history of Bursa after the Ottoman conquest in 1326. It served as the Ottoman capital until 1402, when it was plundered and razed to the ground by Timur's soldiers. It prospered during the reigns of Orhan (r. 1324–62), Murad I (r. 1362–89), and Bayezid I (r. 1389–1402), with the establishment of many public buildings and religious endowments, such as mosques, hospices, baths, and caravanserais.[96] Using the accounts of visitors to Bursa in the fourteenth century, Lowry deduces that it was a relatively large and well-built city, with a population around ten thousand at the turn of the fifteenth century. Bursa's Muslim, Christian, and Jewish populations all enjoyed the benefits offered by the pious establishments in the city.[97] Immediately after the conquest, Bursa began to receive immigrant Turkoman groups from Anatolia. Orhan built a hospice around which immigrants could settle. As the city grew in population, new areas of settlement extended toward the west of the walled city. Until Mehmed II, all Ottoman sultans sponsored the construction of imperial buildings in Bursa and encouraged the elite to build religious establishments.[98]

As early as 1430s, there is evidence that Bursa began to emerge as a thriving commercial center with a resident community of foreign merchants. It was an important market, especially for Florentine and Genoese merchants, who bought silk.[99] Raw silk was brought to Bursa from Persia and processed into cloth in the local industries. Italian merchants bought processed, dyed, and ornamented silk and in turn sold their Florentine woolen cloth at great profit.[100] Besides textiles, other commercial goods, such as spices, sugar, perfumes, soap, and dyes, from Egypt, Syria, and India, were also to

---

[95] For the rise and development of urban centers in the sixteenth century, see Faroqhi, *Towns and Townsmen of Ottoman Anatolia*; Jennings, "Urban Population in Anatolia in the Sixteenth Century."

[96] İnalcık, "Bursa," *EI²*.

[97] Lowry, *Ottoman Bursa*, 6–7.

[98] Abdullah Kuran, "A Spatial Study of Three Ottoman Capitals: Bursa, Edirne, and Istanbul," *Muqarnas* 13 (1996): 116–18.

[99] İnalcık, "Bursa"; Lowry, *Ottoman Bursa*, 8–9.

[100] Lowry, *Ottoman Bursa*, 42, 44.

be found in the markets of Bursa, though the trade of these items was never as extensive as that of silk.

The city continued to grow in the fifteenth century, commensurate with its rising commercial standing. Caravanserais and warehouses were built to assist long-distance trade, especially for cotton and slave trade. Bursa's booming economy greatly benefited from the conquests and the resulting expansion under Mehmed II.[101] In the late fifteenth century, after the expansion of the Ottoman domains along the Black Sea coast, one could also find Russian merchants, who brought fur, woolen cloth, and leather to sell in the markets of Bursa.[102] By the end of the century, visitors described Bursa as the most crowded of Ottoman cities and as the center of silk and cloth trade. According to Bonsignori, more cloth was manufactured in Bursa than in the entirety of Italy.[103] All of these commercial links tied Bursa to the larger economies of a wider region, including the Black Sea basin, the Mediterranean, and the Silk Road. As a point of intersection for multiple trade routes that connected Europe, Anatolia, Syria, Egypt, and Persia, it was most vulnerable to incoming infection. In this composite web of trade connections, plague traveled along caravan routes. In addition to increased human interaction and mobility, these commercial contacts also added potential new channels for the circulation of plague. For example, the woolen cloth trade or the fur trade may have served as potential media for the introduction of new infection, because both woolen cloth and fur are known to harbor fleas for extended periods of time.[104]

The rise of Bursa as a transit trade center in the fifteenth century and its effects on changing patterns of plague are clearly illustrated in early-fifteenth-century outbreaks (e.g., the outbreak of 1429–30).[105] The frequent presence of plague in the city is further testified in the writings of İbn Şerif, a fifteenth-century physician in Bursa. In his discussion of the qualities of clean air, free from pestilence, İbn Şerif complains of the terrible stench in the streets of Bursa in the early fifteenth century and recommends the burning of sandalwood and other fragrant trees and fumigation of the air to ward off plague.[106]

The fact that Bursa was infected by plague along with places in Syria, Egypt, and Italian cities[107] may be taken as some indication about the city's standing as hub of trade in the early fifteenth century. As a matter of fact, the

[101] İnalcık, "Bursa"; Lowry, *Ottoman Bursa*, 8–9.

[102] İnalcık, "Bursa and the Commerce of the Levant," *JESHO* 3, no. 2 (1960): 139–40.

[103] Borsook, "Travels of Bernardo Michelozzi and Bonsignore Bonsignori," 163. Also see Lowry, *Ottoman Bursa*, 9–10.

[104] See Chapter 1.

[105] See Chapter 3.

[106] İbn Şerîf, *Yâdigâr*, 1:36.

[107] Dols, *Black Death*, 204–12; Biraben, *Les hommes et la peste*, 1:395. For instance, plague was in Venice (1427–29) and Florence (1429–30).

importance of Bursa as a transit point in trade connecting Persian lands in the east to Europe in the west is confirmed in the accounts of travelers who visited the city. By the mid-fifteenth century, the city was described as being twice as large as Pera, the Genoese colony in Constantinople.[108] In fact, its population was probably within the same range as that of Constantinople in the mid-fifteenth century. The commercial dynamism of Bursa can also be traced in Ottoman court records, which highlight the nature of commercial transactions in detail.[109]

The case of the 1429–30 outbreak in Bursa illustrates several features of an emerging pattern of plague spread in relation to urban setting, trade, and conquest. First of all, it illustrates that already in the early decades of the fifteenth century, a major Ottoman urban center functioned within international trade networks and was thus exposed to an increased risk for plague outbreaks. Second, it points to the development of Bursa as a center for commerce and burgeoning industry. Such an urban economy required an urban labor force, fed by a constant influx of immigrants from the countryside seeking employment. The investments made to urban space by dynastic patronage seem to have rendered Bursa even more attractive to the incomers. Inevitably, the crowded urban space provided the essential conditions for devastating plagues to break out. Third, it illustrates the effects of conquest, though indirectly, on trade and urban development. As new areas were conquered, new elements were added to trade networks, which brought an impetus to the circulation of humans, rodents, goods, and, thus, the plague. Conquest also provided increased resources for urban investment, which attracted more immigrants, thus assuring the availability of a replenished pool of human hosts that lacked immunity to be swept off with every recurrence of the plague. Nevertheless, Bursa is not the only example that illustrates this complex web of relationship between plague and urban growth, conquest, and trade.

Edirne was another Ottoman city that prospered during the fourteenth and fifteenth centuries. Many of the emergent features illustrated in the example of Bursa can be observed in the case of Edirne as well. Although conquered in 1362, Edirne does not seem to have achieved precedence until the end of the century. At the time of its conquest, Edirne had the appearance of a Roman garrison town. For about a half-century, it housed its residents in the old walled area. As early as the fifteenth century, however, new residential areas began to spring up outside of the walled city.[110] The

[108] Lowry, *Ottoman Bursa*, 8–9, 64.
[109] Lowry estimates the population of Bursa in the mid-fifteenth century as 27,500. Gradually increasing, it exceeded thirty-five thousand in the late fifteenth century. It was more than forty-two thousand in 1530 and near ninety thousand in the late sixteenth century. Lowry, *Ottoman Bursa*, 22–23, 26, 28, 37. Also compare with figures presented for Istanbul in İnalcık, "Istanbul"; İnalcık, "Bursa and the Commerce of the Levant," 131–47.
[110] Kuran, "A Spatial Study of Three Ottoman Capitals," 121–22.

emergence of these new residential quarters suggests, most probably, that the city had begun receiving an influx of immigrants and that it had economic resources to offer to those immigrants, such as trade and industry. Among the industries practiced in the city were dyeing, tanning, soap making, distillation of rose extract, carriage building, and bookbinding.[111] The fact that it was situated on the main trade route connecting Istanbul to the Balkans certainly contributed to its thriving as a major hub. In fact, Edirne attracted Venetian, Genoese, Catalan, and Florentine merchants starting from early fifteenth century, a number of whom began to reside in the city permanently.[112] At the end of the century, Edirne is reported as being equal in size to Florence.[113]

The rising economic importance of Edirne was solidified when it began to serve as the seat of the Ottoman throne under Süleyman Çelebi in the interregnum period, and later for Mehmed I (r. 1413–21). The rising importance of the town was also owed to its relatively safe location, especially given the destruction Timur had exacted upon Bursa. Edirne soon benefited from charitable activities: it witnessed the construction of new buildings and pious establishments, including mosques, hospices, dervish lodges, bridges, bathhouses, hospitals, and madrasas. The extensive clearing and building activities in and around it, undertaken by Sultan Murad II (r. 1421–51) and Bayezid II (r. 1481–1512), are mentioned in the Ottoman chronicles of the time. For example, Aşıkpaşazade tells how Murad II cleared the forests, dried up marshy lands outside the city, and built a bridge there. Furthermore, he also writes that the Ottoman sultans built mosques, hospices, bathhouses, and other welfare institutions there. The alms given and food delivered in the hospices attracted many poor to the city.[114] Similar accounts about the construction of public works can also be found in the chronicle of Oruç.[115] Visitors, who were struck by the many architectural beauties of Edirne, also noticed its growth and development in the late fifteenth century. For instance, the mosques, water system, and beautiful fountains impressed aforementioned Florentine traveler Bonsignori in 1497.[116] By the end of the sixteenth century, Edirne acquired the full silhouette of an Ottoman city, not only for the imperial mosques at its three corners, but also by virtue of being a lively economic center that embodied a large number of khans and two major marketplaces.[117]

---

[111] Tayyip Gökbilgin, "Edirne," *EI*².
[112] W. Heyd, *Histoire du commerce du Levant au moyen-âge* (Amsterdam: Hakkert, 1983), 2:352.
[113] Borsook, "Travels of Bernardo Michelozzi and Bonsignore Bonsignori," 158.
[114] Aşık Paşazade, *Osmanoğulları'nın Tarihi*, 187–88, 286–87, 455–56, 559–60.
[115] There are many such references in the chronicle of Oruç. See, e.g., Oruç, *Tarih*, 33, 47, 77–78, 135, 140.
[116] Borsook, "Travels of Bernardo Michelozzi and Bonsignore Bonsignori," 158.
[117] Kuran, "A Spatial Study of Three Ottoman Capitals," 118–22.

Even after the conquest of Istanbul, Edirne did not lose its prime importance as an imperial city, and many sultans continued to hold court there.[118] In fact, Ottoman sources give the impression that the city was considered as a retreat area where sultans would reside when they did not want to stay in Istanbul, in times of crises such as fire, earthquake, or plague. It is rather curious that Edirne is depicted in these sources as being preferred by sultans for "hunting" or for its "clean air," despite the fact that it suffered as heavily from plague as Istanbul did. As a matter of fact, every time plague hit Edirne, the sultan, as well as all those who could, left the city.

The development of Edirne, its thriving economy and industry, and rising population prepared ideal conditions for outbreaks of plague. Starting from the mid-fifteenth century, almost every plague outbreak that infected Istanbul also affected Edirne. Especially during the First Phase, when plague was introduced to Ottoman lands primarily from the west through the overland route connecting the Adriatic to Istanbul, Edirne was infected every time a new plague broke out. This was clearly illustrated in the case of the first wave between 1466 and 1476, as discussed earlier. Like Bursa, Edirne attracted immigrants starting in the early fifteenth century because of its booming economy and its charitable establishments. In addition, it may perhaps be stressed that its industries, such as dyeing and tanning, could expose laborers to increased risk of handling plague-infected material and/or attract rat colonies.

The case of Istanbul also illustrates this complex dynamic between the expansion of plague and the processes of conquest, trade, and urbanization. At the time of the Ottoman conquest, Byzantine Constantinople was a city that had greatly shrunk in population, for reasons including the plague, which continued after the conquest as well. Even before the major wave of plagues between 1466 and 1476, there occurred outbreaks of plague in Ottoman Istanbul. For example, shortly after the conquest, a plague was recorded in southeastern Europe, lasting from mid-summer to mid-fall 1456. Sources confirm the presence of plague in Istanbul and Edirne, as well as in Novi Brdu, Smederevo, and Belgrade in the Balkans. Plague's recorded presence on the island of Crete, in Venice, and along the Dalmatian coast suggests a maritime transmission as well.[119] Although the demographic effects of this outbreak in Istanbul are not well known, it certainly diminished an already reduced population. Mehmed II's consecutive efforts at forcible repopulation of Istanbul might have been an attempt to compensate for this outbreak's death toll. The repopulation of the city had been of primary concern for its conqueror. For this purpose, right after the conquest, he announced that any fugitive who returned would be allowed to live freely again. This

---

[118] Gökbilgin, "Edirne."
[119] Babinger, *Mehmet the Conqueror*, 146; Biraben, *Les hommes et la peste*, 1:396, 441.

was accompanied by practices of compulsory resettlement.[120] According to Halil İnalcık, despite the loss caused by plague, the census of 1477 shows that the population of Istanbul was still as numerous as any city in the Mediterranean.[121]

The sixteenth century, however, was a time of exceptional growth for the population and economy of Istanbul because of the rising importance of the city as the capital of a centralizing empire. It witnessed a rapid population increase in the sixteenth century. This was a general trend in Ottoman cities in this period, when the population of most cities grew by 80 percent. The rate of population increase for Istanbul was even higher than that. During this period, new neighborhoods were formed and old ones became more heavily populated. Istanbul received immigrants, mainly for economic reasons. Merchants and craftsmen as well as simple urban laborers came from near and far. Beyond economic enticements, the welfare of the city provided for by pious foundations made Istanbul attractive for immigration. These foundations served to meet the needs of city folks in water supply, paving of roads, public security, hospitals, street cleaning, and shelter and food for the poor and travelers. At times of crisis in the provinces, such as crises caused by famine, flood, earthquake, locust attacks, and plague, more people immigrated to Istanbul to make a living.[122] Finally, Istanbul was an important point of intersection of maritime routes connecting the Black Sea and its hinterland, the Aegean, and the Mediterranean. It was situated on the main overland route connecting the Balkans to Anatolia and beyond. Owing to the high traffic of commercial goods, the city was susceptible to the introduction of recurrent plagues, perhaps even more than Edirne and Bursa. Especially in the sixteenth century, it received a flood of immigrants, a certain number of whom shared the fate of those in Bursa and Edirne and were swept off periodically by recurrent plagues.

Conclusion

In reconstructing the historical narrative of plagues of the First Phase (1453–1517), three important themes have demanded our immediate attention: new Ottoman conquests, the development of trade and communication networks, and urbanization. As a result of conquests and vassalages won through military superiority, the Ottoman power gained control over established trade networks. Industry also developed in rising urban centers, such as Bursa, Edirne, and Istanbul. Smaller Ottoman towns, especially those along trade routes, grew as thriving urban centers, both in the Balkans and

---

[120] İnalcık, "Istanbul." For a detailed account of Mehmed II's policies of resettlement after the conquest, see Lowry, "Pushing the Stone Uphill," 11–25.

[121] İnalcık, "Istanbul."

[122] Ibid.

in Anatolia. Furthermore, heavy building activities were common in urban centers, in the form of construction of mosques, schools, hospitals, bath-houses, and hospices. Ottoman urbanites began to enjoy the benefits of those institutions in this period. These benefits turned cities into magnets, which constantly attracted population from their hinterlands. The influx of new immigrants was periodically checked by recurrent waves of plague, two of which we have closely studied in this chapter. Overall, out of the sixty-four years of the First Phase, plague is recorded in at least twenty-eight years for core Ottoman areas, which covers about 40 percent of this period. If the vassal states are also included, this number amounts to thirty-two years, which gives a rate of 50 percent. In other words, plague was present in at least one location under Ottoman control between four to five years for every decade. During the First Phase, several Balkan towns in Bosnia, Herzegovina, Macedonia, and Thrace, as well as Edirne, Istanbul, Gallipoli, Bursa, and central Anatolia, seem to have suffered from plague outbreaks. Plague waves recurred with an average interval of ten years. This is roughly equivalent to the average interval between outbreaks in both eastern and western Mediterranean cities in the post–Black Death era (Table 1). More specifically, without suggesting that they had the same length of duration, and the same intervals between durations, this means that the patterns of waxing and waning in the eastern and western Mediterranean cities were similar in longevity. However, the year 1517 seems to stand as a caesura, marking not only the beginning of Ottoman control over Syria, Egypt, and the Muslim holy cities of Mecca and Medina but also changes in plague epidemics with regard to size and frequency. After 1517, plague outbreaks affecting Ottoman areas seem to diverge from those affecting the western Mediterranean: the plague outbreaks in the Ottoman areas started to recur more frequently and spread to a wider area. Hence, both the extensive scale and the frequent recurrences of outbreaks after 1517 make it necessary to discuss them in the next chapter.

5

The Second Phase (1517–1570)

Multiple Plague Trajectories

This chapter is an account of plague outbreaks during the Second Phase (1517–70). As in the previous phase, plague came and went in waves. Though fragmentary in nature, sources still make it possible to identify three waves of epidemic activity: the first wave (1520–29), the second wave (1533–49), and the last wave (1552–68). However, unlike in the First Phase, the infection no longer spread along the east-west axis only. What characterizes the outbreaks of this phase is the emergence of multiple trajectories along which plague propagated. As is shown in the following pages, between 1517 and 1570, Ottoman dominions saw the formation and mutual integration of new trade and communication networks as well as the revival of those that had lost their vitality in the preceding centuries. The formation of these new avenues of exchange and mobility was related to ongoing conquests and urbanization. Ultimately, the result of this process was increased plague activity, which gradually transformed the disease from an occasional visitor to a permanent resident of the Ottoman healthscape.

The conquest of Syria and Egypt (1516–17), which doubled the size of Ottoman dominions and its subject population, also resulted in more plague activity. A new trajectory of contamination emerged along the north-south axis in the eastern Mediterranean, following the conquests of Syria, Egypt, and Rhodes, connecting Istanbul to Egypt. This connection was especially important for the provisioning of Istanbul by the supplies of Egypt as well as securing the pilgrimage route to the Muslim holy cities. What is interesting for our purposes here is that, from the first wave of the Second Phase, plagues began to circulate between Cairo and Istanbul directly, an unmediated exchange of infection that was not possible in the First Phase. When this new north-south axis was integrated into the east-west axis of the First Phase, the result was a wider distribution of the infection between western and eastern Mediterranean ports and Istanbul (Map 4).

In addition to this north-south axis, the Second Phase also witnessed the formation of channels through which plague could spread along the

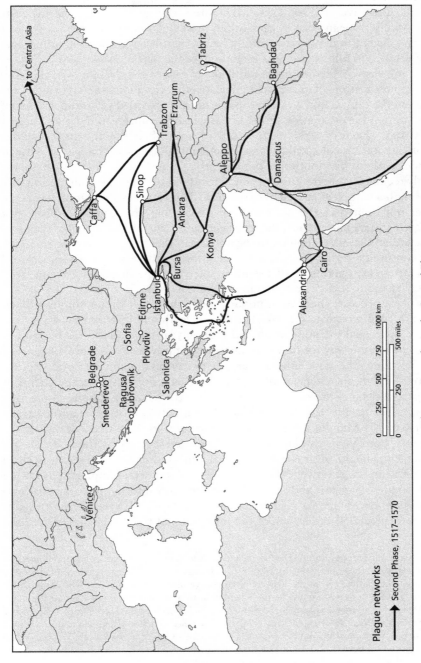

MAP 4. Plague networks in the Second Phase, 1517–70.

Plague networks

→ Second Phase, 1517–1570

newly emerging connections between the Persian Gulf and Istanbul, which entailed the overland road systems connecting Anatolia, Iraq, and the eastern Mediterranean ports to each other. In a similar vein, with the integration of the Black Sea network to Istanbul and Anatolia, the infection found new trajectories to follow from the hinterland of the Black Sea to Anatolia, Istanbul, the eastern Mediterranean and as far east as the Persian Gulf. Finally, an intensification of piracy that developed throughout the sixteenth century in the central and western Mediterranean provided yet another channel facilitating the circulation of the disease and its transfer to these mentioned networks. Each of these plague networks and their subsequent consolidation facilitated ecological exchanges, including disease exchange, on a much wider scale of distribution. Consequently, plagues in the Second Phase not only recurred more frequently than before but also were disseminated swiftly through a complex pattern of expansion. This time the circulation of plague was not limited to the Mediterranean basin but connected the Black Sea region and its hinterlands, the Caucasus and Central Asia, the Red Sea, and the Indian Ocean. It should also be noted that there emerged a greater degree of continuity during this phase bridging the disease ecologies of coastal and inland areas, making it all the more likely for the infection coming from local enzootic foci to be disseminated far and wide.

These processes need to be understood in the larger context of post–Black Death Mediterranean history. The Black Death and its recurrent waves not only exhausted the population and economy of the states in the region but also paved the way for new configurations of power. To be sure, plague did not produce the same effects everywhere it visited; some societies seem to have been more adversely affected than others. For example, the effects of repeated plagues proved to be dramatic for the Mamluk Empire in the long run.[1] This meant that the pre–Black Death network of international trade between the Mamluks, Venice, and Genoa was in the process of dissolving. In fact, both Venice and Genoa were impacted severely by the Black Death, but Genoa could never recover fully from this blow, which in the end helped Venice gain more power.[2] These changes had important implications for the Ottoman expansion and its gradual integration into the international networks of exchange. As Nicola di Cosmo has aptly observed, the Ottomans fully appreciated the legacy of the international trade that united the land

---

[1]   David Neustadt [Ayalon], "The Plague and Its Effects upon the Mamluk Army," *Journal of the Royal Asiatic Society* 66 (1946): 67–73. He argues that the negative effects of epidemics were cumulative; i.e., in the long term, successive plague epidemics after the Black Death were even more destructive for the Mamluk army than the initial epidemic of the Black Death. For a general assessment of the demographic effects of the Black Death in Egypt and Syria, see Dols, *Black Death*, 143–235. For a detailed analysis of the effects of the plague on Egypt's population and a comparison to the case of England, see Borsch, *Black Death in Egypt and England*.

[2]   Abu-Lughod, *Before European Hegemony*, 102–31.

routes of Pax Mongolica to the Italian trade networks that connected the Black Sea to the Mediterranean.[3] The late-fifteenth-century Ottoman conquests of key ports of international trade on the Black Sea clearly indicate a vision directed to taking over that legacy.

Reconfiguration of power in the Mediterranean world continued in the sixteenth century between the competing forces of the Ottomans, Venetians, and the Portuguese as well as the Spanish and the French. Among these, Venice was one of the most important commercial and political forces in the Mediterranean, though this power hardly went unchallenged. The Ottoman conquest of Venetian colonies resulted in a series of wars to establish control over the Aegean and Adriatic seas throughout the fifteenth century. The advent of the Portuguese into the picture at the turn of the sixteenth century further challenged the commercial power of Venice by preparing the subsequent fall of the Mamluks to the Ottomans.

Until the Ottoman conquest in 1516–17, the slave Sultanate of the Mamluks was in need of a constant flow of manpower, which was met by Venetian merchants. Egypt was also an important center for textiles and sugar as well as goods brought from India and China, such as spices, porcelain, and silk. As a result of the catastrophic effects of the Black Death on the population and economy of the Mamluk Empire, long-distance trade remained the only viable source for Egypt's economy. Europeans had been trying for a long time to gain access to the Red Sea, but the Mamluk power was blocking them by rigidly regulating the access of European merchants to Alexandria. Through its partnership with Venice, the Mamluk power was in control of the trade of goods coming from India and China. However, the primary importance of this trade route was disrupted by the circumnavigation of Africa by the Portuguese. In 1497, Vasco da Gama circumnavigated Africa and thus prepared the end of the monopoly over the eastern trade of the Venetian-Mamluk partnership. As early as the turn of the sixteenth century, the Portuguese began to challenge severely the primary importance of the Mediterranean as the main channel of trade goods from the east to Europe. Under these circumstances, when the main source for the Mamluk economy had collapsed, it did not take long for the Ottoman conquest to follow.[4] The victory of Ottoman Sultan Selim I (r. 1512–20) over the Mamluk Empire resulted in the conquest of Syria in 1516 and of Egypt in 1517. Ottoman conquests of northern Iraq and Hijaz, Baghdad in 1534, Basra in 1546, Yemen (1538–39 and 1547–48), and the eastern Mediterranean port cities, as well as those in the Red Sea, enabled them to have

---

[3] Nicola Di Cosmo, "Black Sea Emporia and the Mongol Empire: A Reassessment of the Pax Mongolica," *JESHO* 53, nos. 1–2 (2010): 83–108.

[4] Abu-Lughod, *Before European Hegemony*, 230–44; Andrew C. Hess, "The Ottoman Conquest of Egypt (1517) and the Beginning of the Sixteenth-Century World War," *IJMES* 4, no. 1 (1973): 55–76.

access to and exert control over the Persian Gulf and its Indian Ocean trade connection. The Portuguese, even though they held the great advantage of having access to the Indian Ocean, did not succeed in establishing a monopoly over this trade. Generally speaking, then, the oceanic route and the Mediterranean competed for eastern trade throughout the sixteenth century. The Ottoman conquest and presence in Egypt, Syria, and the Arabian Peninsula, and its effects on the expansion of plague, can be best understood in this wider context.[5]

The First Wave (1520–1529)

What appears to be a new wave of infection can be documented in the sources by 1520, if not earlier.[6] This epidemic wave affected a vast area, including the Mediterranean, Europe, England, Scandinavia, Russia, and the Balkans. In the Ottoman-ruled areas, it was first documented in Istanbul and Edirne in 1520 as well as in the area between the two.[7] Although it is not clear where this outbreak originated, its presence in Hungary and the southeast Balkans might indicate an eastward spread. What is clear is that the epidemic's spread did not follow the patterns of expansion discernible in the pre-1517 outbreaks (e.g., from Venice and Ragusa through the Mediterranean maritime route or via the overland route of the Balkans). This time plague started in Italian port cities two years after it struck Istanbul. This seems to suggest that Istanbul might now be part of another network of contamination that was not limited solely to the former connection with the Italian port cities.

What makes this outbreak even more interesting is that it was witnessed at the time of the death of Ottoman Sultan Selim I and the ascension of his son Süleyman to the throne. When Selim left Istanbul for Edirne, plague was raging in the area.[8] An encrypted letter sent from the Venetian *bailo* on

---

[5] For this context, see Giancarlo Casale, *The Ottoman Age of Exploration* (Oxford: Oxford University Press, 2010).

[6] Venetian sources suggest that plague was in Istanbul and Thessaloniki in summer 1516. See *Sanudo*, 22:541, 547; 23:41, 116. There were further reports of plague having broken out again in the capital in summer 1518, lasting until the end of the year. See *Sanudo*, 25:687; 26:66, 133–34, 162, 296. Moreover, an Ottoman document from late July to early August 1519 shows the registration of the death of a novice janissary boy from plague in the Kalburcu village of Gebze, some fifty miles east of Istanbul. Even though this may be taken as some evidence for the presence of plague before 1520, it is not possible to determine exactly when the death took place. See *İstanbul Kadı Sicilleri*, ed. Mehmet Âkif Aydın, Rıfat Günalan, and Coşkun Yılmaz (Istanbul: ISAM, 2010), 2:160. These outbreaks do not seem to belong to a continuous wave of plague, as they appear to be sporadic cases.

[7] *Sanudo*, 28:230, 232, 596. Biraben does not mention the presence of plague in the *sud-oriental* region (North Africa, Southeast Balkans, north of Black Sea, Asia Minor, and the Levant) between 1513 and 1520 but notes the plague in Edirne and Bosphorus (Istanbul) in 1520–21. See Biraben, *Les hommes et la peste*, 1:442.

[8] *Sanudo*, 29:304.

September 17 reported the news that the sultan was already suffering from two infectious boils but that a plague boil also appeared over his shoulder, which caused him great pain; it was feared for his life.[9] When the latter died in Çorlu, halfway between the two cities on September 21, 1520, some early reports suggested that he died from plague.[10] A letter written by the Venetian ambassador Lorenzo Orio in October confirmed that the news of Selim's death from plague was true.[11] Other reports reaching Venice soon afterward seem to further confirm this account.[12]

Ottoman sources seem to agree that an infectious boil called *şir-pençe* (literally "lion's claw," possibly anthrax) caused Selim's death. Given the evidence, it may be difficult to determine whether it was indeed bubonic plague, anthrax, or another disease that killed Selim.[13] It is possible that the Ottoman sources did not want to attribute the Sultan's death to plague and instead fabricated a narrative of another fatal disease. Whatever the real cause of his death may have been, the story of an infectious boil that killed him was circulating in Istanbul. This version of his death news could be found soon after the Sultan's death, as mentioned in the report of *bailo* Tomà Contarini to Venice.[14] The sixteenth-century Italian historian Paolo Giovio (d. 1552) also seems to echo this version of the story. According to the latter, Selim died of the "French pox." He narrates that Selim was lying quietly in his home when he noticed an aching boil in his back, which grew to cover all his body like a cancer. This changed the disposition of his body little by little. Soon thereafter, he had a pestilential fever. He died of this fever in September 1520 in the same place where he had fought against his father, between Edirne and Istanbul.[15]

Shortly after Selim's death, his son Süleyman ascended the throne on September 30, 1520, while plague was still going on in Istanbul. News that reached Venice suggested that plague was lessening in the capital by October.[16] The outbreak most likely died out that fall, perhaps soon after Süleyman's accession to the throne. The claim that plague ended after Süleyman ascended the throne was used by some of his contemporaries to

[9] Ibid., 29:323.

[10] Ibid., 29:303.

[11] Ibid., 29:341; İnalcık, "Selim I," *EI²*; Peter Schreiner, *Die byzantinischen Kleinchroniken*, 554–55.

[12] *Sanudo*, 29:341–42.

[13] It has been claimed that Selim died of plague in Jan Schmidt, *Pure Water for Thirsty Muslims: A Study of Mustafā Âli of Gallipoli's Künhü'l-ahbar* (Leiden: Het Oosters Instituut, 1991), 322. It is not clear how Schmidt deduces that this was caused by plague, because his source, Mustafa Ali, mentions the disease as *yanıkara* ("black complaint," possibly anthrax).

[14] *Sanudo*, 29:359.

[15] Paolo Giovio, *A shorte treatise vpon the Turkes chronicles* (London: Edvvarde VVhitchurche, 1546), 146b–147aff.

[16] *Sanudo*, 29:361.

instill the much-needed legitimacy in the early years of his rule. For example, Tabib Ramazan, a physician hoping to serve in Süleyman's court, wrote that plague came to an end when the latter ascended the throne. He tried to explain this by depicting Süleyman as a just ruler, whose justice he compared to the seventh-century Muslim caliph 'Umar ibn al-Khattāb.[17] Soon after his accession, Süleyman undertook an expedition to Hungary, which resulted in the conquest of Belgrade (1521). The fact that plague was reported there may have been related to the expedition of Ottoman armies to the city. Biraben suggests that the Ottoman army might have carried plague to Hungary.[18] Ramazan also mentions plague in conjunction with the siege of Belgrade.[19] However, on the basis of available evidence, it is not clear whether the infection was indeed carried by Ottoman armies to Hungary.

The next year, the Ottomans laid siege to the island of Rhodes. Fully aware of the necessity of establishing direct communication between Egypt and Istanbul, they acknowledged that Rhodes had to be conquered. This communication was important not only for trade and the provisioning of the capital but for the protection of the Muslim pilgrimage route as well.[20] After a long siege, the island surrendered in 1522.[21] The conquest of Syria (1516), Egypt (1517), and Rhodes (1522) meant that the intended connection between the center and these provinces could now be established. Commercial, administrative, and military links were forged rapidly, and ecological ramifications soon became visible. Both maritime and overland communication between Istanbul and Syria and Egypt quickly developed. Although the journey from Istanbul to Alexandria lasted more than two months overland, sources note that a fully equipped vessel only took twelve days to make the journey.[22] Cairo was a great metropolis, connected to both Alexandria and Damietta through Rosetta and the Nile. The pilgrimage-caravan routes to Jerusalem, Mt. Sinai, and Mecca also started in Cairo. Now the richest Ottoman province, Egypt supplied many important staples

---

[17] Tabib Ramazan, *Al-Risalah al-Fathiyyah al-Ungurusiyyah al-Sulaymaniyyah*, Topkapı Palace Museum Library, ms. Revan 1279, 26–27ff. For a detailed discussion of this reference, see my "From '*Bête Noire*' to '*le Mal de* Constantinople.'"

[18] Biraben, *Les hommes et la peste*, 442.

[19] Ramazan, *Al-Risalah al-Fathiyyah*, 89ff.

[20] The Knights of St. John based in Rhodes inflicted heavy losses upon the ships of Muslim merchants and pilgrims traveling from Istanbul to eastern Mediterranean port cities and the Red Sea and captured many Muslims. See Nicolas Vatin, "La conquête de Rhodes," in Veinstein, ed., *Soliman le magnifique et son temps*, 435–54.

[21] Svat Soucek, "Rodos," *EI².*

[22] Ships arriving from Istanbul and from non-Ottoman areas disembarked at Alexandria and from this port could have overland access to Rosetta (Rashid), where one could take a small boat to travel to Cairo through the Nile. Ships arriving from Tripoli, Jaffa, or Cyprus disembarked at Damietta, which was more of a port for internal commerce. They brought silk, carobs, and wine to Damietta and loaded sugar and rice from there. See Yerasimos, *Les voyageurs*, 67, 76–77.

for Istanbul, especially grain. In reality, grain trade was one of the most favorable channels for the spread of plague. As elsewhere, grain trade between Alexandria and Istanbul would have involved the movement of rat populations. During the process of transportation of grain from Egypt to Istanbul by ships and during the processes of loading, unloading, and storing the grain, black rats (and their fleas) must have been present in large numbers. Grain transport was most favorable for the spread of rats and the increase in the number of rat colonies.[23]

As soon as this new north-south channel of communication opened up in the eastern Mediterranean between Istanbul and Egypt, a new trajectory of plague contamination started to surface, as evidenced in this wave of plague (1520–29). Before 1517, plague did not spread directly from Cairo to Istanbul, or vice versa, even when both cities were infected through their links with European port cities, in particular, Venice. This was the case during the episode of 1511–14, for instance, discussed in the previous chapter. Because there was no established direct connection between Istanbul and Cairo, plague did not spread from one to the other but instead was introduced to both from Venice through maritime and/or overland routes. However, starting in the 1520s, because of this newly formed direct link between them, whenever plague broke out in Istanbul, it spread to Egypt, or vice versa.

Hence, the conquests of Rhodes, Syria, and Egypt helped the Ottomans forge a north-south connection in the eastern Mediterranean. The island became an important point in this newly forged connection between Istanbul and Cairo.[24] A court record testifying to the death of a military commander from plague may be helpful to consider in this context. According to this document, the commander fell victim to plague while returning from Rhodes to the capital.[25] Since the long siege of the island ended in December, soldiers were transported back to the mainland and continued overland back to Istanbul, arriving in the early days of 1523.[26] In fact, that was when this soldier succumbed to plague in İznik, on his way back. This document, which would otherwise be an isolated reference, is in fact significant as it

---

[23] McCormick, "Rats, Communications, and Plague."

[24] The vessels leaving Alexandria headed toward one of the two ports on the island, one military and the other commercial; afterward, they continued to Istanbul. Yerasimos, *Les voyageurs*, 67–69.

[25] Yvonne J. Seng, "The Üsküdar Estates (Tereke) as Records of Everyday Life in an Ottoman Town, 1521–1524," PhD diss., University of Chicago, 1991, 45.

[26] After landing at Marmaris, the troops marched north through Muğla, Sultanhisar, Alaşehir, Akhisar, and Mihalıç and continued northeast to Istanbul through Mudanya, Gemlik, and Üsküdar. See Donald Edgar Pitcher, *Osmanlı İmparatorluğu'nun Tarihsel Coğrafyası*, trans. Bahar Tırnakcı (Istanbul: Yapı Kredi Yayınları, 2001), 162, Map 25. This itinerary was different than the route the army took from Istanbul to Rhodes. They marched through Gebze, İzmit, İznik, Yenişehir, İnönü, Kütahya, Sandıklı, Denizli, Bozdoğan, Muğla, and Marmaris and crossed the sea from Marmaris to Rhodes.

may highlight a trajectory for the distribution of plague. The evidence about this soldier might be representative of others who could have suffered the same fate, yet it would be difficult to determine whether they could contract the disease in Rhodes or at another point of their return journey. What is clear, however, is that there was now improved communication between Istanbul and Egypt and that the island of Rhodes played an important role in the chain of mobilities.

This north-south connection was quickly integrated into the previous east-west network, which resulted in a wider dissemination of plague. The effects of this integration became quickly observable. The appearance of plague in places that do not seem to be directly related to each other can be much better understood when these trajectories of contamination are established. The presence of plague in the coastal cities of Greece is especially well documented at this time. For example, in spring 1523, plague was in Thessaloniki[27] and in other parts of the Aegean and Ionian seas. Between 1522 and 1523, the infection was in the Ottoman towns of Narda (Arta) and Yanya (Ioannina) in Epirus, in Morea, Athens, and in the island of Rhodes. Plague had already reached Ragusa by October 1522.[28] It affected several islands in the Mediterranean, including the Venetian colonies in the Ionian Sea, such as Corfu, Zakynthos, and Crete, as well as the Archipelago.[29] Before the formation of the north-south axis between Istanbul and Egypt, we do not see such complex patterns of distribution of the disease.

The other end of the north-south axis, obviously, was Istanbul, which was struck by plague around the same time. Venetian sources document the sustained presence of the plague in the capital starting in summer 1522. On July 21, a letter written by Andrea di Priuli, the Venetian *bailo* in Istanbul, noted that the outbreak was very severe and that twenty-three thousand died in twenty-two days. The letter also said that this was when Süleyman left for Rhodes.[30] On August 13, the latter wrote that plague in the capital continued in a most terrible manner.[31] The next day, he sent another letter to report that the galley that the former *bailo* Tomà Contarini had boarded had many deaths from plague.[32] Two weeks later, the *bailo* reported that plague was still very severe in the capital.[33] No further news from the capital

---

[27] Plague was in Thessaloniki on May 23, 1523. See Schreiner, *Die byzantinischen Klein-chroniken*, 563.
[28] *Sanudo*, 33:508.
[29] Schreiner, *Die byzantinischen Kleinchroniken*, 564n78; Biraben, *Les hommes et la peste*, 1:442.
[30] *Sanudo*, 33:422.
[31] Ibid., 33:447.
[32] Ibid., 33:448. The news of plague in the galley was also confirmed by a letter sent to Venice from Crete dated August 22, 1522. See ibid., 33:467–68.
[33] Ibid., 33:462.

pertaining to plague suggests that the outbreak may have ended some time in the fall. However, plague was again reported from the capital the next summer. In mid-July, plague in the capital was reported to be very severe. On July 18, 1523, Andrea di Priuli died from plague, merely two days after contracting the illness.[34] On August 5, Venetian ambassador Pietro Zen reported that plague in the city continued severely, whereupon five hundred died daily. He also noted that the Sultan would neither leave the palace nor grant audience to anyone.[35] Plague seems to have continued into the fall, as suggested by the testimony of Pietro Zen's son Francesco, who left Istanbul at the end of October. Francesco also noted that the former *bailo* Andrea di Priuli had contracted the plague after helping a sick man left on the street and carrying him to his own residence.[36] Francesco believed that even though the disease was ubiquitous in the capital, it was different than that in Italy because the majority of the afflicted in Istanbul recovered.[37] A letter sent to Venice from Istanbul on February 14, 1524, indicates that plague was still raging in the capital.[38]

A cluster of death records from court registers testifies to the presence of plague in Üsküdar (on the Asian shore of the Bosphorus) in May 1524. These were records of novice janissary boys whose death from plague was registered at the court.[39] The fact that there is a cluster of such records concentrated around mid- to late May confirms that plague affected the area. This is further supported by the fact that Üsküdar's mortality figures during that month peaked in comparison to the previous three years.[40]

Venetian sources point out that plague was still severe in the fall. In a letter written on November 6, 1524, the Venetian *bailo* Pietro Bradagin reported that plague was everywhere in the city and taking five hundred to six hundred lives every day. He wrote that he was the only Venetian remaining in Pera; all their merchants took refuge in vineyards outside the city.[41] This wave of epidemic activity seems to have lingered in the city,

[34] Ibid., 34:384. Also see Eric R. Dursteler, "The Bailo in Constantinople: Crisis and Career in Venice's Early Modern Diplomatic Corps," *Mediterranean Historical Review* 16, no. 2 (2001): note 64. After his death, his valuable belongings were sent back to Venice. See Jane L. Stevens Crawshaw, *Plague Hospitals: Public Health for the City in Early Modern Venice* (Burlington, VT: Ashgate, 2012), 211.

[35] *Sanudo*, 34:399.

[36] Ibid., 35:257.

[37] Ibid., 35:260.

[38] Ibid., 36:117–18.

[39] *İstanbul Kadı Sicilleri*, 3:75–77.

[40] Yvonne Seng suggests that out of the eighty-nine deaths between March 1521 and May 1524 registered in the courts of Üsküdar, one was caused by murder and another was due to an accident. Causes of death are not always explicitly remarked in the registers, but the concentration of deaths in summer months suggests that plague outbreaks could be a factor. See Seng, "The Üsküdar Estates," 43–45, 284.

[41] *Sanudo*, 40:515.

on and off, until the end of the decade. There are a series of references to its presence in the capital in the mid-1520s. Venetian sources suggest that plague was believed to be lessening toward the end of 1525. In a letter dated December 29, the *bailo* wrote that the epidemic was seemingly coming to end,[42] although there were still reports of deaths from plague in early January 1526.[43] The *bailo* stated that he nearly caught the disease himself because of coming into frequent contact with the plague-stricken around his residence.[44] In November 1526, news of the death of Süleyman's young son (presumably Abdullah) from plague was reported to Venice.[45] In early 1527, the outbreak must have been severe enough to generate false rumors that Süleyman himself died of plague, which even found their way into Venice.[46] In early May 1527, Venetian reports from Istanbul suggest that plague was once again increasing in intensity.[47] In July, *bailo* Pietro Zen wrote that plague was taking two hundred lives per day.[48] Toward the end of the decade, news of plague from Istanbul starts to appear anew in Venetian records. In late summer 1529, it was noted that the outbreak was abating,[49] which testifies to its presence, as usual, in the spring and summer months.

Given the sustained presence of the disease in the Mediterranean basin through the 1520s[50] and Istanbul's new position at the intersection of newly forging plague axes, this wave lasted until the end of the decade, with short intervals. An interesting connection can be noted between plague outbreaks in Istanbul and those experienced by the Ottoman army in Hungary. Venetian sources suggest there was plague in the Ottoman army encampments in 1526.[51] As a matter of fact, Süleyman was again on a military expedition

---

[42]   Ibid., 40:826.
[43]   Ibid., 40:894.
[44]   Ibid., 41:534.
[45]   Ibid., 43:473.
[46]   Ibid., 44:263.
[47]   Ibid., 45:291.
[48]   Ibid., 45:620.
[49]   Ibid., 52:60.
[50]   Plague continued in Continental Europe and in European port cities of the Mediterranean between 1522 and 1529. Between 1522 and 1528, it was in Ragusa and Spalato (Split) on the Dalmatian coast, as well as in all Italian cities. See Biraben, *Les hommes et la peste*, 1:397, 442; Sticker, *Abhandlungen*, 1:90. Further west, the epidemic continued to affect French and Spanish cities both on the Mediterranean coast and inland and occurred sporadically in North Africa between 1521 and 1522. See Biraben, *Les hommes et la peste*, 1:382, 391; Sadok Boubaker, "La peste dans les pays du Maghreb: attitudes face au fléau et impacts sur les activités commerciales (XVIe–XVIIIe siècles)," *Revue d'Histoire maghrébine* 79–80 (1995): 314. Plague was also seen in Herzegovina in 1529. See Biraben, *Les hommes et la peste*, 1:442.
[51]   *Sanudo*, 42:653.

to Hungary in 1529.[52] It has been suggested that the infection was carried there by Ottoman troops.[53]

Overall, it is clear that this wave displays major differences from the outbreaks of the First Phase. The simultaneous presence of plague in several locations in western Anatolia littoral and on the Aegean coast, as well as in Epirus, Morea, the Ionian Sea, and the Archipelago, is certainly indicative that a new plague network was forged in the 1520s and fast integrated into the existing east-west network. This new interconnectedness of Istanbul to the eastern Mediterranean ports made outbreaks of plague occur simultaneously in various locations of the empire, not necessarily in a linear pattern of spread. This pattern became even more complicated as the century progressed, as seen in the analysis of the following waves of epidemic activity.

The Second Wave (1533–1549)

In this new wave, plague spread quickly around the Mediterranean, creating interesting connections between seemingly disparate places, such as Venice, Syria, and Cyprus (under Venetian control). For example, the infection was in Venice in 1532 and 1533 with all its strength,[54] before it moved to Ragusa, where it continued until 1534.[55] On the eastern end of the Mediterranean, it was in Cyprus, as evidenced by letters sent to Venice. A report dated March 28, 1533, suggested that the pestilence came from Syria, killed two hundred in Famagusta, and continued through the spring. A second report (dated May 5) reported that the outbreak was very severe and killed eight hundred there, and that it had devastated Syria. A third report written three days earlier recorded that out of nine thousand inhabitants of the island, two thousand had already fled.[56] Plague's effects on the island seemed to be grave, despite the inconsistencies in the reports.[57]

While the pestilence was traveling in the Mediterranean, it did not take long before it reached Ottoman territory. Spreading eastward by way of

---

[52] Gilles Veinstein, "Süleyman," *EI²*.

[53] Plague was in Istanbul, Hungary, and Herzegovina. See Biraben, *Les hommes et la peste*, 1:109, 442.

[54] Ibid., 397. Sticker reports that in 1532 in Venice, thirty thousand people were stricken in one day, and a great majority of them died. Sticker, *Abhandlungen*, 1:91.

[55] *Sanudo*, 58:301; Biraben, *Les hommes et la peste*, 1:397, 442. At the same time, on the western end of the Mediterranean, plague was in Fez in 1533. See Boubaker, "La peste," 314.

[56] Ronald C. Jennings, *Christians and Muslims in Ottoman Cyprus and the Mediterranean World, 1571–1640* (New York: New York University Press, 1993), 184.

[57] Reports seem to disagree on the death toll. Whereas a letter indicates that 5,500 died in Famagusta, another letter informed Venice that 1,073 people died in five months. A third letter dated June 22 reports that two thousand died from plague. See Jennings, *Christians and Muslims*, 185.

sea, it was documented in the capital in mid-summer 1533.[58] Venetian reports noted that plague broke out with great severity, taking five hundred lives daily.[59] Repeated reports testify to its ruthless progress later that summer, forcing the Sultan to take refuge in Beykoz.[60] Despite the fragmentary nature of the data and the evident lacunae in them, it is still possible to observe that this wave of outbreaks displayed different characteristics than the waves before it. This wave of infection was intimately connected to Ottoman expansion and its immediate results. Once plague broke out in Istanbul in 1533, it quickly spread to the Balkans, Anatolia, Egypt, and Persia. The next year, it was in Athens, Morea, and Anatolia and in Egypt.[61] In 1535, while still in Istanbul, it was also in the Gilan province on the southern shores of the Caspian Sea.[62] This pattern of plague spread was quite unprecedented and as such deserves further elaboration.

First, the initial outbreak in Istanbul may be taken as indicative of its newly forged position as the prime recipient of infections circulating in the Mediterranean world. Unlike the previous episodes in which plague was introduced from the Balkans or at least via an intermediary point in the Aegean, the prime target of this wave was Istanbul. This implies its appearance at the nexus of east-west and north-south axes of the Mediterranean. Second, Istanbul emerges as the distributor of infection. For instance, the fast spread of plague to Egypt should hardly come as a surprise after the establishment of the north-south link in the eastern Mediterranean, connecting the two important metropolises of the empire. Third, Anatolia seems to have worked as a conduit between Istanbul and Persian lands. Such a function would not be possible in the absence of a unified network to enable the transmission of the infection to the adjacent networks. Fourth, it may be worth noting that plague most likely spread eastward from Anatolia to the Gilan province. Interestingly, this coincides with an eastern Ottoman campaign that was undertaken between 1533 and 1535, which supports a possible movement of plague along with the army. Venetian sources reported that plague broke in the Ottoman army encampments in summer 1533.[63] Istanbul was now forging a variety of commercial, administrative, and military links to Tabriz and further to the Persian Gulf, and beyond.

This wave of plague seems to have continued in Ottoman lands and adjacent regions.[64] In 1538, plague was in Istanbul and in Bursa, as testified

---

[58] *Sanudo,* 58:577; Sticker, *Abhandlungen,* 1:92.

[59] *Sanudo,* 58:625.

[60] Ibid., 58:636, 692, 699.

[61] McNeill, *Plagues and Peoples,* 334; Biraben, *Les hommes et la peste,* 1:431, 442–43; Dols, "Second Plague Pandemic," 186.

[62] Sticker, *Abhandlungen,* 1:92; Biraben, *Les hommes et la peste,* 1:443.

[63] *Sanudo,* 58:632.

[64] In the *sud-oriental* region, there was a time of renewed plague activity, after a period of remission of more than a decade between 1533 and 1545. See Sticker, *Abhandlungen,* 1:95.

by a cluster of plague deaths in court records.[65] The next year, Ayas Pasha, Süleyman's grand vizier, succumbed to plague on July 11, 1539.[66] Following this, the pestilence seems to have lingered in Istanbul for a few more years, where it has been recorded in 1541 and 1542.[67] In summer 1544, plague was again in the capital, as testified by the account of Jérôme Maurand, a French priest who accompanied the Ottoman fleet. When he went to the city in August, plague was killing about five hundred a day, which caused many to take refuge in the vineyards outside Galata.[68]

Plague can also be documented in Anatolia and the Balkans around that time.[69] An order issued on March 4, 1545, confirmed the flight of soldiers from the fortress of Hınıs (in the Erzurum province) on account of plague.[70] Plague continued to appear around the Mediterranean in the first half of the decade.[71] Toward the end of it, mortality was clearly in decline, with outbreaks only seen in Istanbul, Sofia, and Thessaloniki in 1547, as testified by the accounts of travelers.[72] The last recorded presence of plague in this wave

Plague seems to have paused for about a decade in Europe. Plague in France was weak between 1535 and 1541. No plague in Spain between 1533 and 1540. No outbreak in Italy between 1537 and 1547. Overall, there was a period of decline or remission of plague in Europe between 1532 and 1542, in general. See Biraben, *Les hommes et la peste*, 1:367, 383, 391, 398, 443; Boubaker, "La peste," 314.

[65] Evidence from the court registers of Bursa attests to the registration of deaths of novice janissary boys due to plague. For example, for the death of Davud in the village of Çavuş, see Bursa Şeriye Sicilleri, A 40/45, 29a, 19 Ramazan 944/February 19, 1538 [cited in OS 2:40, doc.62]; for the deaths of Hızır and İlyas in Bursa, see Bursa Şeriye Sicilleri, A 40/45, 29b/1, 19 Ramazan 944/February 19, 1538 [cited in OS 2:40–41, doc.63]; for the death of Hüseyin in Bursa, see Bursa Şeriye Sicilleri, A 40/45, 29b/2, 19 Ramazan 944/February 19, 1538 [cited in OS 2:41, doc.64]. Also see Sticker, *Abhandlungen*, 1:92; Biraben, *Les hommes et la peste*, 1:443.

[66] Ünver, "Türkiyede Veba (Taun) Tarihçesi Üzerine," 74; Biraben, *Les hommes et la peste*, 1:443.

[67] Sticker, *Abhandlungen*, 1:93; Biraben, *Les hommes et la peste*, 1:443; Orhan Kılıç, *Genel Hatlarıyla Dünyada ve Osmanlı Devleti'nde Salgın Hastalıklar* (Elazığ: Fırat Üniversitesi Rektörlüğü, 2004), 47n10.

[68] Jérome Maurand, *Itinéraire de Jérome Maurand d'Antibes à Constantinople* (Paris: E. Leroux, 1901), 204–5, 224–27, 236–37.

[69] In the Balkans, plague was reported in Bosnia, Skopje, and Herzegovina in 1541. Plague was in Bosnia in 1543 and in Ragusa from 1543 to 1545. In 1545, it was in Herzegovina, Mostar, Neretva, and Thessaly. See Biraben, *Les hommes et la peste*, 1:443.

[70] Halil Sahillioğlu, ed., *Topkapı Sarayı Arşivi, H. 951–952 Tarihli ve E-12321 Numaralı Mühimme Defteri* (Istanbul: IRCICA, 2002), 235–36, 272.

[71] In western Mediterranean regions, plague was seen in Oran every year between 1542 and 1545. See Boubaker, "La peste," 315; Sticker, *Abhandlungen*, 1:93; plague in Oran in 1542; Biraben, *Les hommes et la peste*, 1:431.

[72] In 1547, plague was in Sofia. See Jean Chesneau, *Le Voyage de Monsieur d'Aramon ambassadeur pour le Roy en Levant escript par noble homme Jean Chesneau l'un des secrétaires dudict seigneur ambassadeur* (Paris: E. Leroux, 1887), 12–13. Also see Biraben, *Les hommes et la peste*, 1:443. He notes plague in Istanbul and Sofia in 1547. Belon noted the plague in Thessaloniki. See Yerasimos, *Les voyageurs*, 34.

seems to be in Tabriz in the year 1549, where it caused great mortality. Yet it is difficult to establish its connection to other outbreaks. One possibility, as suggested by chronicler Hasan Rumlu, was that it was brought there by the Ottoman army.[73]

Outbreaks of this wave continued assuming new patterns of dissemination, most heavily in Istanbul but also elsewhere in the empire and sometimes simultaneously in regions as far away as Persia and the Balkans. Owing to lack of information, it is not always easy to trace the precise itinerary of each year's plague. It is possible, however, to see the new patterns of plague spread, the effects of the multiple new trajectories, and new areas that opened up for infection. Perhaps the most complex and central of these networks was in Anatolia.

The Anatolian Urban Network

With the eastern conquests of Selim I, an important part of southeast Anatolia, Syria, and the eastern Mediterranean coast was incorporated into Ottoman dominions. Eastward expansion also continued under his son Süleyman, whose first eastern military expedition was undertaken in 1533–36, which resulted in the capture of Bitlis, Erzurum, and Van[74] in eastern Anatolia and in the short-lived conquest of Tabriz and Baghdad. Consequently, by the 1530s, Anatolia had become a relatively integrated area under Ottoman rule. Anatolia also experienced an overall population increase (especially a dramatic rise in its urban population) and the rise of an urban network. All of these factors contributed to the spread of plague much more effectively than before. In the First Phase, as we have seen, plagues diffused relatively sparsely into central and eastern Anatolia; but starting with the Second Phase, Anatolia began to suffer more intensely from widespread outbreaks.

To discern how plague might have spread in Anatolia, it may be useful to examine the development of urban centers and the networks that connected them. The scholarship has already highlighted the significant rise of an urban network in Anatolia in the 1520s, accompanied with a surge in urban population that roughly doubled in about a half-century. It has been demonstrated that the sixteenth century was a time of unusual growth for Anatolian towns, in which most towns almost doubled their taxpaying populations.[75] Nevertheless, it is important to consider the population

---

[73] Hasan Rumlu, *A Chronicle of the Early Ṣafawīs*, ed. and trans. C. N. Seddon (Baroda: Oriental Institute, 1931–34), 153.

[74] Van was lost to the Safavids the following year, only to be conquered again in 1548. See Veinstein, "Süleyman."

[75] In 1520, Bursa and Ankara were the only cities of large size, with populations of more than ten thousand. By 1580, eight more cities had reached that size: Konya, Kayseri, Kastamonu, Tokat, Sivas, Urfa, Ayntab, and Aleppo. See Faroqhi, *Towns and Townsmen*, 1, 14; Jennings, "Urban Population in Anatolia in the Sixteenth Century," 21.

growth in Anatolia in conjunction with that of Istanbul. A city of about half a million people in the mid-sixteenth century, Istanbul had a substantial transforming economic impact on Anatolian towns. As its economy depended on the industries of its hinterland, Istanbul had a power in shaping the crafts and industries, and thus the size, of Anatolian towns. Yet the increase in Istanbul's population was sometimes caused by migrations from Anatolia, especially in times of crises, such as during epidemics.[76]

In the sixteenth century, the Anatolian towns became closely connected, with administrative, military, and commercial contacts with each other, on one hand, and with the capital, on the other. By the mid-sixteenth century, mainland Anatolia was administratively divided into provinces, which were further divided into administrative-military districts – all tied to the central administration in the capital.[77] This was essential for a steady flow of information back and forth between the provinces and the center. The towns and cities of Anatolia were connected with a web of maritime and overland routes to the capital. Official couriers ran back and forth between the center and the provinces, especially for confidential communication. The center sent state officials and administrators to look after various types of duties in the provinces. There were merchants accompanying caravans loaded with goods going back and forth between the provinces and the center. Travelers, envoys, pilgrims, and imperial troops also followed these routes. All this movement and mobility could only be possible on a well-maintained network of roads.

The Anatolian road system in the sixteenth century comprised roads followed by caravans and armies as well as alternative routes used by couriers, ambassadors, travelers, and pilgrims.[78] Drawing from campaign records and travelers' itineraries of the sixteenth century, Stefanos Yerasimos produced a detailed study of roads. According to this, the Anatolian network linked Istanbul to the cities of northern Persia, which can be analyzed in four main segments. The first segment of the land road connected Tabriz to Erzurum in multiple trajectories. An important city in the east, Tabriz was where caravans left westward. Upon reaching Erzurum, caravans had to pay customs there before moving further west. Erzurum was connected to Istanbul via three different trajectories constituting the second, third, and fourth segments of the land-road system of Anatolia: a northern, middle, and southern route. The northern route, though shorter, was not preferred by the military because of its high altitude and rugged terrain. It was the couriers

---

[76] Faroqhi, *Towns and Townsmen*, 14–15; İnalcık, "Istanbul."

[77] Halil İnalcık, *The Ottoman Empire: The Classical Age 1300–1600*, trans. Norman Itzkowitz and Colin Imber (London: Weidenfeld and Nicolson, 1973), 106. Also see Pitcher, *Osmanlı İmparatorluğu'nun Tarihsel Coğrafyası*, Map 25.

[78] The earliest systematic study of Ottoman roads was undertaken by historian Franz Taeschner, based on the accounts of Evliya Çelebi and Katip Çelebi, and on military campaign records. Faroqhi, *Towns and Townsmen*, 63n94, 63–64, notes 95, 97–99.

who preferred to follow this shorter route. The middle route was mostly preferred by caravans going to Istanbul and Bursa, connecting three of the most important commercial centers of sixteenth-century Anatolia, namely, Tokat, Ankara, and Bursa. The southern route was the military road, one of the most important routes that crossed Anatolia, with frequent caravanserai stops, especially on its northwestern part. That part of the road was also used as a pilgrimage route, which continued southeast toward Aleppo. As the third largest Ottoman city after Istanbul and Cairo, Aleppo's connection to the capital was important. This was a principal artery of the sixteenth-century road system of the Ottoman Empire because it united commercial, military, and pilgrimage routes, used as much by Christian visitors to Jerusalem as by Muslim pilgrims to Mecca and Medina.[79]

The roads that crisscrossed Anatolia were vital for the commercial, administrative, military, and religious mobilities of the empire. Even though land routes were notoriously dangerous (robbers, abusive tax collectors, administrators, madrasa students, and rebels), the Ottoman administration took great care for their safety and maintenance. For this purpose, the inhabitants of certain villages located on the main roads were appointed as pass guards, responsible for the security of roads in return for exemption from certain taxes and holding the privilege of carrying firearms. On a presumably safe and well-maintained web of roads, local, regional, and long-distance trade flourished in Ottoman Anatolia starting in the second half of the sixteenth century. The backbone of regional and long-distance commerce was the overland caravan trade, which consisted of camels for transporting loads and of horses reserved for the use of people. Mules, donkeys, and oxen were also used to carry people or cargo. Wheeled carts were limited to local transportation, as they were not suitable for long distances. The movement of a caravan in Anatolia was rather slow but unobstructed. For example, once a caravan paid the customs, then it could freely travel as far west as Bursa, Istanbul, and in some cases even to the Balkans.[80] Hence, caravans facilitated long-distance movement of people, animals, and goods. In doing so, they bridged different ecological zones. They also stopped in designated locations along the way and acquired food and other necessities for themselves and for their animals. In various ways, they interacted with local people and also likely facilitated the movement of plague. In this context, it may be important to remember that camels can host plague.[81]

[79] Yerasimos, *Les voyageurs*, 59–66. As discussed in Chapter 3, plague moved along this trajectory during the Black Death.
[80] Faroqhi, *Towns and Townsmen*, 50–51, 52–54, 56–57; Faroqhi, "Sixteenth-Century Periodic Markets in Various Anatolian *sancaks*, İçel, Hamid, Karahisar-ı Sahib, Kütahya, Aydın, and Menteşe," *JESHO* 22, no. 1 (1979): 71; Xavier de Planhol, "Le boeuf porteur dans le Proche-Orient et l'Afrique du Nord," *JESHO* 12, no. 3 (1969): 317–18.
[81] See Chapter 1.

In addition to overland caravan trade, there was a limited degree of maritime commercial activity in sixteenth-century Anatolia. Despite the apparent urban growth, there were no major port cities, except Trabzon, Sinop, and Antalya, all of which were of moderate size. Generally speaking, in the sixteenth century, the Ottoman port cities were almost exclusively involved in regional, but not in international, trade. This was mostly due to the fact that Istanbul served as a hub both for overland and maritime trade and for distribution of goods, which made other ports dependent on it. At this time Ottoman port cities did not have a resident foreign merchant community, which would have fostered opportunities for international trade. It was only in the late sixteenth century that new port cities started to emerge on the Mediterranean coast of Anatolia, such as İskenderun and Silifke, and they were quickly connected to the existing networks of land routes.[82]

The Eastern Mediterranean Network
The military expeditions undertaken by Süleyman in the second third of the century resulted in expanding the Ottoman control in the east significantly. Most important, they secured Iraq for Ottoman rule, which now extended over Baghdad, Basra, and the Persian Gulf. This meant that the Ottomans had direct access to the Indian Ocean. This moment had political, economic, and ecological implications. For our particular purposes here, it is important because it opened up a new channel for the communication of plague.

The route that connected the Persian Gulf to the Mediterranean had been of prime importance for trade since antiquity. However, it lost its vitality in the mid-thirteenth century as a result of Mongol conquests. Hence, the bulk of the trans-Asian trade shifted to either the northern route through Central Asia or the southern route from the Indian Ocean to the Red Sea and Egypt. After three centuries of relative inactivity, this route was revived under Ottoman rule and restored, once again, to prime importance. This was also in tandem with the development of ports on the eastern Mediterranean coast (e.g., Tripoli, İskenderun). This new route was quickly integrated into the urban network of Anatolia, largely as a result of the connection provided by the main pilgrimage and caravan route between Istanbul and Aleppo. As a hub, Aleppo was connected by caravan routes to Baghdad, Basra, and the Persian Gulf, on one hand, and to Tabriz by military and commercial routes, on the other. Aleppo was also connected to other major centers, such as Damascus, Jerusalem, and, more important, Cairo, which was a major hub.[83] Cairo was the starting point of the pilgrimage and caravan route that connected it to Jerusalem, on one hand, and to Mecca and Medina, on the other. In this context, it may be helpful to remember that the Ottoman administration, with claims to be the protectors of Muslim holy cities, took

---

[82] Faroqhi, *Towns and Townsmen*, 76n9.
[83] Yerasimos, *Les voyageurs*, 72–76, 80–84.

great care to maintain safety along the pilgrimage route. It worked to secure the roads and provide food and water for pilgrims in places where these were not available. Safer pilgrimage routes attracted more pilgrims and also stimulated trade, which made this route also a caravan route. As a result, Mecca and Medina became active markets with goods brought along this trade and pilgrimage route as well as exotic goods brought from India.[84]

The integration of the eastern Mediterranean network into the other networks of the empire has important implications for plague. This integration allowed an increased degree of interconnectedness in a vast region that extended from the Persian Gulf to the Mediterranean ports of Europe and North Africa. A tightly knit network of land and sea routes enabled the unobstructed flow of people, animals, and goods, and of plague between different ecological zones that were not in direct contact with each other previously.

The Black Sea Network

The Ottoman conquests along the Black Sea coast (e.g., Trabzon, Crimea) brought some degree of connection in the second half of the fifteenth century. This was further solidified in the sixteenth century by the annexation of lower Moldavia and the conquest of the coastal strip of the lower Danube. This was of great significance militarily because it allowed land contact with the vassal Khanate of Crimea and an easier overland passage of cavalry for joining the Ottoman army at times of campaign.[85] Further attempts to unite the region under Ottoman rule helped consolidate the Black Sea network by the mid-sixteenth century. This network secured not only diplomatic and commercial connections but also the pilgrimage route that came from Central Asia. To be sure, the effects of the unification became rapidly visible in the distribution of plagues in the Second Phase.

As elsewhere, new areas brought together with conquest and ruled by a centralized empire facilitated the flow of people, animals, and goods. In particular, the link between Caffa and Istanbul was the proverbial link of the Black Sea, already firmly in place before this era, as testified in the spread of the initial wave of the Black Death in the mid-fourteenth century. The was the main channel for the shipment of cotton goods, mohair, and silk as well as olives, olive oil, wine, and raisins to Crimea in return for wheat, tallow, clarified butter, fish, salt, and slaves. This connection overpowered the contacts between other Black Sea ports of secondary importance. In the sixteenth century, the ports along the northern Anatolia forged improved maritime links with Istanbul. Customs registers of 1533–34 show that three-fourths

---

[84] Faroqhi, *Towns and Townsmen*, 55; Yerasimos, *Les voyageurs*, 77–78, 84–87; Pitcher, *Osmanlı İmparatorluğu'nun Tarihsel Coğrafyası*, Map 34.

[85] Caroline Finkel, *Osman's Dream: the History of the Ottoman Empire, 1300–1923* (New York: Basic Books, 2006), 129; Veinstein, "Süleyman."

of all maritime traffic at the port of Amasra, for example, was directly with Istanbul. Those ports were instrumental for supplying the capital with major trade items like wood and various types of foodstuffs, including honey, butter, and walnuts, as well as beeswax and linseed oil.[86] Commercial links seem to have triggered urban development as well. For example, the Anatolian port cities on the Black Sea coast, such as Trabzon and Sinop, benefited from these newly emerging connections, especially with their links to the capital. Eventually they both became important urban centers and served as trade entrepôts.

The Black Sea network emerged as a tightly knit system of connections comprising not only the port cities along its shores but also their hinterlands, which meant the integration of a wide variety of disease ecologies. With respect to plague, this meant that possible enzootic foci in Moldavia and Wallachia, the Caucasus, and along the shores of the Caspian Sea were connected to port cities of the Black Sea and those along the Danube. However, most important, this system was integrated into other plague networks of the empire. For example, the link between Caffa and Istanbul was now integrated into the north-south link between Istanbul and Egypt. Therefore, with the integration and consolidation of these new plague networks, an uninterrupted connection between the Black Sea region and Egypt and the eastern Mediterranean was possible. This system of networks came to replace the late medieval trade partnership between the beneficiaries of the Pax Mongolica and the Genoese, Venetians, and Mamluks.[87] Now, the Black Sea region was also integrated into the Anatolian network, especially through the Anatolian port cities on the Black Sea coast and their overland links to the Anatolian road system. All of these connections showed their effects on more diverse and complicated trajectories and wider dissemination of plague for the rest of the century. This second wave (1533–49) demonstrates many of the new features of plague spread, in particular with regard to its coverage of a wider area, its influence over previously unexposed places, its decreased intervals, and its complex patterns of propagation.

The Third Wave (1552–1568)

The third wave is the best documented in the Second Phase. An unmistakable feature of the outbreaks in this wave is their increased frequency – perhaps an artifact of better documentation. Between the 1550s and 1570s, outbreaks began to be ever more recurrent, paving the way for patterns of plague persistence of the Third Phase (1570–1600) and beyond. Especially North Africa's experience of plague is illustrative of this wave's nature and span. A new wave of epidemics introduced to North Africa in the early 1550s lasted

---

[86] Faroqhi, *Towns and Townsmen*, 77, 92.
[87] Di Cosmo, "Black Sea Emporia and the Mongol Empire."

there for about two decades.[88] Examining the nature of sixteenth-century maritime interactions in the western Mediterranean promises to offer some clues about how this activity may be related to the plagues in other Ottoman areas.

Establishing a north-south communication in the eastern Mediterranean was important for the Ottomans in securing their power in the region. The increased Ottoman maritime presence in the Mediterranean in the sixteenth century was not limited to the building of an armada. It also entailed assisting and sponsoring piracy activities – an integral part of seafaring in the early modern Mediterranean.[89] Even though the links between plague and early modern piracy in the Mediterranean are largely unexplored, Biraben suggested that the Mediterranean Sea served as the principal medium of epidemiological exchange between different disease ecologies. He stressed that the maritime propagation of the plague in the Mediterranean increased considerably in the sixteenth century as a result of the expansion of the region in which pirates were most active, starting from 1518.[90] As a matter of fact, there does seem to be a link between Ottoman conquests and piracy in the Mediterranean. After the incorporation of the Mamluk Empire into Ottoman domains, Selim I appointed Hayreddin Barbarossa (d. 1546) as the governor of Algiers, who would later be appointed as the naval captain of the imperial fleet during the reign of Süleyman. Over the course of the sixteenth century, the Ottoman navy under his command attacked several coastal towns in central and western Mediterranean. The rise of Ottoman sea power in the Mediterranean, the sponsorship of piracy activities, and the interaction and competition with other political and commercial actors of the Mediterranean world showed their effects especially in the outbreaks between 1552 and 1568 in North African port cities.

Such being the case, the plague in the western Mediterranean rapidly found its way to core Ottoman areas. In 1553–54, a series of outbreaks affected Istanbul, Bursa, Edirne, the Balkans, and the Black Sea area.[91] According to Hans Dernschwam, plague was in Istanbul in spring 1554.[92] It seems to have affected Bursa in the summer months.[93] Busbecq mentioned

---

[88] Biraben, *Les hommes et la peste*, 1:432. Boubaker, "La peste," 315; Sticker, *Abhandlungen*, 1:96–97.

[89] So much so that toward the end of the century, the piracy activities caused great losses to the Venetians and gradually ruined their commercial supremacy in the early decades of the seventeenth century. See Alberto Tenenti, *Piracy and the Decline of Venice, 1580–1615*, trans. Janet and Brian Pullan (Berkeley: University of California Press, 1967).

[90] Biraben, *Les hommes et la peste*, 1:106, 109. However, he thinks that 1536 marks a demarcation line in the epidemics of the region *nord-occidental*. He suggested that the frequency of plague outbreaks between 1347 and 1536 was different than the frequency after 1536. See Biraben, *Les hommes et la peste*, 1:121.

[91] Ibid., 428, 443; Sticker, *Abhandlungen*, 1:96.

[92] Dernschwam, *Seyahat Günlüğü*, 104–5.

[93] Hızır, a novice janissary, died of plague in Bursa in summer 1554. See Ünver, "Buğdan Voyvodası Oğlunun Vebadan Ölümü," *Türk Tıp Tarihi Arkivi* 12 (1939): 147–50.

that a man from his retinue contracted the plague near Edirne and died, probably in the early days of 1555, which then spread among others in his service and caused great terror.[94] It is possible that they acquired the infection in one of the places they passed through on their way.[95] The same year, plague was also said to be in Aleppo and its surroundings, killing a great number of people.[96] In 1556, Edirne continued to suffer from plague. Victims included the court pages of the imperial palace. When a number of them fell ill, they were assigned a daily allowance of food.[97] In addition to Edirne, plague was also recorded in several Balkan and Mediterranean towns around that time.[98] In 1559, perhaps even earlier, the presence of plague in the Balkan towns located on the main route connecting Istanbul to Buda is attested in *mühimme* orders. Had it not been due to the difficulty experienced by the local villagers of Popost and Kekenç in providing two courier horses as a result of the flight of the local population on account of plague, we would not have heard about this outbreak.[99] In 1560 and in summer 1561, plague was in Istanbul, as testified by the account of Busbecq. His account relates how plague killed one of his servants and his doctor, upon which he became anxious and left the city for Princes' Islands, where he stayed for almost three months to be secure from the outbreak.[100] According to another eyewitness, there were eighty thousand deaths in the month of August alone in and around Istanbul.[101] The outbreak of 1561 also affected the Balkans.[102] It was probably around this time that the local market in the town of Salona, in southern Thessaly, ceased to meet because of plague and the flight of the locals.[103] In 1562, plague was in Edirne and Budapest as well as in Istanbul.[104] In 1564, it was recorded in Aleppo,[105] Istanbul,[106] and Thessaloniki,[107] and in 1565 in the province of Karaman in Anatolia.

---

[94] Busbecq, *Turkish Letters*, 68–69.

[95] Biraben, *Les hommes et la peste*, 1:443. In 1554, plague was in Transylvania, Istanbul, Edirne, and Athens; in 1555, it was in Buda, Hungary, Athens, Sofia, and Serbia.

[96] *Albèri*, 1:219.

[97] MD 2, 21/188 (3 Rebiülahir 963 H./February 15, 1556).

[98] Biraben, *Les hommes et la peste*, 1:443; Sticker, *Abhandlungen*, 1:99.

[99] Kılıç, *Genel hatlarıyla*, 45–46n6.

[100] Biraben, *Les hommes et la peste*, 1:443; Busbecq, *Turkish Letters*, 180, 182–90.

[101] *Albèri*, 3:208.

[102] Biraben, *Les hommes et la peste*, 1:443.

[103] MD 4, 192/2009 (29 Cemaziyelahir 968 H./March 17, 1561).

[104] Biraben, *Les hommes et la peste*, 1:443; Gülgün Üçel-Aybet, *Avrupalı Seyyahların Gözünden Osmanlı Dünyası ve İnsanları (1530–1699)* (Istanbul: İletişim, 2003), 528.

[105] Kılıç, *Genel hatlarıyla*, 46n8.

[106] Biraben, *Les hommes et la peste*, 1:443.

[107] Considerably more detail is known about the outbreak of plague in Thessaloniki, which was an important hub in the Balkans for the production and distribution of woolen cloth. The town was especially vulnerable to infection coming from outside because it was located at the intersection of overland trade routes of the Balkans and the maritime routes of the Mediterranean and the Aegean. A series of documents help identify the plague experience of Thessaloniki in conjunction with its woolen-textile industry. See my "Plague, Conflict,

A *mühimme* order sent to the governor of Beyşehir commended him to seek out some criminals in central Anatolian towns. During these investigations, the latter heard news of plague in the province of Karaman and sent a letter to the center asking for permission to postpone the search on account of plague. He reported that the inhabitants of the province had fled to areas they heard were safe from the plague.[108] Another case of plague in the same year comes from Istanbul. The butchers had fled, leaving the city's means for producing and processing meat in disarray. The *kadı* of Istanbul was asked to have them found and brought back to duty.[109]

Plague and flight from it also caused problems in Trabzon during 1565 and 1566. As an important port city on the eastern Black Sea coast and an entrepôt on the route connecting Istanbul to Tabriz, Trabzon was repeatedly exposed to the infection. Evidence from local court records suggests that plague started at least a few months before the first recorded cases in the registers dating from early spring 1565, lasting into the next year. Most of the records point to plague's disruptive effects on trade and the flight of the local population in fear, including members of the *askeri* class.[110] Another testimony of plague in December 1565 comes from the region south of Lake Van in eastern Anatolia. According to the account of Affonso, who was traveling from India to Portugal through Ottoman domains, Edremit and surrounding villages south of Lake Van were deserted due to plague.[111] In spring 1566, plague must have been so widespread in the Aegean that the island of Sakız (Chios) requested that merchant ships wait before entering its port on account of the plague.[112] Shortly afterward, plague made a big spectacle in the capital. Evliya Çelebi mentions a plague with exceptional mortality during the reign of Selim II (r. 1566–74). The fact that he mentions Beşiktaşi Yahya Efendi (d. 1571) preaching for relief against plague makes it

and Negotiation: The Jewish Broadcloth Weavers of Salonica and the Ottoman Central Administration in the Late Sixteenth Century," *Jewish History* 28, nos. 3–4 (2014): 261-88.

[108] MD 5, 156/369 (22 Rebiülevvel 973 H./October 17, 1565).

[109] Kılıç, *Genel Hatlarıyla*, 48n13. Plague was in Thessaly and Volos the same year. See Biraben, *Les hommes et la peste*, 1:443.

[110] Jennings, "Plague in Trabzon."

[111] Yerasimos, *Les voyageurs*, 83, 270–71.

[112] It was stated that merchants suspected of coming from plague-infested places were incarcerated in Chios for twenty-five days and charged two *akçes* for each day. An order sent from Istanbul commanded that detaining Muslim merchants was not acceptable; instead it recommends keeping them waiting in a different location. See MD 5, 492/1334 (4 Ramazan 973 H./March 26, 1566). Ships coming through Istanbul had an easier option of obtaining bills of health from the Venetian *bailo* in Istanbul. To avoid waiting in Venetian and other ports, ships or travelers were asked to obtain bills of health from the Venetian *bailo* in Istanbul before leaving the city. Such a document was accepted not only in Venice but also in other ports of the Mediterranean, including the Ottoman ports. See Eric R. Dursteler, "The Bailo in Constantinople: Crisis and Career in Venice's Early Modern Diplomatic Corps," *Mediterranean Historical Review* 16, no. 2 (2001): 7.

likely to date the outbreak to some time between 1566 and 1571,[113] possibly to the year 1567.[114] It appears that the infection moved west from Istanbul to Edirne and then spread to various places in the Balkans. Shortly before it broke out in Thessaloniki in early summer 1568, there is evidence for its appearance in the Black Sea town of Vize.[115]

Conclusion

Of the three phases examined here, the second is least well documented by contemporary sources with respect to plague; documentation only becomes more prolific after the mid-century. In the three waves of this phase – the first (1520–29), the second (1533–49), and the last (1552–68) – plague was present in at least one, sometimes multiple locations during forty-four years out of the total fifty-three years of this phase – a presence that yields a ratio of 83 percent. Stated differently, during the Second Phase, plague can be documented in the empire for eight years in every decade. Compared to the figures of the First Phase, it becomes clear that the overall presence of plague in the Ottoman Empire doubled in the Second Phase. It may nevertheless be useful to remember that this increased presence cannot be attributed to better documentation; except for the last decade of this phase, documentation is rather scant. In addition to overall increased incidence, it seems that plague also became more frequent in the Second Phase. The intervals between recurring waves decreased to an average of about three years in this phase, as opposed to an interval of about ten years in the First Phase.

In the Second Phase, plague spread to a greater area. In some years, the presence of the infection in places that may seem entirely unrelated makes it necessary to explore the larger constellations of links connecting those areas for making epidemic spread possible. This era witnessed the emergence of multiple networks of trade and communication in Ottoman lands or the revival of those that had lost their vitality in the preceding centuries. This phenomenon was related to new conquests of the period and the development of new urban centers. After the conquests of Egypt and Syria in 1516–17 and of Rhodes in 1522, a north-south connection in the eastern Mediterranean emerged – a connection that facilitated the provisioning of

---

[113] Evliya Çelebi, *Seyahatnâme*, 1:56–57.

[114] The date of this outbreak can be accepted as 1567, which is the only date recorded by Biraben for plague in Istanbul between 1566 and 1571. See Biraben, *Les hommes et la peste*, 1:443.

[115] The outbreak seems to be already over in Vize by the middle of May 1568. See *7 Numaralı Mühimme Defteri (975–976/1567–1569): özet-transkripsiyon-indeks*, ed. Hacı Osman Yıldırım et al. (Ankara: T. C. Başbakanlık Devlet Arşivleri Genel Müdürlüğü, 1998), 122 (May 13, 1568), 228 (June 29, 1568). In 1569, it was also seen in Herzegovina and Plevlje. Biraben, *Les hommes et la peste*, 1:443.

Istanbul from Egypt in particular. This north-south connection was immediately integrated into the east-west axis profiled in the previous chapter. Other newly forged networks, that is to say, an Anatolian network, an eastern Mediterranean network, and a Black Sea network, joined this complex system of interconnectedness. The rise of competitive piracy, which developed throughout the sixteenth century in the central and western Mediterranean, also seems to have contributed to the further dissemination of epidemics. All of these new trajectories were quickly integrated into one another and consolidated during the Second Phase to produce a more complex pattern of epidemic distribution and more frequently recurring outbreaks.

These networks not only connected port cities and their urban populations to one another. In fact, the ecological implications of these connections are much beyond that. What is more or less visible in the sources is the movement of people, animals, and goods. Yet the invisible protagonists of plague (e.g., commensal rodents, ectoparasites, and the plague bacterium itself) also moved along the very same connections. The resulting total effect is not an unexpected one: the capital effect, in other words, in working as a magnet, Istanbul attracted more plagues. As we will see in the next chapter, starting in the 1570s, Istanbul became the plague hub of the empire. As the point of convergence of the empire's plague networks, the capital received, magnified, and distributed outbreaks of plague.

6

The Third Phase (1570–1600)

Istanbul as Plague Hub

At Constantinople fire devours your goods, plague takes your wife, and women your wit.[1]

In Pera sono tre malanni: peste, fuoco, dragomanni.[2]

This chapter explores the emergence of Istanbul as the plague hub of the empire in the Third Phase – a phenomenon that left its legacy on the empire's post-1600 plague history. As the empire's "plague hub," Istanbul received and redistributed plague across the wide span of the empire. This may be considered in analogy with airline hubs, in which the airline transmits passengers, goods, and information from place to place only through the hub. In other words, the best explanation of the spread of epidemics throughout the empire is not that they arose in isolation from one another, or that they spread pell-mell from one place to another without a central nexus. Instead, the hub of the empire permitted plague, along with trade and even information about the plague, to spread rapidly between otherwise unconnected regions. Nevertheless, Istanbul was not a simple conduit for the passage of the infection. By virtue of its having one of the largest populations in the early modern Mediterranean world, it very likely amplified the infections that it received as well. The large number of human (and perhaps equally large number of rodent) hosts likely led to faster bacterial reproduction.[3]

---

[1] A proverb that comes from a nineteenth-century Ottoman house in Cyprus; quoted in Netice Yıldız, "Ottoman Decorative Arts in Cyprus," *Proceedings of the 11th International Congress of Turkish Art, Utrecht, the Netherlands, August 23–28, 1999*, ed. Machiel Kiel, Nico Landman, and Hans Theunissen (Utrecht: Universiteit Utrecht, 2001), 8.

[2] "The three perils in Pera are plague, fire, and interpreters." See M. L. Shay, *The Ottoman Empire from 1720 to 1734 as Revealed in Dispatches of the Venetian Baili* (Urbana: University of Illinois Press, 1944), 38, quoted in Nigel Webb and Caroline Webb, *The Earl and His Butler in Constantinople: The Secret Diary of an English Servant among the Ottomans* (London: I. B. Tauris, 2009), 22.

[3] See Chapter 1.

The rise of Istanbul as the hub of the empire was a gradual process that took shape over the course of the long sixteenth century. During the Second Phase, the capital fully developed in significance as a trading center as well as a political, administrative, and cultural center. However, perhaps most important, it was sustained by a constant influx of foodstuff, raw materials, livestock, and immigrant labor that came from its hinterland, near or far. The empire's administration took great care, for example, that staple food items (e.g., bread) would be available to the public. In a similar manner, it regulated the bringing of livestock to the capital so as to ensure the availability of meat in the market. In effect, the flow of all types of raw material – ranging from wood to metal, and finished products, both for common use and luxury consumption – was regulated by this centralized empire. Istanbul, as the center, was always the beneficiary of such regulations. However, the regulated flow of goods, animals, and even people (as seen in cases of forced resettlements) sometimes brought along "unwelcome companions" – to borrow a term from archeologist Philip Armitage.[4] In this case, the outcome of such experimental ecological engineering was the plague.

As the epigraphs to the chapter stress, Istanbul's plagues and fires were notorious. Many contemporary observers of the early modern era emphasized the city's frequent exposure to epidemic disease and other misfortunes. But how did Istanbul earn this unenviable reputation? Even though the strategic location of the city at the intersection of maritime and overland trade routes made it always vulnerable to the introduction of new waves of infection, the transition of Istanbul from a city with sporadic outbursts of disease to the plague hub of the empire is an interesting historical process that deserves close scrutiny. Stated differently, the periodic visitations of plague to Istanbul in the First and Second phases turned this disease into a permanent – perceived as "endemic" – presence in the city starting in the 1570s, something that continued at varying degrees until the nineteenth century, giving the imperial city its notorious reputation. From the point of view of historical epidemiology, the sustained presence of the plague in Istanbul may require an explanation. What we seem to identify in the case of Istanbul is that it assumed the function of an urban plague focus, that is, an ability to sustain the infection without the need for the infection being introduced and re-introduced each time from outside. However, without incoming infection, even if the city functioned like an urban focus sustaining the disease, plague would recur in predictable periodic cycles. Such periodicity was more or less the case for about the two centuries that followed the initial wave of the Black Death. Yet plague started to break out in Istanbul nearly every year in the second half of the sixteenth century – something that demands an explanation beyond locally sustained infections. Early modern

---

[4]   Philip L. Armitage, "Unwelcome Companions: Ancient Rats Reviewed," *Antiquity* 68, no. 259 (1994): 231–40.

Istanbul's experience of plague complicates historical processes of plague transmission, both locally and long distance. It may be necessary to explain such a persistent presence with a combination of transmission from local enzootic foci and the introduction and reintroduction of the infection from distant epidemic areas. The possibility of all of these factors seems to be have been present in Istanbul, which likely produced intensive results.

A number of sources testify that a new wave of plague came in 1570 and lasted, with brief periods of intermission – untraceable because of the lacunae in the sources – as a single wave until 1600, and may even have persisted well into the early decades of the seventeenth century. This chapter focuses on this wave of plague activity until the end of the sixteenth century. It studies the plague trajectories of the Third Phase in conjunction with those of the earlier phases to explore the factors that sustained the disease. It demonstrates that the multiple networks of trade and communication that developed in the previous phases were gradually integrated into each other and were eventually consolidated throughout the empire, with Istanbul at the center.

During this phase, every outbreak that took place in one part of the empire was carried either to or from this most powerful of cities, demonstrating the interconnectedness of the center to other parts of this massive but centralized empire. Whether an outbreak was in the Balkans or North African port cities, or in one of the Black Sea ports, it would then immediately be introduced to Istanbul. Similarly, as soon as the infection was in the capital, it would not take long to transmit to other parts of the empire. In the pre-1570 period, the networks of mobility had started undergoing a process of integration and consolidation. Yet it is after 1570 that they were in full contact with each other, via Istanbul, now the plague hub of the empire (Map 5).

Thanks to better documentation dating from the last decades of the sixteenth century, it is possible to follow the circulation of information about the plague throughout the empire, in addition to that of the plague itself. These documents demonstrate that the flow of information within the empire traveled along paths similar to those followed by plague, confirming Istanbul's position as the center of information. In respect of the evidence provided by these documents, the Third Phase is considerably different from the first two phases: they reveal so much more about the spread of plague and the circulation of information about it. In contrast to the earlier phases, it is possible to trace the presence and movement of plagues in this phase almost exclusively through Ottoman archival sources. At the core of these archival sources are *mühimme* registers (registers of important affairs), which are collections of orders sent from the central government in Istanbul to provincial administrators. As a result of the growing centralization and bureaucratization of the empire, these documents started being registered systematically in the second half of the sixteenth century. Typically, each document includes a brief summary of the petition received from a provincial administrator,

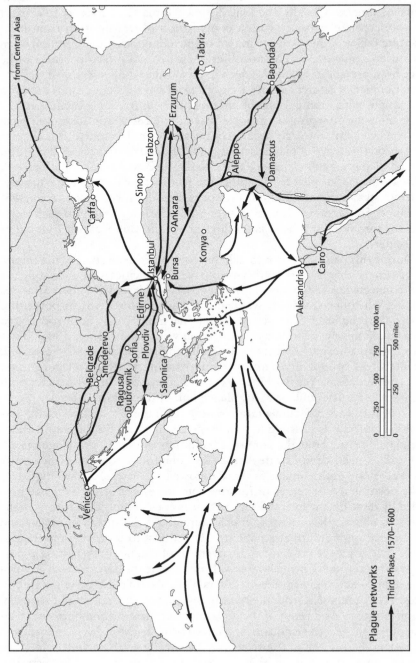

Plague networks

→ Third Phase, 1570–1600

MAP 5. Plague networks in the Third Phase, 1570–1600.

which is followed by the decree issuing from central administration. These orders are particularly useful for our purposes here. First, they facilitate tracing the movement of plague because they provide information about the local presence of the disease in the provinces from where they were sent. This piece of information can be found in the section in which the provincial administrator's petition is paraphrased. Second, the presence of these dated documents makes it clear that there was an active and prompt flow of information throughout the empire, both to and from the center. Receiving information about what is happening in the provinces enabled the center to effectively monitor needs and respond to them in a timely fashion. Last, the study of these documents reveals important clues about the response of the center. Depending on the nature of the petition, these responses could generally take the form of temporary exemption of local populations from certain taxes or other services for the empire. In addition to Ottoman archival documents, published cases from Islamic court registers were also used in this chapter, whenever a case related to plague occurred. The chapter also draws from Ottoman chronicles and travelogues in an effort to reconstruct as complete a temporal and spatial narrative of plague outbreaks between 1570 and 1600 as possible.

A Single Wave of Plague (1570–1600)?

The year 1570 marked the beginning of a series of relentless outbreaks. This time, plague affected a very large area in Europe, the Balkans, and the Mediterranean with unsurpassed severity.[5] For example, between 1571 and 1575, its presence in the Mediterranean and in Persia is known. In 1571 it was both in the west and in the east: in North Africa, in Dalmatia, and in Ardabil, southwest of the Caspian Sea.[6] During this outbreak, plague expanded to countless places that were untouched for some time. It also reached others for the first time. Lasting unremittingly for more than three decades in both European and Ottoman regions, this wave's most dramatic peaks were probably 1578, 1586–87, and 1597–99.[7]

At the outset, when plague started circulating in the Mediterranean in summer 1570, the first Ottoman areas affected were the fortresses in southern Peloponnese, which most probably received it from infected places on the Dalmatian coast.[8] The outbreak was reported to Istanbul, especially stressing the difficulty of maintaining the security of the fortresses because of mortality and the flight of soldiers. What seems to be the first appearance of this outbreak in Ottoman regions is documented in an imperial order

---

[5] Sticker, *Abhandlungen*, 1:105.
[6] McNeill, *Plagues and Peoples*, 334; Biraben, *Les hommes et la peste*, 1:432, 443.
[7] Biraben, *Les hommes et la peste*, 1:368–69.
[8] Ibid., 1:443.

dated July 23, 1570, sent to the governor of Morea. In his petition, the governor reported to Istanbul that plague had broken out in the fortresses of Methoni and Nafplio, located at each end of southern Peloponnese. Noting the high mortality caused by plague in both fortresses, the governor commented on the difficulty of maintaining a minimum number of guards in the fortresses. Istanbul cautioned him against the dangers of leaving the coastal fortresses unprotected and emphatically ordered that the fortresses should not be left short of guards.[9] Another document issued five months later ordered the dispatching of additional guards to Methoni and Koroni.[10] The infection also seems to have spread to the fortress of Mani. An order sent to the governor of Morea strictly prohibited the flight of troops from the fortress, even under the threat of an enemy attack.[11]

Once the disease had reached important points on the maritime routes of the eastern Mediterranean and the Aegean, ships then swiftly carried it from one port to another. The Ottoman central administration was clearly informed about the presence of plague in the region and understood that the infection was being spread by ships, and warned governors of the impending threat. An order dated September 3, 1570, written to the *kadı*s of Rumeli's coastal towns, informed them that infected ships were traveling in the Aegean.[12] Another order sent to the governor of Kavala on September 28, 1570, confirmed the presence of the infection on the ships.[13] It is not clear what exactly this meant for the local governors of these coastal cities and what precautions, if any, were taken at these locations. For example, were they warned against the danger so they would apply some precautionary measures? Or could they refuse the ships coming to their ports, on the grounds that they could be potential carriers of the disease? Unfortunately, it is difficult to answer these questions with certainty given the paucity of textual evidence. Yet it is still possible to say that Ottoman central administration, informed of the infection and its dissemination, spread the word to provincial administrators and informed them about the problem. It may be observed that, like the plague, information about it also had to go through the hub to circulate.

Plague continued to spread from coastal towns to the interior via overland routes in the Balkans. There is evidence for a devastating outbreak that

---

[9] MD 14/1, 125/177 (19 Safer 978 H./July 23, 1570).

[10] MD 14/2, 847/1234 (27 Receb 978 H./December 25, 1570).

[11] MD 14/1, 121/171 (19 Safer 978 H./July 23, 1570).

[12] MD 14/1, 480/680 (2 Rebiülahir 978 H./September 3, 1570). Also see another *mühimme* order issued on the same day confirming the same news: MD 14/1, 486/686 (2 Rebiülahir 978 H./September 3, 1570).

[13] MD 14/1, 388/544 (27 Rebiülahir 978 H./September 28, 1570). Also see another *mühimme* order, which has the same date confirming this news and reports that the navy of the enemy suffers not only from disease but also from famine: MD 14/1, 496/698 (27 Rebiülahir 978 H./September 28, 1570).

continued into fall 1570 in the Morea.[14] Moving north, the infection seems to have reached other Ottoman cities in the Balkans. For example, the presence of the disease in the town of Samokov is attested to in an imperial order sent from Istanbul in September 1570. Southeast of Sofia, Samokov was located on the route connecting Sofia to Istanbul, through Philippopolis and Edirne. It was also known for its rich iron mines. The iron processed for the Ottoman navy in Samakov was then transported to Black Sea ports. Unfavorable effects of the plague distressed both the ironworking industry and the navy. When plague broke out in 1570, ironworkers fled,[15] and people were still away from their homes in the winter.[16] This caused a delay in the preparation of iron needed for ships, which was still not supplied as late as spring 1571. Repeated imperial orders issued in March 1571 stated that the required iron from Samokov had still not been sent to Anchialos (Ahyolu), on the Black Sea coast, to be used in shipbuilding.[17]

Given its wide circulation in the area, it is hardly surprising to see the plague in Crete, an important stop for eastern Mediterranean and Aegean maritime routes under Venetian control. However, the presence of plague in Crete could also be related to military conflict. While Cyprus fell to the Ottoman siege, an allied Christian fleet was on its way to attack the Ottomans in Cyprus via Crete. A *mühimme* order mentions that the Ottoman spies reported a disease spread among the soldiers of the enemy fleet in Crete.[18] It is also stated that when Venetian ships of this fleet arrived at Cyprus, they were disease ridden and were thus kept in isolation in spring 1571.[19]

Spreading both overland and by sea, plague soon reached the Anatolian coast. The devastating effects of the epidemic are testified in a *mühimme* order dated December 5, 1570, which states that the number of households in the village of Lapseki, on the Anatolian shores of the Dardanelles, was reduced from forty-five to nineteen as a result of deaths and flight.[20] A few months later, in spring 1571, the infection was in the Black Sea area, most likely through the overland route connecting Samokov to the Black Sea port of Anchialos. Once the infection started circulating in the Black Sea ports, Caffa was not spared. Plague was reported in the fortress of Caffa in spring

---

[14] MD 14/1, 461/651 (22 Cemaziyelevvel 978 H./October 22, 1570).

[15] MD 14/1, 469/661 (2 Rebiülahir 978 H./September 3, 1570).

[16] MD 14/2, 842/1224 (27 Receb 978 H./December 25, 1570).

[17] MD 14/2, 936/1386 (22 Şevval 978 H./March 19, 1571); MD 14/2, 940/1391 (25 Şevval 978 H./March 22, 1571).

[18] MD 14/1, 368/521 (23 Rebiülahir 978 H./September 24, 1570). In fact, four days later than this *mühimme* order, a new one was issued confirming the news of the terrible disease among the soldiers of the Christian allied forces: MD 14/1, 382/539 (27 Rebiülahir 978 H./September 28, 1570). But the documents do not specify what disease it was.

[19] MD 14/2, 1116/1639 (13 Şevval 978 H./March 10, 1571).

[20] MD 14/2, 628/904 (7 Receb 978 H./December 5, 1570).

1571, which caused massive flight. A *mühimme* order issued on May 13, 1571, to the governor of Caffa prohibited the taxpaying population from leaving the fortress on account of the plague.[21]

The spread of the plague like a wildfire continued into the next year, reaching Poland and northwest Russia.[22] Initially, the infection moved simultaneously along the east-west and north-south axes of the First and Second phases. Although the east-west network alone could only circulate the infection within a limited zone stretching from the Adriatic to Istanbul, its intersection with the south-north network produced a more extensive spread. There is clear evidence for the integrated state of these axes facilitating the spread of the infection. However, this initial distribution of the infection took a much more complicated trajectory after 1571, that is, after plague reached Istanbul.

The earliest indication of plague in the capital dates from June 1571. A *mühimme* order points out that a number of soldiers who were appointed for the protection of Egypt had to stay in Istanbul owing to disease and other causes.[23] Plague could be introduced to Istanbul via several routes: the maritime route from the Aegean ports, the overland route from the Balkans, or from the Black Sea ports. Whatever the case may have been, plague was in Istanbul in summer 1571, which was perhaps the reason for the departure of Sultan Selim II for Edirne. However, what is really important for our discussion here is that from Istanbul, plague spread to every direction. As is shown in the following pages, Istanbul worked truly as the plague hub of the empire, distributing it to faraway places through the networks forged in the First and Second phases.

The infection immediately spread to a large area in the Balkans. The presence of plague in Wallachia and around the Danube is attested in a *mühimme* order dated June 30, 1571. The order is about the flight of the local population to the Danube shores, probably to avoid the infection.[24] Meanwhile, the epidemic continued to linger on the coastal towns of the Adriatic through the end of 1571. Owing to casualties or flight, new artillerymen were needed for the fortresses of Herceg Novi on the Adriatic coast and Lefkada, an island off the western coast of the Greek peninsula. An order dated December 27, 1571, was issued to dispatch these much-needed forces.[25] The following year, however, plague's spread to a much broader area in the Mediterranean and the Aegean can be best understood by the newly assumed role of Istanbul

---

[21] MD 14/2, 1048/1543 (18 Zilhicce 978 H./May 13, 1571).

[22] Biraben, *Les hommes et la peste*, 1:368.

[23] MD 14/2, 1066/1570 (26 Muharrem 979 H./June 19, 1571); MD 17, 27/39 (Gurre, Safer 979 H./June 24, 1571). This order, which is issued a few days later, confirms the previous one.

[24] MD 14/2, 1073/1578 (6 Safer 979 H./June 29, 1571).

[25] MD 18, 83/180 (10 Şaban 979 H./December 27, 1571).

as the plague hub. On one hand, the infection spread along the east-west axis to many places in the Balkans, including Ragusa, Kranj, Constadt, and Transylvania, in 1572. On the other, it seems to have spread along the north-south axis to Alexandria, Cairo, Rosetta, and Damietta in Egypt.[26] It is clear that Istanbul could efficiently and swiftly distribute the infection along several conjoined networks and trajectories. Spreading along the north-south axis, the infection soon reached Cyprus, which now was a newly integrated stop point. After the conquest of the island, a number of households from central Anatolian towns were sent there, in addition to garrisoned troops. An order dated July 1572 documents that soldiers from the province of Karaman fell victim to plague.[27] Another example for plague's propagation along the north-south axis was its appearance in Thessaloniki. In July 1572, Thessaloniki was hit by plague, evidence for which is to be found in a petition given by the Jewish woolen cloth weavers of the town requesting authorization to leave the city, which was granted by the Ottoman central administration on the condition that they finish their weaving duties on time.[28] A month later, in August 1572, plague was still continuing.[29]

Now distributed in all directions from Istanbul, the infection gained further momentum. There were repeated visitations of plague in the Balkans throughout the decade. Moreover, the number of places touched increased steadily. For instance, in 1573 alone, plague was in Istanbul, in the Balkans (Skopje, Livno, Kosovo, Bosnia, and Ragusa), in Wallachia, and on the Mediterranean shores (Algiers, Tunis, Alexandria, Cairo, Rosetta, and Damietta). It was also present in Cyprus though fall 1573.[30] During this outbreak, the renowned Ottoman scholar Birgili Mehmed Efendi contracted the disease in a visit to Istanbul and died in September 1573,[31] The dissemination of plague can easily be traced: for instance, the east-west axis for the spread in the Balkans, the north-south axis for the spread to Egypt and environs, and the Anatolian network for the spread to Damascus. Such a wide scale of distribution would surely have not been possible in the absence of those necessary trajectories for the circulation of infection and a center connecting them to one another.

The outbreaks of 1573 severely affected many regions, causing death and destruction and disrupting social life. Two examples from this year demonstrate how plague led to social disorder. In the spring, plague was reported in the villages between Edirne and Hasköy, which caused many

[26] Biraben, *Les hommes et la peste*, 1:432, 443.
[27] de Groot, "Kubrus," *EI²*; MD 19, 196/407 (28 Safer 980 H./July 9, 1572).
[28] MD 19, 201/417 (Gurre, Rebiülevvel 980 H./July 11, 1572).
[29] MD 19, 301/610 (2 Rebiülahir 980 H./August 11, 1572).
[30] Biraben, *Les hommes et la peste*, 1:432, 443; MD 23, 176/372 (28 Receb 981 H./November 23, 1573).
[31] Emrullah Yüksel, "Birgivî," *TDVİA*.

to flee. As this region was on the main route from Edirne to Philippopolis and Sofia, abandoned villages and the ensuing banditry alarmed the central administration. An order issued on May 25, 1573, urged those who fled to return to their villages.[32] Another example for banditry in conjunction with plague comes from Damascus, located on the main pilgrimage route from Istanbul to the Muslim holy cities. An order dated November 23, 1573, documented that bandits attacked and robbed the pilgrims, who had contracted the disease en route.[33]

In 1574, plague is documented in new locations. A *mühimme* order reported heavy mortality in the district of Üzeyir, in the province of Aleppo. Located on the pilgrimage route, this town seemed to be severely affected by plague as suggested in the mortality of pass-guard households, responsible for maintaining the safety of roads. Out of 236 households, only 60 were left – an overall 75 percent mortality rate.[34] The effects of plague were detrimental not only for the local population but also for maintaining the safety of roads. Other cases of plague come from Wallachia, Bosnia, and Herzegovina.[35] The infection was on the western shores of the Peloponnese in spring 1574, as suggested by an order about the difficulty in finding rowers for the navy because of plague.[36] Another order dated September 17, 1574, warned the governor of Smederevo against the oppressions of officials who inspected towns and villages surrounding Zvornik, southwest of Belgrade, for recording the inheritance of those who died recently, most probably caused by plague.[37] Later in the fall, plague in Edirne affected not only common people but also the Sultan himself, possibly causing Selim II's decision to cancel his plans to winter there.[38] Especially because this seems like a last-minute change of plans, it may have been due to plague in or around Edirne. Another example of plague's disruptive effects in the fall comes from Thessaloniki, where the woolen cloth weavers were again late in sending their output to Istanbul. In this case, as before, the delay was caused by plague and the flight of the laborers.[39] As these examples suggest, plague's effects were felt in every segment of Ottoman society in the Balkans. Plague was also seen elsewhere in the Mediterranean in 1574.[40]

---

[32] MD 22, 38/82 (23 Muharrem 981 H./May 25, 1573).

[33] MD 22, 164/344 (28 Receb 981 H./November 23, 1573).

[34] MD 24, 96/262 (14 Zilhicce 981 H./April 6, 1574).

[35] Biraben, *Les hommes et la peste*, 1:443.

[36] MD 24, 3/7 (16 Zilkade 981 H./March 10, 1574).

[37] MD 26, 218/618 (1 Cemaziyelahir 982 H./September 17, 1574). More than a year later, another order was issued on the same problem, perhaps referring to continued deaths due to plague and the oppression caused by officials who tried to take advantage of it: MD 27, 246/571 (5 Zilkade 983 H./February 5, 1576).

[38] MD 26, 276/767 (28 Cemaziyelahir 982 H./October 14, 1574).

[39] MD 26, 320/922 (1 Şaban 982H./November 15, 1574).

[40] Biraben, *Les hommes et la peste*, 1:432, 443: Plague in Algiers, Oran, and Cairo.

The next year, plague was in Istanbul, Wallachia, the area around the Danube, and Italian cities,[41] as well as in Tabriz, Algiers, and Cairo[42] and in the Crimea.[43] In 1576, it was still causing high mortality and problems for maintaining safety.[44] For instance, in February, plague was seemingly so grave in the Thracian town of Vize, halfway between Istanbul and Edirne, that even a murder could go unnoticed when it was registered as caused by plague.[45] Another instance shows how plague endangered the route connecting Istanbul to main destinations in the Balkans. A *mühimme* order dated February 26, 1576, mentions the case of an Ottoman official, Hüsrev Çavuş, who was en route to Istanbul from Thessaloniki bringing four hundred thousand *akçe*s that he had collected. When he fell sick and died before he could make it to Istanbul, the money in his possession was plundered. The epidemic that ravaged the area must have rendered the highways completely unprotected and vulnerable to the danger of robbery. Although it is not explicitly mentioned in this particular order whether the latter succumbed to plague or another disease, his sudden death may have been due to plague.[46] Perhaps he had contracted the disease when he was still in Thessaloniki, where the presence of plague can be documented a week before this unfortunate incident. This time, woolen cloth weavers of Thessaloniki were granted permission by the central administration to leave the city and take refuge in the countryside on account of the plague. It is reported that the epidemic caused a considerable number of deaths and that the work force had decreased to a great extent.[47] As always, the weavers were allowed to leave the fortress on the condition that they finish the weaving duty on time.[48] In the spring, plague was causing severe mortality in the capital, including among the novice janissary boys.[49] Another piece of evidence for

---

[41] Ibid., 398; Schreiner, *Die byzantinischen Kleinchroniken*, 593. Gerlach indirectly documents the presence of plague in Istanbul in November 1575. In June 1576 he visits the church in Arnavutköy, on the Bosphorus, a place renowned for its water well, believed to protect from infectious diseases. While there, he notes the presence of gold and silver plates that were provided by a woman who had caught the plague seven months before and had prayed to St. Athanasius for a cure. Upon recovering from her illness, she donated these plates to the church. Gerlach, *Türkiye Günlüğü*, 1:361.

[42] Biraben, *Les hommes et la peste*, 1:432.

[43] Gerlach mentions receiving the news of plague in a letter received from Andrzej Taranowski, the former Polish ambassador to the Porte. Gerlach, *Türkiye Günlüğü*, 1:197.

[44] Biraben, *Les hommes et la peste*, 1:443.

[45] MD 27, 261/612 (12 Zilkade 983 H./February 12, 1576).

[46] MD 27, 300/721 (26 Zilkade 983 H./February 26, 1576).

[47] Suraiya Faroqhi, "Textile Production in Rumeli and the Arab Provinces: Geographical Distribution and the Internal Trade (1560–1650)," *Osmanlı Araştırmaları* 1 (1980): 68.

[48] MD 27, 275/655 (20 Zilkade 983 H./February 20, 1576).

[49] Gerlach mentions several deaths in spring 1576, including those of prominent individuals (e.g., the daughter of Piyale Paşa on April 28 and of the son of Ahmed Paşa on April 29), without referring to an outbreak in the city. Also, he records other deaths that summer, though there is no direct mention of plague. A similar allusion to plague is when he writes

heavy plague mortality comes from the eastern Thracian town of Ferres, located on the southern route of the Balkans connecting Thessaloniki and Istanbul. In the summer, plague seems to have caused heavy losses in Ferres, as a result of which twenty households were dead in the villages of Sarı Meşe and Yahnecik. In response to the petition they sent to Istanbul, these villages were kept temporarily exempt from providing the four horses, a duty imposed by the center.[50]

When plague was so widespread in the Ottoman towns of the Balkans, it may be viable to question links regarding the propagation of the infection to non-Ottoman regions in central and eastern Europe. Biraben suggests that plague was brought to Austria and Bavaria in 1576 by the Ottoman troops, from where it spread to Switzerland the following year.[51] Given the fragmentary nature of the evidence at hand, it is hard to establish the direction of spread in the area. As a matter of fact, Austria had been free from infection for more than a decade, until plague was reintroduced in 1576. However, Switzerland had already been exposed to the infection in the preceding years.[52] The absence of a major Ottoman campaign to the region in this specific year makes it even harder to establish whether the infection was indeed carried there by Ottoman troops. Nonetheless, the spread of plague across the Transylvanian border can be better documented. For instance, the bordering town Hoybersin reported a loss of about eight thousand to plague in November.[53] Plague was also in Hungary at this time.[54]

Only a few moths later, in January 1577, more deaths were reported from Ereğli, a town on the northern shore of the Marmara Sea, close to Istanbul. When a number of novice janissary boys were reported dead, Istanbul required the investigation of their cause of death. Although the document does not clearly state the death cause, it is not a remote possibility that they succumbed to plague.[55] Furthermore, plague visited several other locations that winter, including Hungary, Ragusa, Modica, Noto, and around the Danube.[56] North of the Danube, in the Ottoman province of Temesvár

---

that the sultan offered sacrifices and distributed meat, sugar, honey, and other food to the needy in late July to please God, for hundreds of people and numerous novice janissary boys had died. Gerlach, *Türkiye Günlüğü*, 1:329–31, 381, 386–87, 389.

[50] MD 42, 489/1981 (18 Rebiülahir 984 H./July 15, 1576). Also see Machiel Kiel, "Ottoman Building Activity along the Via Egnatia, the Cases of Pazargah, Kavalla and Ferecik," in *The Via Egnatia under Ottoman Rule (1380–1699)*, ed. Elizabeth A. Zachariadou, 145–58 (Rethymnon: Crete University Press, 1996).

[51] Biraben, *Les hommes et la peste*, 1:109.

[52] Ibid., 1:412.

[53] MD 28, 334/843 (13 Şaban 984 H./November 4, 1576).

[54] Gerlach, *Türkiye Günlüğü*, 1:453.

[55] MD 29, 127/313 (17 Şevval 984 H./January 7, 1577).

[56] Biraben, *Les hommes et la peste*, 1:443.

(Temeşvar), mortality was so high that the taxpayers petitioned the governor by January 1577.[57] Further evidence of plague comes from Thessaloniki in 1577. Owing to high mortality that winter, there was a scarcity of weavers, which by the summer caused a dramatic increase in the price of weaving and of the woolen cloth.[58] In the very same year, plague also spread east from Istanbul, underscoring the role of the Anatolian network. In December, plague was in Erzurum, a main hub on the overland caravan route between Istanbul and Tabriz. Although it is not clear through which route the infection was introduced, it was most likely via the overland caravan route. A letter written by the *kadı* of Erzurum reported the news of plague and mortality it caused and petitioned that the survey tax register be postponed to a later date, which was granted.[59] In a related order, it is mentioned that a great many people left the fortress because of the outbreak.[60]

Shortly after the reported outbreak in Erzurum, one can find evidence for plague in the mines of Çaniçe (Canca) in Gümüşhane. A *mühimme* order dated January 16, 1578, testifies that the mines of Çaniçe and the imperial minting house were closed down owing to plague.[61] Gümüşhane, located on the main route connecting the Black Sea port of Trabzon to Erzurum, was open to infections spreading along the Anatolian network and those introduced from the Black Sea. Perhaps this time, plague spread from Istanbul to Trabzon via their direct maritime connection and proceeded overland to Gümüşhane and Erzurum – if not in the opposite direction – because it was also in Istanbul in that year, as well as in Transylvania, Hungary, and Illyria.[62] In August, plague was reported in the fortress of Bakras, near the port of İskenderun. As a result of the death of guards in the fortress, replacements were requested from Istanbul.[63]

Likewise in 1579, plague was documented across the empire. It was in Belgrade and Thessaloniki, where some of the woolen cloth weavers found the solution in maintaining looms outside the fortress where they could work in times of plague.[64] The infection was also reported from Ergani, in the district of Amid in eastern Anatolia, that summer.[65] Shortly after it, Cyprus may have been infected. A *mühimme* order issued on November 3, 1579, mentions that eleven out of fourteen people sent to Cyprus

[57] MD 29, 111/269 (undated).
[58] MD 31, 48/124 (4 Cemaziyelevvel 985 H./July 20, 1577).
[59] MD 33, 177/352 (17 Şevval 985 H./December 27, 1577).
[60] MD 33, 181/360 (17 Şevval 985 H./December 27, 1577).
[61] MD 33, 198/401 (8 Zilkade 985 H./January 16, 1578).
[62] Biraben, *Les hommes et la peste*, 1:443–44.
[63] MD 35, 152/388 (13 Cemaziyelahir 986 H./August 17, 1578); MD 35, 166/423 (15 Cemaziyelahir 986 H./August 19, 1578).
[64] MD 36, 281/738 (27 Rebiülevvel 987 H./May 23, 1579).
[65] MD 37, 268/3190 (3 Cemaziyelevvel 987 H./June 28, 1579).

died because allegedly their constitution did not adapt to the island's "air." Even though the cause of death is not specified, the possibility of plague can be considered.[66] Around the same time, plague was documented in Egypt on account of the delays it caused for pilgrimage and the return trip to Istanbul.[67] Plague was also in southern Iraq at this time. That the infection reached Basra and its environs in November 1579 is attested in a *mühimme* order. The people of Basra petitioned the central administration regarding the great difficulty caused by plague and complained that merchants did not come to their town on account of the epidemic.[68] The locals also suffered as a result of military expedition. The Ottoman army had undertaken an expedition against the Safavids between 1578 and 1580, which seems to have put people in the area in a difficult situation, as these places were already drained of resources by the epidemic. The people of Baghdad, Basra, Şehrizol, and Lahsa, who had all suffered from a famine in 1578 and from plague, found themselves burdened with the imposed duty to provide provisions for the army. Under these circumstances, the people of the region were given exemption from extraordinary (*avarız*) taxes with an order issued in December 1579.[69] Simultaneously, plague is reported from the Crimean ports on the Black Sea. A *mühimme* order dated December 1, 1579, reported the death of soldiers from disease in the fortress of Toprakkale, part of Azak, in the Crimea.[70]

The year 1580 was perhaps lighter in terms of epidemic activity; at least we do not learn of as many cases as had occurred the year before. Plague was reported in Vlorë, on the Adriatic coast.[71] A *mühimme* order dated September 19, 1580, reported that soldiers assigned to Niš in Serbia fell sick because of the "air" of the region, petitioning for their transfer to Sofia.[72] By October 1580, plague caused such great mortality in the town of Zvornik that a new survey tax register was needed.[73]

---

[66] MD 40, 246/568 (13 Ramazan 987 H./November 3, 1579).

[67] MD 40, 285/654 (27 Ramazan 987 H./November 17, 1579). As a matter of fact, plague continued to affect Cairo in 1580 and lasted until the following year. See Biraben, *Les hommes et la peste*, 1:432.

[68] MD 40, 289/662 (27 Ramazan 987 H./November 17, 1579).

[69] MD 40, 135/296 (20 Şevval 987 H./December 9, 1579). Also, a few years later, the people of Basra petitioned again because of repeated outbreaks in their city. They complained that no merchant came to the city because of plague, and they decided to move outside the fortress. They were granted permission to move out. See MD 49, 42/149 (16 Rebiülahir 991 H./May 9, 1583).

[70] MD 40, 67/152 (12 Şevval 987 H./December 1, 1579).

[71] Biraben, *Les hommes et la peste*, 1:444.

[72] MD 43, 242/450 (9 Şaban 988 H./September 19, 1580).

[73] MD 43, 288/547 (16 Ramazan 988 H./October 25, 1580). The great death toll caused by the outbreak is also confirmed in a related order. See MD 43, 288/548 (16 Ramazan 988 H./October 25, 1580).

Plague was reported in Bosnia and Herzegovina in February 1581.[74] Varna, on the Black Sea coast, also suffered in the same year.[75] Once introduced to the Black Sea ports, the infection swiftly reached Istanbul. Plague was reported in the capital in the summer months.[76] By the fall, it was in eastern Black Sea ports. The fortress of Faşe, in Batumi, was almost deserted due to deaths and flight. New guards for the fortress were requested, which was approved by the Porte in an order dated December 31, 1581.[77] In a related order, additional guards were requested from Erzurum.[78]

Over the next two years, sparse documentation does not support heavy epidemic activity. Nevertheless, plague was in the southern Balkans in summer 1582. It was reported in Morea, where the mortality was heavy.[79] The following year, it was in Ragusa[80] and Philippopolis, whose residents were said to have deserted the town in May 1583 for the "fresh air of the mountains" on account of "fever" and "bad air."[81] Later that year, plague can be documented in Ankara, as we find in a court case about the death of a certain Akkoca, which was recorded as caused by plague, even though a petition given to the court claimed it was a murder.[82]

Toward the end of the century, there are detailed accounts about the plague in Istanbul, especially in the chronicle of Selaniki Mustafa Efendi, who recounts the outbreak of 1584, during which a Persian envoy to Sultan Murad III (r. 1574–95) lost his entire retinue to the epidemic.[83] High mortality in Istanbul required a systematic effort to register the inheritance of those who died. In May 1585, the *kadı* of Istanbul was ordered to register the inheritance of the dead and the division of property between inheritors and the treasurer.[84] The following year, a similar order was sent to Egypt for proper registration of the inheritance, most probably following another outbreak of plague.[85]

---

[74] MD 46, 313/715 (4 Muharrem 989 H./February 8, 1581).

[75] Biraben, *Les hommes et la peste*, 1:444.

[76] Schreiner, *Die byzantinischen Kleinchroniken*, 594.

[77] MD 46, 268/605 (5 Zilhicce 989 H./December 31, 1581).

[78] MD 46, 269/609 (5 Zilhicce 989 H./December 31, 1581).

[79] MD 48, 88/238 (3 Şaban 990 H./August 22, 1582).

[80] Biraben, *Les hommes et la peste*, 1:432, 444.

[81] MD 49, 38/137 (13 Rebiülahir 991 H./May 6, 1583).

[82] Halit Ongan, ed. *Ankara'nın 1 Numaralı Şeriye Sicili* (Ankara: TTK, 1958), 115. The exact date of the case is unknown, but the register includes cases between May 1583 and February 1584. Also see Chapter 8.

[83] Selânikî, *Tarih-i Selânikî*, 146–48.

[84] MD 58, 61/180 (15 Cemaziyelevvel 993 H./May 15, 1585); MD 58, 77/224 (17 Cemaziyelevvel 993 H./May 17, 1585).

[85] MD 60, 246/576 (25 Cemaziyelevvel 994 H./May 14, 1586). This outbreak affected a wider area: in 1584, the North African towns of Constantine and Algiers were affected; in 1585, plague was in Serbia and Herzegovina. See Biraben, *Les hommes et la peste*, 1:432, 444.

In summer 1586, we learn of the plague in the capital. One eyewitness testimony was the Fugger report (dated June 25, 1586), according to which there was a major outbreak causing mortality even greater than that of 1584. More than one hundred were said to have died in İbrahim Pasha's palace alone. The report also mentioned that many left the city, and rumors spread that the sultan was planning to leave shortly with his family and children for a summer retreat on the Black Sea coast.[86] On this occasion, Selaniki writes that Istanbul always suffered from plague in the summer months before he goes on to write about the death of Ahmed Sadık of Tashkent, a Naqshbandi mystic, from plague on August 2, 1586.[87] In mid-August, ships bringing provisions to Istanbul headed toward other Black Sea ports instead. To avoid provisioning problems in the capital, such ships were ordered to bring their loads to Istanbul.[88] Toward the end of the month, plague was said to be lessening in the capital.[89] But still in November, it most likely caused 150 young boys working in the imperial gardens to either die or flee.[90]

Plague continued in the capital over the winter months as well. Vizier Cafer Pasha died of plague on January 29, 1587.[91] In the spring, plague was in Egypt.[92] In the fall, it was in Erzurum.[93] It was once again recorded in Istanbul in December 1587. This time, the testimony of pharmacist Reinhold Lubenau, from the Habsburg imperial mission, offers detailed information about the disease's impact in the city.[94] In 1588 plague was in Transylvania, Wallachia, and Herzegovina,[95] and in Istanbul, as observed by Michael Heberer von Bretten.[96]

In 1589, plague was still in Istanbul[97] as well as in the eastern Mediterranean. Its presence is documented in Famagusta (Magosa) on the eastern coast of Cyprus and in Tripoli and Syria. The next year, it was in Algiers, where it continued for three years.[98] In 1590, the infection was still in the capital. Selaniki mentions that the outbreak intensified during the months of

---

[86] Victor Klarwill, *Fugger-Zeitungen; ungedruckte Briefe an das Haus Fugger aus den Jahren 1568–1605* (Vienna: [Rikola], 1923), cited in Metin And, *16. Yüzyılda İstanbul: Kent, Saray, Günlük Yaşam* (Istanbul: Yapı Kredi Yayınları, 2009), 90.

[87] Selânikî, *Tarih-i Selânikî*, 173.

[88] MD 61, 67/176 (3 Ramazan 994 H./August 18, 1586).

[89] Selânikî, *Tarih-i Selânikî*, 174.

[90] MD 61, 131/315 (28 Zilkade 994 H./November 10, 1586).

[91] Selânikî, *Tarih-i Selânikî*, 178–79.

[92] MD 62, 59/135 (16 Cemaziyelevvel 995 H./April 24, 1587).

[93] MD 62, 125/277 (Şevval 995 H./September 4–October 3, 1587).

[94] Reinhold Lubenau, *Beschreibung der Reisen des Reinhold Lubenau*, ed. W. Sahm (Königsberg: Beyer (Thomas and Oppermann), 1915), 2:25–28.

[95] Biraben, *Les hommes et la peste*, 1:444.

[96] Johann Michael Heberer, *Aegyptiaca servitus* (Graz: Akademische Druck und Verlagsanstalt, 1967), 303–5.

[97] Biraben, *Les hommes et la peste*, 1:444.

[98] Ibid., 1:432.

November and December, though shortly after that, it began to abate and the afflicted began to recover.[99]

Over the next few years, plague was still observed in the capital, in addition to its appearance in the archipelago of the Aegean[100] and in the Venetian colony in Crete, which was hit in the spring and summer months of 1592 (from March to July).[101] This time, the presence of the disease in the Mediterranean ports, such as Algiers and Tunis, indicates wide-scale epidemic activity.[102] Selaniki noted that the plague once more broke out in July and was especially devastating in September. For the lifting of the epidemic, communal prayers and processions were held; animals were sacrificed and distributed to the needy as alms; prisoners were let free in the hope that God would accept and respond to their prayers. According to Selaniki, prayers did bring beneficial results for the city, as mortality decreased dramatically.[103] Another eyewitness account to this outbreak was the Bohemian Baron Wenceslas Wratislaw, who was in Istanbul between 1591 and 1596. According to the latter, eighty thousand died in three months during this outbreak, including six people from his retinue.[104]

In fall 1592, we hear that plague was in Antalya, a Mediterranean port of Anatolia, on account of the delay it caused in the construction of ships.[105] Soon after that, reports from Edirne point to high mortality. Young boys were needed to work at the imperial palace's gardens, because a great many of them had either fled or succumbed to plague by November.[106] Adana, in the eastern Mediterranean, also seems to have suffered seriously this time around, as evidenced by the death of those responsible for supplying horses for imperial service.[107]

Plague's presence in Istanbul and in Crete until mid-August 1593 is suggested by Greek sources, in addition to a "pestilential disease" in the year of 1594 in Crete and in the Ottoman fortress of Monemvasia in Peloponnese.[108] The infection was also recorded in Tunis between 1593 and 1595. The presence of the disease in Cyprus or the Mediterranean is hinted at in a *mühimme* order issued on September 13, 1595.[109]

---

99 Selânikî, *Tarih-i Selânikî*, 229.
100 Biraben, *Les hommes et la peste*, 1:444.
101 Schreiner, *Die byzantinischen Kleinchroniken*, 595. Although it is mentioned as an unspec-ified epidemic, the source hints at an unedited work on the plague in the year of 1592 in Crete.
102 Biraben, *Les hommes et la peste*, 1:432.
103 Selânikî, *Tarih-i Selânikî*, 285–87.
104 Wenceslas Wratislaw, *Adventures of Baron Wenceslas Wratislaw of Mitrowitz*, trans. A. H. Wratislaw (London: Bell and Daldy, 1862), 107.
105 MD 69, 63/125 (1 Muharrem 1001 H./October 7, 1592).
106 MD 69, 72/145 (17 Safer 1001 H./November 22, 1592).
107 MD 71, 10/20 (21 Zilhice 1001 H./September 17, 1593).
108 Schreiner, *Die byzantinischen Kleinchroniken*, 595.
109 MD 73, 358/786 (8 Muharrem 1004 H./September 13, 1595).

In 1596, plague was in Syria, Egypt, Azerbaijan, Baghdad, and the Arabian Peninsula.[110] An eyewitness to the outbreak in Istanbul, the unfortunate Baron Wratislaw, describes the fear and terror of people when plague hit Thrace, Istanbul, and the nearby islands. During this outbreak, he was imprisoned in the Rumeli fortress on the Bosphorus, where people in a nearby neighborhood learned about the presence of a surgeon in his retinue and successfully petitioned to have the surgeon let out of prison every day to treat the locals.[111]

The next plague mentioned by Selaniki was in the years 1597 and 1598. After the outbreak in spring 1597, Sultan Mehmed III (r. 1595–1603) ordered the viziers to be prepared for communal prayer, and many in Istanbul met in Okmeydanı for that purpose. Communal prayers were held for the deceased for three weeks until late August; among the victims were members of the dynasty and statesmen. The outbreak seems to have lasted until the fall of the next year or perhaps later.[112] Plague was across the Mediterranean during the last years of the century: for example, it was in Fez, Marrakech, and the port cities of Morocco in 1598 and 1599 and Aleppo the next year.[113]

Conclusion

This chapter has examined plague activity in the Third Phase (1570–1600), which can be studied as one single wave. Owing to its devastating and long-lasting effects, this wave seems to have been the deadliest of the century. As we have seen here, plague was present in at least one location of the empire during these thirty years. Most often, this presence was felt in multiple areas. Even though the outbreaks of this phase appear to have caused higher mortality, this may be an artifact of the sources. Plague was clearly much better reported in the late sixteenth century than in any other period examined here.

The chapter has offered a narrative of the outbreaks during these thirty years, making an effort to trace the trajectories of plague spread. When possible, it has drawn from the plague networks highlighted in the First and Second phases. More important, it has illustrated the wild dissemination of plague with reference to the integration and consolidation of these networks. Eventually, the role of Istanbul as the plague hub of the empire was underscored in the dissemination of plague across regions and networks.

---

[110] Ünver, "Türkiyede Veba," 77; McNeill, *Plagues and Peoples*, 334; Selânikî, *Tarih-i Selânikî*, 545; Biraben, *Les hommes et la peste*, 1:432, 444.

[111] Wratislaw, *Adventures*, 162.

[112] Selânikî, *Tarih-i Selânikî*, 759, 762–63, 768; İnalcık, "Istanbul"; Biraben, *Les hommes et la peste*, 1:444.

[113] Biraben, *Les hommes et la peste*, 1:432.

Simultaneously, it has been shown that the periodic visitations of plague to the capital in the First and Second phases turned plague into a permanent presence in the city in the late sixteenth century. This presence continued to affect Ottoman regions in more or less the same manner in the early decades of the seventeenth century and beyond. Istanbul's experience of plague, as highlighted here, had a critical and transformative impact on Ottoman perceptions, attitudes, and responses to plague, which are discussed in the next part of this book.

PART III

EMPIRE OF PLAGUE

7

Plague Transformed

Changing Perceptions, Knowledge, and Attitudes

Müsülmanlar meger āḫır zamāndur
Ḳıyāmet mi ḳopar bu ne nişāndur
. . . .
Ecel n'olur ki taḳdīr-i ezeldür
Vebā n'olur, ḳażā-i āsumāndur

O' Muslims, as if this were the End Times
Is this the Doomsday, what a sign this is
. . . .
What is death, it is the eternal judgment
What is plague, it is the decree of the heavens
    – Şeyyad Hamza[1] (fourteenth century)

Be-kavl-i hukemâ tâ'ûn nâ-pâklıkdan olur derler.
(In the opinion of the wise, it is said that the
plague is caused by uncleanliness.)
    – Evliya Çelebi[2] (d. after 1683)

Not unlike other societies of the late medieval and early modern era, the Ottomans maintained a broad range of beliefs, ideas, and knowledge about plague. Their experience with repeated waves of plague since the Black Death certainly shaped the notions they held, images they conceived, and cognizance they formed from these conceptions. These in turn molded the norms and principles by which they positioned themselves vis-à-vis the plague as well as their attitude, affect, and response. It is argued here that the Ottoman perceptions of plagues and attitudes toward them changed dramatically in the sixteenth century. As the Ottomans watched plague persist in their lands to the extent that it came to be seen as a problem endemic to their cities, the

---

[1] Akar, "Şeyyad Hamza," 3.
[2] Evliya Çelebi, *Seyahatnâme*, 6:21.

late medieval plague paradigm gradually gave way to something different. This process of change will be surveyed here in terms of three key transformations: *naturalization, medicalization,* and *canonization,* corresponding to the changes in perceptions, knowledge, and attitudes, respectively.

By *naturalization* is meant here a process by which plague came to be integrated into the Ottoman cultural landscape. This process of transformation can be traced in the manner plague is imagined, moving away from an exclusive reference to the supernatural realm toward the natural, which is embodied in a symbolic shift of the locus of the disease from the heavens to the city. As such, this process produced a vision of the plague as something that belonged to a place, a problem that is endemic to a city. Similarly, whereas the former vision of plagues conjured up supernatural images (e.g., apocalyptic apparitions, angels) and thus called for supernatural powers (e.g., miracles, intercession of saints), the latter could be drawn from the natural realm (e.g., the air of the city, filth).

Concurrently, a process of *medicalization* took hold. A new body of knowledge about diagnosis, prognosis, and prophylaxis of plague started to take form in the sixteenth century. In the late medieval era, the plague episteme was a perplexing amalgamation of knowledge and myth, perhaps more illustrative of the perceived feelings of vulnerability than anything else. Heralding this transition was the rise of a new genre of writing (plague treatises) among the Ottoman literati in this era, which became the main medium for the discussion, circulation, and elaboration of the plague episteme. This can be characterized as a process of *medicalization,* in the sense that plague moved away from being characterized as a celestial disaster toward being recognized as a distinct disease, the causes and treatment of which had to be sought in medical means and methods.

In conjunction with these processes, this new body of perceptions and knowledge prompted changes in formulating the norms and principles to guide the conduct of the Ottomans. This effort dictated not only how people had to see plagues but also how they ought to carry themselves in facing them. It was this set of principles that came to be promoted and circulated for future generations to come, as the mainstream position to be adopted vis-à-vis the plague, hence the process of *canonization.*

This chapter revolves around these three processes, highlighting the major turning points in the way plague was imagined, discussed, and understood from the late medieval into the early modern era. First, each of these processes is surveyed, emphasizing the major changes with evidence from the sources. Then the broader context of the changes is discussed with a view to relate them to other transformations that the Ottoman society was going through in the same era. Yet before moving on to a detailed analysis for reconstructing plague mentalities, a word of caution on methodology and sources is in order. First, it should be noted at the outset that this chapter privileges the plague experience of Istanbul over other Ottoman cities. When possible, examples from other cities are provided, but the case of Istanbul, by virtue of being better documented in the historical sources and being critical to comprehending the processes of transformation, is the centerpiece of the argumentation here. Why Istanbul, in particular? As the following pages make clear, Istanbul's experience of plague is key, not only because of the city's constant exposure to this disease, but also because it was this experience that shaped the Ottoman perceptions, attitudes, and responses to plague to a large extent.

Second, the chapter maintains a distinction between "popular" and "learned" receptions of plague, even though such a distinction may not always be straightforward. Imposing this distinction carries the risk of being artificial, anachronistic, and exogenous to the sources used. At times, sources used do not neatly belong to one of these; rather, they may complicate such categories. Being fully aware of these problems, the chapter seeks to reconstruct the kinds of beliefs, images, metaphors, and prophecies about plague that circulated widely across different sections of Ottoman society. To this end, chronicles, hagiographies, medical treatises, and works of poetry are used.

Third, it should be remembered that all of these processes outlined here were *gradual* and *incomplete*. Even though the overall transformation is unmistakable, the argument cannot be overstated. It is true that new ideas about plague opened up new possibilities of thinking about it, but this did not mean that the old ways were entirely eliminated. On the contrary, many of the old discourses were resilient enough to continue over time, though it becomes more difficult to trace them in the sources as they are displaced from the mainstream view. Such examples will be pointed out as they appear in the following discussion. While the processes of *naturalization* and *canonization* seem to manifest their full effects by the end of the sixteenth century, the process of *medicalization* – in comparison – was slower; the full effects of the latter should be sought in the post-1600 era, which is beyond the scope of this study.

Late Medieval Ottoman Perceptions of Plague

At the outset, it should be noted that late medieval Ottoman perceptions of plague remain largely unknown. As discussed earlier, plague is mostly absent in the early Ottoman chronicles. The silence of the sources makes plague a black hole in the early Ottoman history-writing tradition and a bête noire in modern Ottomanist historiography of the early Ottoman era. As such, this black hole, void of meaning, does not figure in the written narratives of the early Ottoman centuries. Only when plague acquired a certain meaning did we see it develop as a discursive theme in those narratives. Stated differently, the dearth of references to and the near-total absence of descriptions of plague in early Ottoman historical sources are products of a mind-set in which plague was understood. Thus, it becomes even more critical to identify the particular set of beliefs, images, and metaphors used in reference to it. Before delving into a detailed analysis of the sources, however, it may be helpful to situate late medieval Ottoman mentalities of plague in a larger historical context.

Generally speaking, the Ottoman mentalities of plagues can be understood within the general outlines of an *Islamic plague cosmology*, a *systématique* of causal and contextual explanations, which had God and divine agency at its very core. According to this, God inflicted epidemic diseases upon humankind, and only he had the power to lift this ill. Within this general framework, other supernatural powers and the intercession of saints could be legitimately sought for relief against such misfortunes. In its broadest outlines, the vision of divine origins and agency prevailed in the Islamic world throughout the ages and as such remained the predominant discourse, circulating both orally and in written texts.[3] In the main, as Muslims and as heirs to Islamic traditions, members of Ottoman society entertained this vision of plague and pestilence. Yet this is not to mean that there is one universal and monolithic Islamic tradition that can explain all notions and beliefs about plagues in all Muslim societies across all ages. On the contrary, there is a multiplicity of differing – and often competing – discourses that Ottoman society simultaneously drew from and strove to reshape as it produced a distinct body of knowledge with which to understand and explain this phenomenon.

The continuities and similarities of the Ottoman perception of plague to the Islamic tradition notwithstanding, there may be a larger late medieval Mediterranean context to study it. As the recent literature indicates, there

---

[3] For a discussion of the medieval Islamic religio-legal interpretations of plague, see Jacqueline Sublet, "La peste prise aux rêts de la jurisprudence: le traité d'Ibn Ḥaǧar al-ʿAsqalānī sur la peste," *Studia Islamica* 33 (1971): 141–49; Michael W. Dols, "Plague in Early Islamic History," *Journal of the American Oriental Society* 94, no. 3 (1974): 371–83; Dols, "The Comparative Communal Responses to the Black Death in Muslim and Christian Societies," *Viator* 5 (1974): 269–87; Dols, "Ibn al-Wardī's *Risālah al-Nabaʾ ʿan al-Wabaʾ*: A Translation of a Major Source for the History of the Black Death in the Middle East," in *Near Eastern Numismatics, Iconography, Epigraphy and History, Studies in Honor of George C. Miles*, ed. D. Kouymjian (Beirut: American University of Beirut, 1974), 443–55; Dols, *Black Death*; Lawrence Conrad, "The Plague in the Early Medieval Near East," PhD diss., Princeton University, 1981; Conrad, "*Ṭāʿūn* and *Wabaʾ*: Conceptions of Plague and Pestilence in Early Islam," *JESHO* 25, no. 3 (1982): 268–307; Irmeli Perho, *The Prophet's Medicine: A Creation of the Muslim Traditionalist Scholars* (Helsinki: Finnish Oriental Society, 1995); Marie-Hélène Congourdeau and Mohammed Melhaoui, "La perception de la peste en pays chrétien byzantin et musulman," *Revue des études byzantines* 59 (2001): 95–124; osef van Ess, *Der Fehltritt des Gelehrten: Die "Pest von Emmaus" und ihre theologischen Nachspiele* (Heidelberg: Universitätsverlag C. Winter, 2001); Anna Akasoy, "Islamic Attitudes to Disasters in the Middle Ages," *The Medieval History Journal* 10, nos. 1–2 (2007): 387–410; Justin Stearns, "New Directions in the Study of Religious Responses to the Black Death," *History Compass* 7, no. 5 (2009): 1363–75; Stearns, *Infectious Ideas*.

may be more in the way of commonalities and shared visions, knowledge and responses, among the Christian, Jewish, and Muslim traditions than once assumed.[4] Such comparative work may offer an understanding of shared knowledge, ideas, themes, and motifs of the larger pool of the late medieval plague episteme of the Mediterranean world. It also promises to afford overarching interpretations, so as to avoid exceptionalizing any particular tradition.

Having laid out the general context in which the late medieval Ottoman perception of plagues can be most fruitfully explored, we can move on to survey some of the salient features and recognizable themes, motifs, and imagery of the plague drawing from works of literature and early Ottoman chronicles (including anonymous chronicles). Needless to say, this is not an exhaustive survey of the examples of these genres. It is instead an attempt to sketch the contours of the plague imaginaries as entertained by the late medieval Ottoman society. In the light of previous discussions, there seems to be no reason to doubt that the first encounter of the mid-fourteenth-century Balkans and Anatolia with plague had shocking effects. The Black Death was like nothing else; its speed of propagation and the high mortality it caused were not comparable to anything known in the recent past. Plague was seen as a celestial disaster, a catastrophe, and a cataclysmic event. For most, it was a sign of the impending apocalypse, the end times themselves.

An elegy composed by fourteenth-century Anatolian mystic poet Şeyyad Hamza (fl. 1348), who lost his children to the plague, is the earliest known piece of poetry written in response to the Black Death in Turkish by an eyewitness (though not necessarily within Ottoman domains).[5] In this poem, the poet makes open references to the end of times and the signs of the impending apocalypse. By likening plague to a "rain of death," the poet establishes it as something that comes down from the skies pouring onto the earth. He similarly likens the plague to a "wind of death"; whomever it touched "fell down to the soil," just like dead leaves falling on the ground in the autumn. In his poem, plague "picks" people, "ripe or unripe," just as we harvest fruit from an orchard. The poet then asks, rhetorically, "what is the plague?" and goes on to answer, "it is the decree of the heavens."[6] In this poem, we have several of the key aspects common to the perception of plague in the late medieval era. First, it is a divine decree, an order sent from the heavens. Second, it is a sign of the impending apocalypse, a portent of the end times. Third, it has moral and social underpinnings. The poet calls the Muslims to repent, urgently, as it is implied that there are moral

---

4 E.g., see Stearns, "New Directions," and the bibliography cited therein.
5 Nothing much is known about the poet's life. For a brief biographical introduction, see Şeyyad Hamza, *The Story of Joseph: A Fourteenth-Century Turkish Morality Play*, trans. Bill Hickman (Syracuse, NY: Syracuse University Press, 2014), 6–8.
6 Akar, "Şeyyad Hamza," 3.

ills in his society. The poet offers a moral and political critique of his own society: greedy kings, oppressive rulers, loss of traditional values, and the hypocrisy of believers and men of religion alike. As we shall see, plague was often associated with social and moral problems in the Islamic traditions.

Given these implications, plague was also open to political associations. One of the earliest examples of its use in this manner comes from the fourteenth-century Ottoman historian Ahmedi's poetry. In a poem written for Prince Süleyman, one of the sons of Bayezid I, Ahmedi likens the prince's rage to a plague that would befall the rivals to the Ottoman throne.[7] Here he uses the plague as a motif of curse or punishment in a political context. Even though other such examples from poetry are scarce, hagiographic literature abounds in such themes.

Like poetry, late medieval Anatolian hagiographies (*menakıbname*) reveal a similar picture, in which plague is seen as divine decree, an apocalyptic portent, having moral and religious overtones. It also figures as punishment or curse, sometimes for individuals, at other times for entire communities. Put into writing from the fifteenth century onward, hagiographies have liberally used the themes of plague and pestilence in addition to other natural disasters.[8] These works were composed to illustrate the supernatural powers of saintly figures, including their ability to inflict plague on others as punishment. For instance, Hacı Bektaş, a thirteenth-century Anatolian mystic, curses Saru so that he would have a carbuncle in his armpit (plague bubo?), whereupon he suffers death as a result of this condition. In a different example, Abdal Musa, a fourteenth-century mystic and contemporary of the Black Death, leaves the community of Genceli to suffer from plague because they did not acknowledge his saintly powers and offended him.[9] To be sure, the motif of the saint cursing his community or his enemies continues as a common trope down to very late examples of the genre.[10]

---

7   Ahmedî, *Dîvân*, 87 [Der-medh-i Emîr Sülmân]: "Bu tâhûn-ı felek altında hışmı / İricek hasma tâ'ûn ı vebâdur" (Under this heaven's mill, his rage / will befall upon the rivals like plague and pestilence).

8   Although historians have long been critical of the historical value of these stories because of the supernatural elements in their narrative, a fresh interest has recently grown for the examples of the genre. Instead of taking these events as literal representations of the past, this new approach interprets them in their historical contexts, with a view to understanding the ideas and beliefs expressed in them. See, e.g., John Curry, "Scholars, Sufis, and Disease: Can Muslim Religious Works Offer Us Novel Insights on Plagues and Epidemics in the Medieval and Early Modern World?," in *Plague and Contagion in the Islamic Mediterranean*, ed. Nükhet Varlık (Burlington, VT: Ashgate, forthcoming).

9   Abdal Mûsâ, *Velâyetnâme*, 140–41. The text does not openly refer to plague but to "a celestial disaster" (*âfât-ı semâviye*). I discuss why I believe this is a reference to the Black Death in Genceli in Chapter 3.

10 For further examples, see my "From '*Bête Noire*' to '*le Mal de* Constantinople.'" Also see Curry, "Scholars, Sufis, and Disease."

Like poetry and hagiographies, early Ottoman chronicles also show a similar picture. In these sources, plague appears as a celestial disaster or a cataclysmic event. As such, it is *timeless* and *placeless*. In other words, it is not imagined to belong to a temporality of this world; rather, it is a sign of the impending apocalypse and the thereafter. Neither is it imagined to take place in a particular worldly locus (let alone Ottoman); its locus is somewhere in the heavens. In this manner, plagues often figured as part of apocalyptic scenarios, especially fueled by expectations on the eve of the turn of the Islamic millennium. Corresponding to the late fifteenth century, this was a time when such scenarios widely circulated in Ottoman society. For example, the chronicler Oruç commented that "the constant presence of plagues in every clime" was a sign of the impending apocalypse.[11] In seeking comfort from these apocalyptic anxieties, stories of the Prophet-Saint Hızır's intercession, among others, found their way into these accounts.[12] Not too long before Oruç, the Yazıcıoğlu brothers, well-known intellectual figures of the fifteenth century, also mentioned plagues in this way. Whereas Mehmed Yazıcıoğlu (d. 1451) briefly mentions plagues and pestilence as signs of the apocalypse, writing a decade later, his brother Ahmed Bican Yazıcıoğlu (d. after 1465) vividly describes the events associated with the Islamic millennial expectations of the apocalypse in his encyclopedic work *Dürr-i Meknun* (Hidden Pearls), including the appearance of the plague as "white death" (*mevt-i ebyaz*), in addition to famine and other causes of deaths.[13]

As briefly mentioned in the case of Şeyyad Hamza, the connection between plagues and perceived moral decay was not peculiar to the fourteenth century. In fact, such associations had a long history in Islamic apocalyptic thought. In Islamic apocalyptic traditions in general, and in fifteenth-century Ottoman apocalyptic thought in particular, plagues and moral decay were considered to be signs of the apocalypse.[14] Moreover, moral decay was seen as the cause of plagues. For example, Ahmed Bican claims that adultery, especially when it was openly practiced, was the main cause of plagues in a society. He commented, "A drop of semen falling on forbidden [*haram*] ground must certainly be plague [*ta 'un*]; if it begets a child, the child must

---

[11] Oruç, *Tarih*, 153: "Şimdiki zamanımızda ta'un her memleketten çıkmaz oldu. Kıyamet günü gelmesine delalet ve işarettir."

[12] As a striking case, Oruç tells the curious story of the encounter between a wagon driver and the Prophet-Saint Hızır, who was chasing black riders (plague and pestilence). I analyze that story closely elsewhere. See my "From '*Bête Noire*' to '*le Mal de* Constantinople.'"

[13] Mehmed Yazıcıoğlu, *Muhammediye*, 313; Ahmed Bîcan Yazıcıoğlu, *Dürr-i Meknun (Saklı İnciler)* (Istanbul: Tarih Vakfı Yurt Yayınları, 1999), 120: "mevt-i ahmer kandır ve mevt-i ebyaz ki ta'undur; zuhur ede." Also see Ahmed Bican Yazıcıoğlu, *Dürr-i Meknun: kritische Edition mit Kommentar*, ed. Laban Kaptein (Asch: privately published, 2007), 307, 556.

[14] Kaya Şahin, "Constantinople and the End Time: The Ottoman Conquest as a Portent of the Last Hour," *Journal of Early Modern History* 14, no. 4 (2010): 317–54.

be evil [*şerli*]."[15] By doing so, he not only strengthened his apocalyptic discourse but also reenacted beliefs about the social and moral dimensions of plagues. In this perspective, plagues broke out, not haphazardly, but for a reason. Notwithstanding its divine origins, pestilence was believed to happen when humans transgressed social and moral boundaries.[16]

Neither Oruç nor the Yazıcıoğlu brothers, however, were lone voices in imagining plagues in this fashion. Plagues were crucial constituents of apocalyptic tales in the anonymous Ottoman chronicles of the late fifteenth century. Composed after the Ottoman conquest of Constantinople in 1453, the examples of this genre included sections on the history of the city, often mentioning plague as an unambiguous sign of the impending apocalypse. The manner in which these accounts used plague and pestilence in the history of the city cannot be dismissed as simply fictitious and mythical, as they suggest the effects of a larger historical process at work.

As is well known, Constantinople had been the celebrated imperial capital city of the Byzantine Empire for more than a millennium when it fell to Ottoman rule in 1453. In the wake of the conquest, the new owners of the city saw that it had long lost its days of glory. As a matter of fact, Byzantine Constantinople had never fully recovered from the destructions of the Latin conquest in 1204 and since then had gradually lost its population, economic vitality, and political power. The Black Death and the successive waves of plague only added to the city's misery. Finally, the sack of the city by the Ottoman troops was the last catastrophe for its population, whereupon many fled, and those remaining were either enslaved or killed. Hence, repopulating and reviving the city immediately became a primary concern for its conqueror, Mehmed II, who took a series of measures to this end. Still, despite these efforts, the increase of the city's population was slow in the beginning, partly because of the check by periodic plagues.[17] Within a century or so, Ottoman Istanbul became one of the most important cities of the early modern Mediterranean. The conquest of the city not only increased Ottoman power and prestige considerably but also gave the new rulers of

---

[15] Ahmed Bîcan, *Dürr-i Meknun*, 109. Also see Ahmed Bican Yazıcıoğlu, *Dürr-i Meknun: kritische Edition mit Kommentar*, 532–33: "haram yere düşen meni elbette taun olsa gerekdir; veled olursa şerli olsa gerekdir." A similar association between the spilled "semen of adultery" and plague is mentioned by Taşköprizade, who wrote that some scholars believed that God creates a group of blind jinn from "semen of adultery" and they pierce whomever God wants to afflict with plague. See Taşköprizade, *Risalah al-shifa' li-adwa' al-waba'* ([Cairo]: al-Matba'ah al-Wahbiyah, 1875), 40.

[16] Adultery and fornication, morally unacceptable behaviors according to Islamic religious principles, have often been mentioned in association with plague in the hadith literature. Taşköprizade discusses this at length. See Taşköprizade, *Risalah al-shifa'*, 29–40.

[17] Following the Black Death in 1347, there were at least ten waves of recurrent outbreaks, as testified by the Byzantine sources. For a more detailed account of these outbreaks, see Chapter 3. For the demographic effects of plague and conquest, see Kafesçioğlu, *Constantinopolis/Istanbul*, 16; İnalcık "Istanbul."

the city an opportunity to extend their ideological claims based on the city's imperial Roman tradition.

The conquest of the city marked important social and political transformations in Ottoman history. Following the conquest, Mehmed's ambitious imperial and centralist political claims, taxation policies, and bureaucratization processes alienated some sections of Ottoman society and caused widespread resentment. These were mostly frontier warriors, religious scholars, and urban classes, who lost their power vis-à-vis the rising power of the central administrative and military structures. These sentiments of resentment and alienation, which could not be expressed during the reign of the latter, began to find a voice during the reign of his successor, Bayezid II. Well aware of the widespread discontent, Bayezid followed a conciliatory policy vis-à-vis the disenchanted military and religious groups. Yet it was no coincidence that this era saw an explosion in the number of historical texts, which reflect the voice of those who were marginalized by Mehmed's centralist policies. These chronicles, generically titled *Chronicles of the House of Osman (Tevarih-i Al-i Osman)*, were composed in Turkish and typically included sections about the history of Constantinople, which are seemingly a recollection of popular Byzantine tales and legends. In the late fifteenth century, popular legends about the foundation of the city, its religious monuments, and especially the imperial church of Hagia-Sophia were circulating widely. As the Ottomans began to familiarize themselves with these tales, the legendary elements soon found their way into these texts.

In these anonymous chronicles, the history of the city is pictured as a series of devastating punishments inflicted by God, like earthquakes, fires, and plagues. According to these narratives, the city was built and successively destroyed three times, each time with cataclysmic events. The narrative of successive thriving of the city and its imminent devastation had the underlying theme of an eternal curse as a trajectory that preserved the memory of Constantinople's multilayered history. Modern scholarship has demonstrated how the anonymous chroniclers attributed strong apocalyptic overtones to the city's past in an attempt to criticize the current centralist political ideology formulated on the basis of the city. The authors of these chronicles used, modified, and re-created the legendary constituents of popular tales of Istanbul's past in such a way as to express their anti-imperial sentiments in the late fifteenth century. In other words, these tales easily turned into ideological tools in the hands of the chroniclers in voicing the resentment of the discontented parties against the Ottoman imperial project.[18]

---

[18] For one version of the story dating from 1468, see Stéphane Yerasimos, *La fondation de Constantinople et de Sainte-Sophie dans les traditions turques: légendes d'Empire* (Paris: Institut français d'études anatoliennes, 1990), 5–48.

In addition to its ideological use, the imagery used in association with plague and pestilence in these accounts is also significant. To exemplify the visual clues with which plague is associated in these texts, consider the reference to the magic column in Constantinople. According to the anonymous chronicles, Constantine, the third founder of the city, had a magic column erected in the Hippodrome. A statue of a bronze dragon with formulaic writings on it, this column was believed to protect the city against snakes, centipedes, and dragons. He also had another column erected on which there was a copper statue of Constantine himself on a horse. It was believed that this column protected the city from plagues.[19]

These narratives and the visual clues they mobilized allow a glimpse into how the city's new owners perceived themselves vis-à-vis the city and its past. The city is portrayed in these texts as a land of enigmatic horrors and perils, and one that embraces all sorts of misfortunes. It is wild, full of unexpected (and divine) punishment. These examples of the genre dating from the late fifteenth century clearly suggest that the Ottomans neither perceived the city and its past as belonging to them nor yet saw themselves as part of it. The imagery used for plagues went hand in hand with sources of other real or imaginary fears, such as dragons, centipedes, scorpions, and snakes. It should also be noted that these texts talked about plagues as a thing of the past, a past with which they did not necessarily associate themselves. In other words, Istanbul had not been yet fully established as part of the Ottoman identity in the popular perception of the late fifteenth century. In this context, plague was imagined as a foreign, mythical, and mysterious presence. Notwithstanding the heavy Byzantine influence,[20] the general framework in which plagues were understood overlaps with the grand divine scheme of the Islamic cosmological discourse, with its strong social and moral implications. In this discourse, as it surfaces in the hagiographic and historical sources, all explanation regarding the origins, causes, and even resolution of this ill were to be sought in divine power, sometimes executed through the intercession of saintly agents. In this configuration, disease is seen as an unfamiliar and unruly presence over which the Ottomans imagined themselves as having no control.

---

[19] Ibid., 23–24, 28. The story of the magic column can also be found in the chronicle of Oruç, though with a slightly different emphasis. See Oruç, *Tarih*, 100–101.

[20] Byzantine perceptions of and responses to plagues and pestilence have been largely shaped by the experience with the Justinianic plague (541–750). Metaphysical-eschatological perceptions (plagues as divine retribution or punishment, as the outcome of human transgression) dominated over rational explanations (epidemics caused by pestilential air) and prevailed across time and genres. See Dionysios Stathakopoulos, "Crime and Punishment"; Congourdeau, "La peste noire"; Congourdeau and Melhaoui, "La perception de la peste en pays chrétien byzantin et musulman."

Changing Conceptions of Plague: Naturalization

Popular perceptions of plagues and pestilence that appear in the historical narratives of the sixteenth century stand in clear contrast to those of the previous era. The mainstream Ottoman historical narratives composed in the sixteenth century gradually eliminated the theme of devastation. During the first half of the century, the cataclysmic and apocalyptic elements that had been much emphasized in relation to the history of Istanbul started to fade away in the chronicles.[21] The city was no longer seen as doomed to destruction. The imagery of wild beasts, dragons, and snakes gradually disappeared from narratives, if not necessarily from popular imagery.

In this narrative context, the long-held bonds of late medieval Ottoman plague imaginaries started to come loose of their apocalyptic implications. To be sure, plague was still seen as carrying out the divine decree, and it mostly retained its former association with morality. However, it came to represent something less fantastical in the Ottoman mentalities. This decreasing component was offset by a new vision, in which the elements drawn from the supernatural realm gradually came to be replaced by those drawn from the natural. Hence, the Ottoman plague imaginaries started going though a process of *naturalization*. By this, I mean that plague was no longer viewed as an alien presence to the Ottomans; it came to be accepted as their own. I think of this cultural process as analogous to the biological process of *naturalization* by which a new species (plant or animal) can become established in places where they are not indigenous. Similarly, in the context of the modern nation-states, a citizen of another country (an *alien*) becomes a *naturalized* citizen. Just like this, plague was domesticated in the Ottoman imagination; it was no longer an alien presence. In this sense, the Ottomans naturalized plague in the sixteenth century.

Having laid out the basic parameters of this transformation, we can shift our attention to the actual transformations in the Ottoman urban context – the very set of transformations that enabled the process of naturalization. In the case of Istanbul, these transformations entailed dramatic changes since the Ottoman conquest of the city, but especially over the course of the sixteenth century, that deserve further consideration. In a nutshell, in the century following its conquest, the former Byzantine capital changed spectacularly. An astoundingly rapid population increase (nearly a tenfold increase within a century), its emergence as a hub of international commerce, and the ensuing civic undertakings turned Istanbul into a cosmopolitan

---

[21] For example, *Ayas Paşa Tarihi* (up to 1534) eliminates many of the cataclysmic elements from the narrative, which turns the text into a series of unrelated legends. Two decades later, *Lütfi Paşa Tarihi* (up to 1554) removes several apocalyptic references. Later, *Rüstem Paşa Tarihi* (up to 1560) tried to interpret the legends within the imperial perspective. See Yerasimos, *La fondation*, 215–23.

metropolis and a cultural magnet, attracting poets, scholars, artists, and mystics. Hence, Ottoman Istanbul was already deep in the process of emerging as the political, economic, cultural center of the Mediterranean world in the mid-sixteenth century.

Indeed, the Ottoman administration followed a conscious policy for rendering the newly conquered Constantinople the likes of a Muslim city. To this end, a heavy program of building activity slowly but surely started to change the city's silhouette. Erecting new edifices, such as a new imperial palace (the Topkapı Palace), and massive building projects, such as impressive imperial mosques (as well as conversion of former Byzantine churches), quickly made an impact on the onlooker, local and visitor alike.[22] These policies not only sought to project the new image of a Muslim city to its present and future spectators, it also sought to reinvent its past. For example, the "discovery" of the tomb of Ebu Eyub el-Ensari, one of the companions of Prophet Muhammad, who was believed to have died during an early siege of Constantinople, proved to be very successful in providing the city with a much-needed source of legitimization – especially in the eyes of those groups who were critical of it. The spiritual power of the dead helped to restore or reinvent Istanbul's pious character. Much like Bursa and Edirne, Istanbul could now be imagined as blessed by Muslim blood. The fact that a mosque was built on the location of the tomb, a public burial ground developed there, and the neighborhood acquired a sanctity as a result shows how successful these attempts have been in the long run.[23] As this example suggests, Istanbul was in the process of acquiring a new legitimacy and being adopted as part of the new Ottoman identity. Above all, this meant that people's perception of the city and their affective position vis-à-vis the city changed. This shift in mentality needs to be understood within the context of the formation of an Ottoman urban culture and identity.

A new Ottoman urban elite that embraced the political culture of the imperial project and that of the imperial city emerged in the sixteenth century. This new elite simultaneously formulated and believed in values such as urban culture, cosmopolitanism, or imperial ideology and enjoyed the ensuing feeling of living in safety and peace. The sentiments of military, political, and religious superiority, the belief in the supremacy of justice and law, the splendor of material riches and beauties, manifestations of new esthetic values in arts and architecture, availability of commodities in the markets and harbor, and the social welfare services at their disposal certainly contributed

---

[22] See, e.g., Gülru Necipoğlu, *Architecture, Ceremonial, and Power: The Topkapi Palace in the Fifteenth and Sixteenth Centuries* (New York: Architectural History Foundation, 1991); Necipoğlu, "A Kânûn for the State, a Canon for the Arts: Conceptualizing the Classical Synthesis of Ottoman Art and Architecture," in Veinstein, *Soliman le magnifique*, 195–216; Kafesçioğlu, *Constantinopolis/Istanbul*.

[23] Edhem Eldem, *Death in Istanbul: Death and Its Rituals in Ottoman-Islamic Culture* (Istanbul: Ottoman Bank Archives and Research Centre, 2005), 16.

to the changing self-perception of the urban population of Istanbul over the course of the sixteenth century and helped redefine the imperial city as a part of its cultural identity.[24]

Those who identified themselves with the imperial project situated Istanbul as a new epicenter of their "Ottomanness." The rise of this new Ottoman urban culture and identity manifested in myriad ways: the rise of court poetry in the Ottoman Turkish language; new genres in literature to express new urban ways, tastes, and pleasures, such as *şehrengiz, surname, tezkiretü'ş-şu 'ara*, and works of etiquette. Over time, this new elite was to develop new tastes for commodities of pleasure (e.g., coffee, tobacco) and to enjoy new social venues and activities in the city, such as chatting in *bozahanes* in the winter, private drinking and poetry reciting gatherings, going to the taverns in Balat, Samatya, and Galata, and taking promenades in the summer in Kağıthane, Bahariye, and Tophane.[25]

It was this new perception of the city that retrospectively changed the perception of its past. This is why the cataclysmic events of the late-fifteenth-century anonymous chronicles came to be retold with a new eye. The theme of the curse in the foundation legend of the city was no longer necessary; neither were the apocalyptic plagues needed. The metaphors and imagery of plagues were also replaced accordingly. For example, to compensate for the dark imagery of the city's past, historical and literary accounts now started to introduce images of beauty and motifs of paradise into their descriptions.[26] Despite the continued and even aggravated presence of epidemic outbreaks in the sixteenth century, the new residents of the city did not write about those outbreaks in the same way as their ancestors had just a few generations before them. Within a few generations, the resentments of the previous century faded away and the people of Istanbul saw themselves as belonging to the city and acknowledged the city as part of their own identity. The perceived threats of the past were traded for sentiments of security of living under the body of a powerful empire.

Taken as a whole, this dramatic change has direct bearings on the treatment of plagues in Istanbul's past. Even though the chroniclers may have preserved the theme of plague in the narrative – perhaps also because it was part of their current experience – they no longer imagined it in apocalyptic terms. The following quotation from İlyas Efendi's *Tarih-i Kostantiniye* (*History of Constantinople*, written in 1562), where he narrates

---

[24] For the development of these new ideas and their embracement by this new elite, see Cornell H. Fleischer, *Bureaucrat and Intellectual in the Ottoman Empire: The Historian Mustafa Âli (1541–1600)* (Princeton, NJ: Princeton University Press, 1986); Necipoglu, "A Kânûn for the State"; Ebru Turan, "The Marriage of Ibrahim Pasha (ca. 1495–1536)," *Turcica* 41 (2009): 3–36; Kafesçioğlu, *Constantinopolis/Istanbul.*

[25] See, e.g., Ebru Boyar and Kate Fleet, *A Social History of Ottoman Istanbul* (Cambridge: Cambridge University Press, 2010), 157–248.

[26] Kafesçioğlu, *Constantinopolis/Istanbul,* 175–76.

the tale of the foundation of the city, seems to encapsulate this vision fully:

They [the people of Istanbul] observed that plague is not absent in the city, and the city dwellers are not free from sorrow and grief.... However, it is a city of fortune and glory, which welcomes (and is full of) fine and rare commodities from all around the world. Considering this nature of the city, its population found comfort to a degree from other calamities.[27]

As we read here, the author does acknowledge the frequent plagues, sorrow, and grief as being deeply embedded in the city. However, the fact that it is a land of glory and prosperity, full of all the rare and fine merchandise of the world, makes it a place worth living in. It seems that the perceived threats of the past are traded for sentiments of security under the body of a powerful empire and its material riches.

The naturalization of plague can be detected in the language and imagery used by Ottoman chroniclers. In particular, the chronicle of the late-sixteenth-century Ottoman historian Selaniki Mustafa Efendi (d. after 1600) is a rich source for illustrating these changes. Selaniki uses allegorical language to convey the *naturalized* view of plagues. For example, he personifies plague as someone who befriends victims who are on the "list of invited guests for the banquet," thus placing it in the very texture of the city's social life.[28] In another instance, our chronicler portrays the disease as the "cupbearer of death" who gently offers the cup.[29] The allegory of the cupbearer – borrowed from the Persian literature and commonly used in Ottoman poetry – generally represents the beloved, sometimes depicted as cruel and vicious.[30] Here, by replacing the beloved with plague, the author cultivates an image of the cupbearer who offers the drink of death gently and irresistibly. His personification of plague was not limited to this; in another instance, plague is a merciful figure. While the author narrates the events of autumn 1590, he says that the plague this time did not last long

---

[27] Yerasimos, *Kostantiniye ve Ayasofya Efsaneleri*, trans. Şirin Tekeli (Istanbul: İletişim, 1993), 244: "gördüler ki ta'un eksik olmıya ve anda sakin olan kimesne gam ve gussadan hali olmaya ve en son halkı zelzeleden kırılub ve harab olması andan ola, amma devlet ve 'izzet yeri ola ve cümle dünyanın malları ve a'la tuhfe ve yadigarları ana celb olunub dolu mal ola. Hala bu haline nazar eylediler ve gayrı belasından bu mikdar bile teselli oldular." Also see Yerasimos, *La fondation*, 228.

[28] Selânikî, *Tarih-i Selânikî*, 283: "while he [Mehmed Beg] was in Istanbul, the blessed [i.e., plague] adopted him as a friend. As he was on the list of invited guests for the banquet, he accepted the invitation."

[29] Selânikî, *Tarih-i Selânikî*, 173.

[30] It is not uncommon to find such depictions of the beloved in Ottoman poetry. For example, the beloved could be depicted as a merciless calamity "with blood-drinking lips" or "murderous, violent, and vengeful." See Walter G. Andrews, *The Age of Beloveds: Love and the Beloved in Early-Modern Ottoman and European Culture and Society* (Durham, NC: Duke University Press, 2005), 266–67.

but had mercy on people and left quickly, leaving behind teary-eyed parents mourning for the loss of their children.[31] In Selaniki's narrative, plague comes across as a regular in Istanbul – a recognized and accepted part of life in the city. Showing such acceptance is testified in the chronicler's use of expressions such as "the blessed plague" (*mübarek ta 'un*) or simply "the blessed" (*mübarek*), "the manifest disease" (*maraz-i zahir*), and "the blessed disease" (*maraz-i mübarek*). Selaniki uses equally allegorical language in reference to the effects of the plague and places this experience on the sensory imaginaries of life in the city. For example, he mentions the plague as having roasted people's livers ("cigerlerin biryan edip") in reference to the intense emotional pain of losing their children to plague.[32] He also uses the cries of the deceased's families to complement the sounds of the sensory map of the pain: "The sighs of people due to separation from and missing of their dear ones was a smoke fogging every corner of the city."[33] In Selaniki's Istanbul, plague is deeply ingrained in the very texture of urban life; it was familiar. Another sixteenth-century historian, Mustafa Ali, voices the same sense of familiarity, albeit in a more ironic manner. Ali said, "Eveything is in scarce supply there; only its plague is ample."[34] The sense of familiarity voiced by chroniclers seems to be shared by other members of Ottoman society as well. When a late-sixteenth-century letter submitted to the Palace during an epidemic stated, "There is no place free from that *blessed* disease," this was an unambiguous reference to plague without even naming it (Figure 2).[35] By the end of the century, plague had taken its place in the cultural landscape of early modern Istanbuliotes.

Occurrences of plague were now ripe for associations with the nature of the city. Sixteenth-century observers to the city seem to display a certain familiarity with the recurrent plagues, drawn from experience. They recognized its seasonal patterns of recurrence, predicted what climatic and environmental factors would precipitate or inhibit it, how the figures of

---

[31] Selânikî, *Tarih-i Selânikî*, 229.

[32] Ibid., 759. Sam White recently argued that this particular reference casts doubt on Selaniki's references to plague. White, *Climate of Rebellion*, 86; White "Rethinking Disease," 556. Although it is true that a literal reading of Selaniki may lead to confusion, this is clearly one of his allegorical references to the plague and the emotional pain it caused for losing loved ones. Reading the sentence in full helps to clarify the confusion: "Ekser halkun semere-i fu'âdın alup, ciğerlerin biryân eyledi." Here Selaniki is unmistakably referring to the pain of losing their beloved children to plague. In addition to its literal meaning as "liver" or "lungs," *ciğer* also meant "a dear; a darling." See, e.g., J. W. Redhouse, *A Turkish and English Lexicon* (Beirut: Librarie du Liban, 1890).

[33] Selânikî, *Tarih-i Selânikî*, 229.

[34] "Zâd u zevâde kılleti öldürdü halkı hep / Her nesne nâdir anda fe'emmâ vebâsı bol." See Kudret Altun, *Gelibolulu Mustafa Âli ve Divânı (Vâridâtü'l-Enîkâ)* (Niğde: Özlem Kitabevi, 1999), 515. For further discussion on how plague appears in Ali's poetry, see Fleischer, *Bureaucrat and Intellectual*, 134.

[35] See the discussion on plague terminology in the introduction.

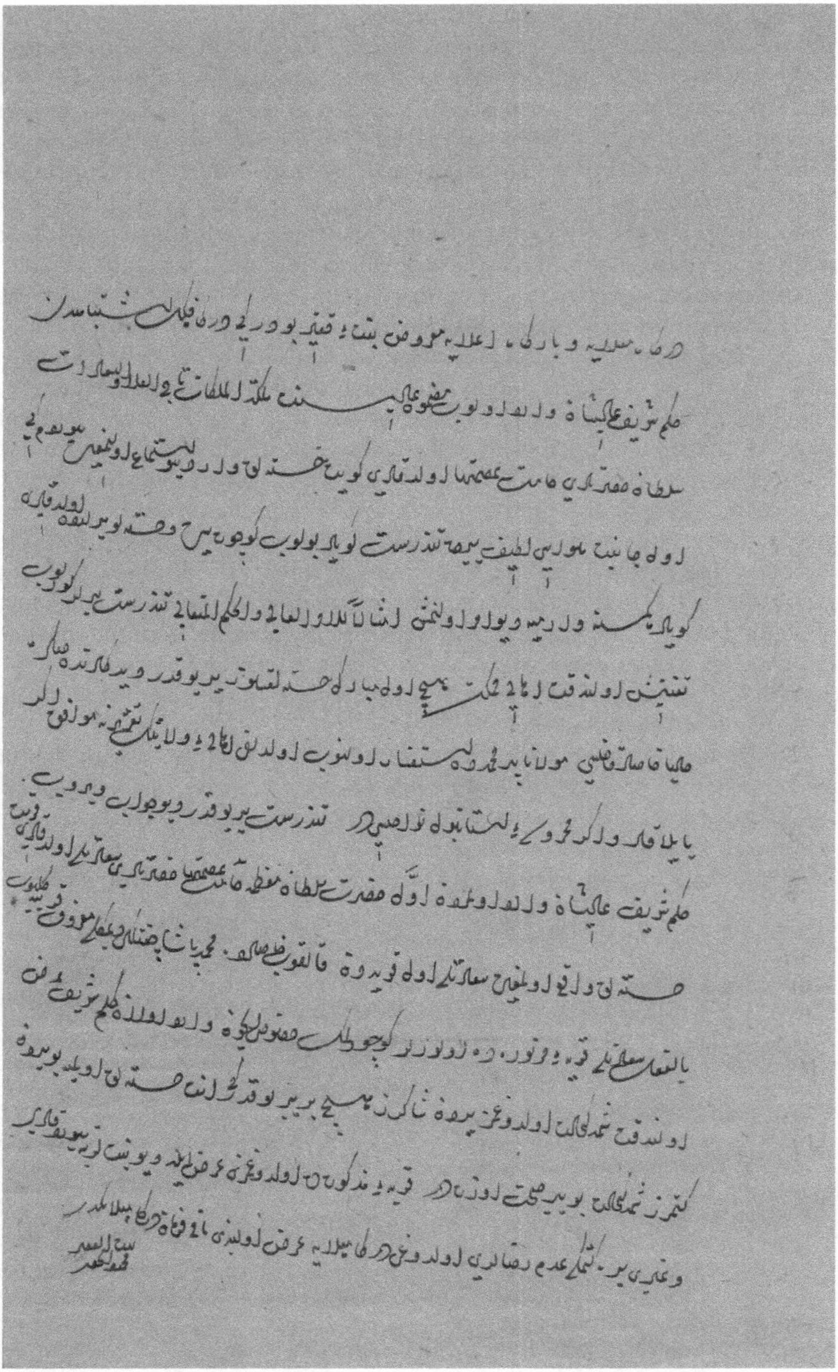

FIGURE 2. Letter submitted to the Palace during an epidemic. Second half of the sixteenth century. E. 4214. Document from Topkapı Palace Museum Archives.

mortality should be interpreted, and so on.[36] For example, Taşköprizade highlighted discussions of plague's seasonality and periodicity. He noted that plague mostly occurred during the spring and fall in areas with moderate climate, and rarely during hot summers and cold winters. He also added that sometimes it continued two years on a row; other times it skipped a year or two.[37] Istanbul's experience informed such localized discussions of plague, in the works of scholars and beyond. For example, Selaniki noted that plague lessened in the months of November and December of 1590, and the infection gradually died down; those afflicted recovered.[38] As firsthand observers to the disease, people of Istanbul recognized plague's established patterns of behavior in their city. Further testimony to discussions of Istanbul's disposition to plague on account of its climate is to be found in the account of Rabbi Moses Ben Barukh Almosnino. Writing in the sixteenth century, Almosnino believed that Istanbul had plagues owing to its climatic and environmental conditions (winds, rains, humidity of the soil, etc.).[39] Just as its climatic conditions or notorious fires, plague was also to be accepted as a problem endemic to the city itself.[40] This vision is expressed perceptively in the words of Jean Gontaut, Baron of Salignac, the French ambassador in Istanbul who, in the beginning of the seventeenth century, referred to plague as "*le mal de* Constantinople."[41] The locus of the disease has now shifted from the heavens to the city, from the domain of the supernatural to that of the natural. Plague was *naturalized* in the Ottoman cultural landscape.

Late Medieval Ottoman Knowledge of Plagues

In the words of Şeyyad Hamza, plague was so terrible that "no cure could heal this ill; even the wisdom of the legendary physician Lokman could not stop this suffering."[42] These lines reflect the widely shared feelings of helplessness of mid-fourteenth-century Anatolia. As has been observed, the intensity with which the disease killed, its swift spread, and the high levels of mortality must have each contributed to such feelings, certainly in the fourteenth century but to a large extent in the fifteenth as well.

---

[36] See e.g., discussion of changes in plague mortality as evidenced in TSMA E.6155 and E.2544 in Chapter 8.

[37] Taşköprizade, *Risalah al-shifa'*, 47–48.

[38] Selânikî, *Tarih-i Selânikî*, 229.

[39] Mosé ben Baruj Almosnino, *Extremos y grandezas de Constantinopla* (Madrid: Francisco Martinez, 1638), 7–8.

[40] Compare with the case of plague in Egypt, which had strong ties with the environment, as discussed in Mikhail, *Nature and Empire in Ottoman Egypt*, 202–21.

[41] Dursteler, "The Bailo in Constantinople," 16.

[42] Metin Akar, "Şeyyad Hamza," 14: "Bu derde diriğä dermān irişmez / Bu rence ḥikmet-i Loḳmān irişmez." In the Anatolian lore, Lokman was held to be a wise man and a legendary physician, renowned for his healing skills and his knowledge of the elixir of immortality. For Lokman in Anatolian belief, see, e.g., folktales 112 and 131 at the Uysal-Walker Archive of Turkish Oral Narrative, http://aton.ttu.edu.

The hagiographies also testify to the same mind-set. Because there was no known method to treat the plague, it would take a miracle to recover from it. This belief led people to seek out the healing power of saints. Only the intercession of saints, it was widely held, could make a difference. In these works, there are copious examples in which the saintly figure cures a sick individual by touching or by other miraculous means and even brings the dead back to life. In one such instance, Pir Ebi Sultan, a fourteenth-century Anatolian mystic and a disciple of Hacı Bektaş, loses two of his sons during a plague epidemic (possibly the Black Death) in Konya. A few days later, when a third son contracts the disease and dies, the deeply mourning wife of the mystic exhorts him to supplicate God to restore his third son's life, which brings him back to life.[43] There are also stories in which the holy man's miraculous cures extend to an entire community. For example, Abdal Musa, a fourteenth-century Anatolian mystic, became renowned for his spiritual powers for predicting plagues and for expelling them from his community, as he was believed to have "the soldiers of plague under his command."[44] Similarly, a fifteenth-century Sufi leader, Cemal el-Halveti (d. 1499), miraculously causes an epidemic in Istanbul to come to an end upon his departure for the holy cities of Mecca and Medina to supplicate for the salvation of the capital from this and other catastrophes.[45]

The medical literature of the time was not very different. Overall, it seems to present an ambiguous attitude toward plague. Even though this literature acknowledges that it was a very severe condition, discussions of plague do not correspond to its affirmed gravity. Taken as a whole, quite a number of medical works were composed in vernacular Turkish in fourteenth- and fifteenth-century Anatolia. These included works on surgery, preventive medicine, and medical compendia.[46] Among these, medical compendia were

---

[43] Hacı Bektaş Veli, *Vilâyetnâme*, 87. For a comparison of this case to the biblical story of Elisha's restoring the dead son of a Shunammite woman to life, see Ahmet Yaşar Ocak, *Kültür Tarihi Kaynağı Olarak Menâkıbnâmeler: Metodolojik Bir Yaklaşım* (Ankara: TTK, 1992), Appendix VI. For Pir Ebi Sultan, also see Chapter 3.

[44] For Abdal Musa being renowned for protecting against plagues, see *Abdal Mûsâ Velâyetnâmesi* (Ankara: TTK, 1999), 55. In addition to protecting or curing people from plague, Abdal Musa was also believed to have supernatural powers for inflicting it upon others. His power over plagues is also confirmed in the hagiography of Kaygusuz Abdal, one of his disciples, in the following way: "ta'un askeri, Allah emriyle Sultan Abdal Mûsâ Hazretlerinin zabtındadur." See Kaygusuz Abdal, *Kaygusuz Abdal (Alâeddin Gaybî) Menâkıbnamesi* (Ankara: TTK, 1999), 134. The metaphor of plague as soldier seems to surface in seventeenth-century accounts. See the following pages for a story recounted by Evliya Çelebi.

[45] John J. Curry, *The Transformation of Muslim Mystical Thought in the Ottoman Empire: The Rise of the Halveti Order, 1350–1750* (Edinburgh: Edinburgh University Press, 2010), 71.

[46] For a general introduction of the medical works composed in Turkish in fourteenth- and fifteenth-century Anatolia, see *OS*, 1:151–56, 165–95.

the most comprehensive genre of medical writing, covering topics ranging from anatomy to pharmaceutics, from preservation of health to various diseases afflicting different parts of the human body. In these works, the organization and classification of diseases followed the conventions of this genre; they were listed according to the body part they afflicted, typically arranged from head to toe. This scheme made it difficult for the authors of these compendia to classify infectious and contagious diseases. For instance, the *Müntahab-ı Şifa* of physician Hacı Paşa (d. circa 1417), one of the early examples of the genre, composed at the turn of the fifteenth century, discusses bubonic plague toward the end of the book.[47] After discussing all body parts and their afflictions, plague is presented along with snake and scorpion bites. This is curious because the author firmly states that plague is the most ferocious of all diseases. Perhaps he did not know how to categorize this disease and which body part to associate it with, and thus in which section of the compendium to discuss it. Because this seems to be one of the earliest surviving descriptions of the symptoms, prognosis, and treatment of plague we have at hand, it deserves further consideration.

Hacı Paşa describes the symptoms of the disease with great precision and accuracy: "Plague [*ta 'un*] is a feverish swelling or pustules that appear behind the ear, in the armpits, or in the groin area. These painful swellings appear when there is an epidemic and produce a burning feeling. The lesion of the swelling is black or green, or red. It gives nausea, vomiting, thirst, and shortness of breath." The author attributes the origin of the disease to the corruption of the air and to miasma but does not discuss it any further. For treatment purposes he suggests a selection of methods, such as bleeding or using laxatives, Armenian clay (*gil-i ermeni*), vinegar, theriacs, and rosewater. He recommends sprinkling vinegar inside the houses and fumigation; moderation in exercise, sex, and food; and avoiding bathing as much as possible. According to *Müntahab-ı Şifa*, while sour pomegranate juice, lemon juice, and other sour drinks are recommended, sweet food and drinks, fish, and yoghurt are to be avoided. In addition, he lists prayers, magic squares, and formulae for preparing amulets.[48] It may be worthwhile to note that what Hacı Paşa presents here is very much in line with other late medieval medical texts on plague in other parts of the Islamic world and in Europe. Having received an education in Cairo, and practiced medicine there, Hacı Paşa showed familiarity with classical texts of ancient Greek and Islamic medicine; he cites frequently from authors such as Hippocrates, Galen, Rufus of Ephesus, Ibn Sina, and al-Razi.

Another compendium in Turkish was Abdülvehhab el-Mardani's *Kitabu'l-Müntehab fi't-Tıb*. Composed in 1420 for Mehmed I, this work follows the same structure as that of *Müntahab-ı Şifa* but is less

---

[47] Hacı Paşa, *Müntahab-ı Şifâ* (Ankara: Türk Dil Kurumu, 1990), 172–79.
[48] Ibid., 172–79, quotation on 172–73.

comprehensive. Even though it includes discussions of other diseases, such as leprosy, scabies, smallpox, and measles, there is no separate entry devoted to plague. The author comments on plague only in comparison to measles and smallpox and concludes that the former is more serious than the latter two.[49] Considering this work in conjunction with the former, one may argue that these authors knew that plague was a very dangerous disease but did not have an established category in which they could discuss it in the compendium genre.

Even when a more extensive consideration was given to infectious diseases, their classification in the genre of medical compendia could still be problematic. For instance, the fifteenth-century Ottoman physician İbn Şerif's *Yadigar* classified fevers and skin diseases separately from diseases affecting body parts, arranged from head to toe. While placing measles and smallpox under fevers, he lists plague, leprosy, and scabies under skin diseases and presents remedies to use against them. His discussion of the symptoms, prognosis, and treatment of plague is largely similar to that of Hacı Paşa. In addition, he recommends carrying a piece of elephant bone on one's body, especially for children, and burning sheep bones at home for protection. He also recommends lancing and cupping plague buboes, as well as branding them or applying worms or leeches to them, which he mentions were methods experimented by the Mamluks with some success.[50]

As these examples suggest, these diseases did not have a clearly defined taxonomy in the Ottoman medical texts of the time. Discussions on etiology, prognosis, or prophylaxis, when they were included, were brief and did not follow a system of organization. In addition, the advice presented in these works was not exclusively medical; the authors did not refrain from offering spiritual methods of treatment, prayers, or use of magic squares. It may be noteworthy to observe that these spiritual methods were more emphasized than medical means for the treatment of plague – ironically enough (and perhaps precisely because) they all spoke of it as the most dangerous of all diseases.

In addition to the more general works of medicine, we also see the earliest examples of the more specialized works devoted solely to plague and epidemic diseases in the first half of the fifteenth century. Abdurrahman Bistami (d. 1455), a leading polymath of the fifteenth century, composed two treatises on epidemic diseases in Arabic.[51] Writing in Bursa in the 1430s, Bistami

49   Abdülvehhâb bin Yûsuf ibn-i Ahmed el-Mârdânî, *Kitâbu'l-Müntehab fî't-Tıb: inceleme, metin, dizin, sadeleştirme, tıpkıbasım*, ed. Ali Haydar Bayat (Istanbul: Merkezefendi Geleneksel Tıp Derneği, 2005), 159 [facsimile: 137a–37b].

50   İbn-i Şerîf, *Yâdigâr*, 2:152–53, 221, 321–22, 365.

51   Abdurrahman Bistami, *Wasf al-dawa' fi kashf afat al-waba'* [Description of the remedy on the discovery of calamities of epidemic], Süleymaniye Library, ms. Şehid Ali Paşa 2811/44; Bistami, *al-Ad 'iyyah al-muntakhabah fi al-adwiyyah al-mujarrabah* [Select prayers on proven prescriptions], Süleymaniye Library, ms. Hacı Mahmud Efendi 4228/1. For a brief discussion of these treatises, see İhsan Fazlıoğlu, "İlk dönem Osmanlı ilim ve kültür

had most likely witnessed the plague there in 1429–30, which took many lives.[52] Unlike Hacı Paşa or İbn Şerif, Bistami was not a physician, so his discussion of plague and epidemic diseases is not exclusively medical. Instead, he treats all forms of pestilence as calamity and discusses them with respect to Islamic sciences, prophetic and folk medicine, magic, and occult sciences. It should be noted that he, too, presents bubonic plague, as well as other diseases, such as smallpox, leprosy, and skin diseases, without a systematic classification. What he offers is an eclectic explanation of epidemic diseases on the basis of knowledge drawn from a mixture of ancient prophetic wisdom, classical works of Greco-Roman and Islamic learned traditions, and pre-Islamic Arab beliefs and customs filtered through the corpus of Prophetic medicine. For example, in his treatment of etiology, while acknowledging the divine origins of plague, he also comments on the natural-environmental causes, such as corrupted or miasmatic air, certain constellations of the stars, and supernatural agents like the jinn.[53] Clearly drawing from these disparate domains of causality did not constitute a problem for him. By the same token, the advice he offers on prevention and treatment is diverse. Bistami recommends using spiritual methods (magic squares, formulae for writing talismans, using the names of God, prayers, and the like), along with preventive and therapeutic recipes made of substances of plant, animal, and mineral origins. In these, he does not necessarily follow a distinction between plague and other diseases. For instance, he recommends a method of protection against bubonic plague that is also believed to guard against a number of completely unrelated ills, ranging from migraine to bed-wetting, from madness to miscarriage.[54] In another instance, prayers or other protective methods against plague are also recommended for other purposes, such as breaking spells and warding off the threat of sudden death, evil eye, nightmares, skin diseases, smallpox, accidents, the devil, burning, drowning in water, and theft. As these examples clearly suggest, Bistami neither used a system of classification of diseases nor distinguished between incongruent methods of prevention and treatment.

The lack of a clear-cut categorization in the knowledge of plagues can also be evidenced in the organization of book catalogs. For example, an early-sixteenth-century book inventory in the Ottoman palace library lists only three treatises on epidemic diseases in the section of medicine and allied sciences.[55] Not listed in the same section of the inventory, however, were Bistami's two treatises. Moreover, judging from the order in which

hayatında İhvânu's-safâ ve Abdurrahmân Bistâmî," *Dîvân: İlmî Araştırmalar* 2 (1996): 229–40.

[52] See Chapter 3.

[53] Bistami, *al-Ad'iyyah*, 4.

[54] Bistami, *Wasf al-dawa'*, 247.

[55] *Treatise on Epidemic Disease* (*Risalah fi al-waba'*); *Treatise on Plague* (*Risalah fi al-ta'un*); *Book of Regimen of Travelers and the Plague* (*Kitab al-tibb fi tadbir al-musafirin wa maradh al-ta'un*). See Atufi, *Defter-i Kütüb*, Hungarian National Library, ms. Török F. 59, 151–72.

these treatises were listed in this particular inventory, they do not seem to be understood as core medical texts. Not appearing until two-thirds into the section on medicine and allied sciences in this inventory, these treatises are listed under the subsection of medical miscellanea, mixed with others books on joint pain and dubious diseases, after the main categories of general medicine, medical theory, and handbooks, and only before works on pharmacology, zoology, and agriculture.

On the basis of this evidence, it can be argued that there was no clear taxonomy of epidemic diseases in Ottoman medical works before the early sixteenth century. Nor was there a clearly defined classification of their knowledge. Barely anything was written on the subject in the fifteenth century – sparing the works of Bistami, for which we have no clear evidence regarding their circulation until the mid-sixteenth century. Medical knowledge of this era included certain causal explanations, such as the corruption of the air or the *miasma*, constellations of the stars, and the jinn. Generally speaking, these explanations were compatible with Islamic cosmological discourses that acknowledged divine agency. In such times, it was recommended to do charitable acts, help the needy, and pray. There was, nevertheless, a set of recommendations for protecting oneself or one's family from the disease, such as the use of moderation, certain foods and drinks, and certain prayers, magic squares, talismans, and the like. However, it should be noted that the very same methods were also recommended for other, unrelated conditions. On the whole, it seems there was a limited pool of knowledge on plague, and that body of knowledge was largely ambiguous and eclectic.

Changing Knowledge of Plague: Medicalization

In the sixteenth century, a much larger body of plague knowledge came into existence in the Ottoman lands. Starting early in the century, Ottoman authors began composing works devoted to this subject in particular. Even the mere fact that we see the composition of these works in this era suggests that an intellectual shift toward the subject was at work. Moreover, these works were written by the leading Ottoman intellectuals – jurists, physicians, historians, and scholars – and as such were credited by their contemporaries, as well as in the later Ottoman eras, with a high degree of prestige. All this suggests that plague as a subject started to find its way into the intellectual world of the Ottoman scholars in the sixteenth century.

Taken as a whole, the body of knowledge represented in this corpus stands in clear contrast with the limited pool of knowledge and observations to be found in that of the fifteenth. But the difference is not only in the number of works composed, nor, for that matter, because plague came to be recognized as a legitimate subject to write about. The contrast, as is argued here, mainly lies in three important differences: first, the organization of plague knowledge; second, the use of plague knowledge; and third, views about authority and expertise over plague. In what follows, I argue that sixteenth-century Ottoman plague knowledge represents a process of (or toward) *medicalization* on the basis of the three criteria listed.

Even though the concept of medicalization is generally understood in modern context, its possible uses for the premodern era might be explored.[56] Here, *medicalization* is used primarily in reference to the changes in both the nature and use of plague knowledge. As new works were composed on the subject, the genre of plague treatises, along with its organizational conventions, started to take shape, contributing to the development of a systematic body of knowledge. The treatises enabled the circulation of knowledge, both among the specialists and beyond, creating possibilities for that knowledge to be put to use. All these, in turn, affected the general perception of who held authority and expertise over plague. That said, this does not imply that medical professionals were necessarily involved in the process of diagnosis or in legal matters related to deaths as a result of plague, even when this involved the Ottoman tax-exempt *askeri* class, whose bodily health was under a higher degree of surveillance by the Ottoman state than that of its taxpaying subjects. In that sense, the process of *medicalization* was not fully accomplished over the course of the sixteenth century.

Before going into a closer analysis of that body of knowledge, it may be useful to make some general observations about the sixteenth-century Ottoman plague corpus. First, it must be noted that this substantial body of literature remains largely unexplored. Until recently, the scholarship has underestimated their value and believed that they were simply unoriginal copies of each other, or of the earlier Arabic corpus. Recent literature suggests quite the opposite. It appears that this corpus involved different opinions and lively intellectual debates.[57] Moreover, these treatises seem to have

---

56 For discussions of "medicalization" in the context of transition to modern medicine, see e.g., Jean-Pierre Goubert, ed., *La médicalisation de la société française, 1770–1830* (Waterloo, ON: Historical Reflections Press, 1982); Colin Jones, "Montpellier Medical Students and the Medicalisation of 18th-Century France," in *Problems and Methods in the History of Medicine*, ed. R. Porter and A. Wear, 57–80 (London: Croom, 1987).

57 Until recently, these treatises have been ignored or discredited by the mainstream scholarship, which maintained that they were simply translations and copies of earlier works in Arabic. For examples of scholarship that discredited Ottoman plague treatises, see Panzac, *La peste*, 48 and Dols, "Second Plague Pandemic," 164. For a brief analysis of the genre of Ottoman plague treatises of the fifteenth and sixteenth centuries, see Nükhet Varlık, "Disease and Empire: A History of Plague Epidemics in the Early Modern Ottoman Empire (1453–1600)," PhD diss., University of Chicago, 2008, 173–204; for a selected list of manuscript copies of the genre, 279–83. Some of the prominent examples of the genre have been analyzed in Bulmuş, *Plague, Quarantines, and Geopolitics*. Also see Nurten Çankaya, "Taşköprülüzade Ahmet İsameddin Efendi'nin *Risaletü'ş-şifa li-edva'il-vebâ* adlı Risalesi Üzerine bir Değerlendirme," in *VIII. Türk Tıp Tarihi Kongresi: Kongreye Sunulan Bildiriler* (Istanbul: Türk Tıp Tarihi Kurumu, 2006), 313–22; Curry, "Scholars, Sufis, and Disease."

functioned as the main media for the production, discussion, and dissemination of the knowledge and ideas of plague and deserve more extensive consideration.

In the main, discussions in the sixteenth-century treatises reflect dramatic changes in the development and organization of plague knowledge. These treatises tried to present, analyze, and synthesize the available knowledge in a systematic fashion. They discussed the causes and origins of epidemics, making clear distinctions between plague and other diseases. They also included medical advice for physical treatment as well as religious and magical means for spiritual treatment. They offered advice for prevention and dealt with the problem of the transmission of disease, and they recommended proper conduct in times of plagues. The tracts typically discuss plague etiology, prognosis, and prophylaxis under separate chapters or headings, which suggests a more systematic and in-depth study of this phenomenon. Oftentimes, treatise writers, or their users, integrated their own empirical observations into the main text or in the margins. It is not at all uncommon to see added comments in those manuscripts, for instance, about remedies that are marked as "tried and proven beneficial" (*mücerrebdir*). Above all, the role of the treatises must be recognized in the production, classification, and circulation of knowledge.

That said, let us study the process of *medicalization* more closely, in three stages. First, plague was identified as a distinct disease, which was followed by the articulation of a set of knowledge about its sign and symptoms, causes, prognosis, and prophylaxis. Second, this knowledge became crystallized and adopted as working knowledge for state policies. Third, the expertise over plague and claims to predict, calculate, or heal it gradually moved from the domain of the saints and Sufis to that of the state and its institutions of health.

To begin with, a precise identification of plague that aimed to differentiate it from other epidemic diseases surfaced in the treatises. An early-sixteenth-century example was a treatise – titled *Majannah al-ta ʿun wa al-waba ʾ* (The Refuge from Plague and Pestilence) – written by İlyas bin İbrahim (Eliahu ben Avraham) (d. after 1512), an Iberian Jewish physician who came to Istanbul around the turn of the sixteenth century and converted to Islam.[58] In this work, plague (*tā ʿun*) is described as follows: "In the human body, the plague appears like an inflamed boil which gives intense pain and suffering. Its surrounding area is black or green. Its inside is red." When the bubo is black, the author added, this indicated that the patient was most likely to expire.[59] This is an example of a precise reference to a

---

[58] İlyas, *Majannah*; İlyas, *Tevfīkāt*; Ekmeleddin İhsanoğlu, "Endülüs Menşeli Bazı Bilim Adamlarının Osmanlı Bilimine Katkıları," *Belleten* 58 (1994): 565–605; Ron Barkai, "Between East and West: A Jewish Doctor from Spain," in *Intercultural Contacts in the Medieval Mediterranean*, ed. Benjamin Arbel (Portland, OR, 1996), 49–63.

[59] İlyas, *Tevfīkāt*, 16–17.

plague bubo, accompanied with description of other symptoms. We know that earlier descriptions in the fifteenth century had also accurately done so. However, there is a major difference. Now, not only was plague identified as a distinct disease, separate from others, but also explanations for its causes and treatment had to be distinct from those of other diseases. Hence, unlike the eclectic body of causes of the fifteenth-century works, we find the articulation of a distinct body of causal explanations in the sixteenth-century treatises. Taken as a whole, the corpus represents a complex systematic of disease etiology. In a nutshell, there was a hierarchy of causes, at the top of which there was God, without whom neither epidemics nor cure would be possible. Next in the hierarchy was celestial powers, cosmic influence of the stars, and other astronomic and astrological events. God, stars, and planets all exercised indirect influences through a more direct agent: the air, a substance that, once corrupted, could damage the vital powers of the living when breathed. The air was understood to be subjected to the specific conditions of different locations. Hence, it was understood to be displaying variations from place to place in terms of the effect of heat, humidity, and seasons. At the bottom of the hierarchy were humans (and animals), who either by their natural dispositions or through their regimen were capable of falling prey to disease. Within the general outlines of this hierarchical scheme of causation, there were individual differences of emphasis between different authors. For example, some authors, such as Taşköprizade, held a distinction between "material" (*ruhani*) and "spiritual" (*cismani*) causes of plague, discussing them separately. According to this, while the spiritual causes involved the power of evil spirits or the jinn, material causes stemmed from putrid air.[60] It should be underlined that these authors did not find it controversial to draw from different pools of etiological concepts. On the contrary, the scheme of hierarchy of causes afforded a combination of factors they could use in conjunction with each other. Stated differently, as long as there was a hierarchy of causal explanations, one could always find a way of explaining plagues; if one causal factor failed to explain it, another would do it. Moreover, a hierarchy of causes allowed explanations to be attuned to local variations. Having the flexibility of using multiple systems of etiology, treatise writers could establish connections between seemingly incongruent notions. For example, İlyas insisted on the possibility of a causal relationship between earthquakes and plague, which he held was due to the unleashing of corrupted air to the surface of the earth. He explicitly stated in his introduction that he composed his treatise following a major outbreak in Istanbul (perhaps that of 1509), fearing that it would lead to a plague outbreak.[61] Similarly, Taşköprizade wrote that the corruption of the air was related to terrestrial and celestial causes: "Corruption usually occurs at the end of the summer and during fall. During summer, bad

---

[60] Taşköprizade, *Risalah al-shifa'*, 29, 39–49. Also see Ünver, "Türkiyede Veba," 70–71.
[61] İlyas, *Tevfikät*, 11–13. For the connection between earthquakes and plague, see Chapter 1.

residues come together and are in close contact with corrupt air." At the same time, he referred to the seasonal character of plague in an effort to explain why sporadic outbreaks affect one area but not others.[62] As seen in these examples, in addition to well-known causes of corrupt air or miasma, such as arising from swamps or soldiers fallen dead on battlefields, these authors have sought to establish a relationship between different pools of etiological explanations and tried to adjust them to the local conditions of sixteenth-century Istanbul.

The very same authors also referred to contagion, as a causal explanation, alongside corrupt air or miasma. Both İlyas and Taşköprizade discuss contagion taking place in different forms to explain the spread of the disease from one person to another, once it broke out as triggered by whatever macrocosmic force they preferred to attribute it to, depending on their choice of environmental flavor. Even more specific to the case of Istanbul's plagues were the statements of Rabbi Almosnino, who suggested that while Istanbul's specific environmental and climatic conditions (its winds, rain, etc.) favored the plague, it was also brought from outside.[63] As these examples suggest, the more direct causes were sought to explain the local spread of the disease, while larger environmental and cosmic forces were used to explain the initial outbreak of epidemic or pandemic plagues. Overall, the ideas of contagion and miasma were like two sides of a coin, tossed and flipped to suit the needs of a particular epidemic and its spectators.[64]

Likewise, a distinct set of knowledge on prevention and treatment surfaced in the sixteenth-century plague tracts. Unlike the mixture of methods recommended in the fifteenth century for a variety of illnesses and other conditions (such as wounds caused by accidents or burning), now we see that plague started to acquire its own set of preventative and therapeutic measures – peculiar to plague only. In general terms, sixteenth-century tracts favored preventive methods over remedial ones, as prevention was understood to be more important than treatment. It was well known, from observation, that plague was mostly fatal; once the disease was contracted, chances of survival were slim.[65] Still, there were recommendations for a host of methods for treatment, ranging from simple herbal recipes to more complex pharmaceuticals like theriacs and complex formulaic prayers.

---

[62] Taşköprizade, *Risalah al-shifa'*, 47.

[63] Almosnino, *Extremos y grandezas*, 7–8.

[64] These explanations did not have a contradictory character at this time. See, e.g., Kinzelbach, "Infection, Contagion, and Public Health."

[65] Even though we do not have data that would help calculate mortality vs. morbidity figures, we do occasionally hear in the sources about people who recover from plague – perhaps the most famous example in the sixteenth century was Aşık Çelebi. See Hatice Aynur, "Kurgusu ve Vurgusuyla Kendi Kaleminden Âşık Çelebi'nin Yaşamöyküsü," in *Âşık Çelebi ve Şairler Tezkiresi Üzerine Yazılar*, ed. Hatice Aynur and Aslı Niyazioğlu (Istanbul: Koç Üniversitesi Yayınları, 2011), 52–53.

Generally speaking, the Ottoman treatise writers distinguished between spiritual and material methods offered for the purposes of prevention and treatment. Some are clearly drawn from the medical paradigm of humors in that they emphasize moderating the six nonnaturals, such as sleep, exercise, and diet. For example, İlyas stressed that the air had to be clean: places with corrupted air had to be avoided, the mouth and nose had to be covered by a handkerchief imbibed with fragrant oils, houses had to be sprinkled with vinegar, and fumigation was recommended. Similarly, one had to keep a well-regimented diet and avoid excesses in sleep, sex, exercise, excretion, and emotions to preserve health.[66] For treatment purposes, İlyas recommended bloodletting, purging, and lancing and cupping the plague bubo. More interestingly, the application of a live chicken or pigeon on top of the plague bubo was also recommended as a method to drain the "poison" of plague. For his part, Kemalpaşazade's (d. 1534) *Risalah fi al-ta'un* (Treatise on Plague) recommended spiritual methods, such as prayer, formulae for preparing amulets, and magic squares, along with material methods, such as consuming sour pomegranate, *terra sigillata*, theriacs, and so on.[67]

On whole, it is possible to observe that a certain cognizance started to take shape for differentiating plague from other diseases and for classifying and categorizing different bodies of knowledge about its diagnosis, prognosis, and prophylaxis. Even the mere proliferation of plague tracts can be taken as evidence for the process of the articulation of that knowledge. However, it may be important to keep in mind that this body of knowledge did not develop in a vacuum. On the contrary, the social and intellectual contexts in which it was produced, circulated, received, and applied are critical to understanding the crystallization of this body of knowledge and its use by members of Ottoman society. Yet, before addressing where this knowledge stood in relation to its use, it may be necessary to point out some methodological problems. First, this emerging body of knowledge – be it about etiology, prognosis, or prophylaxis – was mostly prescriptive in nature. As such, it included information about what *ought* to be done but not about what actually *was* done. It is difficult, for example, to find out about what medicinal substances were available and what people actually used to ward off the plague. This shortcoming can be partly compensated by using them in conjunction with other sources. Hence, it may be possible to catch glimpses of what medicinal substances circulated in the Ottoman market and what was available for sale in the herbalist shops of Ottoman cities. For example, sources suggest that a range of theriacs (such as *tiryak-ı faruk* or *tiryak-ı kebir*), *terra sigillata* or Lemnian earth (*tin-i mahtum*), bezoar stone, balsam, and some fragrant oils were much-sought-after substances in

---

[66] İlyas, *Tevfikāt*, 28.

[67] Kemalpaşazade, *Risalah fi al-ta'un* [Treatise on plague], Süleymaniye Library, ms. Aşir Efendi 430/36, 160–61.

the late sixteenth century.[68] For example, French priest Jérôme Maurand and his friends took a certain powder with a glass of Lesbian wine, as prescribed by their physician, to be protected from plague.[69] Similarly, Stephan Gerlach's account mentions the use of *terra sigillata* and other substances at times of plague among the members of Habsburg ambassadorial mission in Istanbul. Yet, most of these substances or pharmaceuticals were costly and probably not easy to acquire for the majority of the Ottoman population. Sources refer to their limited availability and circulation as well as their acquisition through a network of individual contacts.[70] Hence, it may be difficult to believe that these substances circulated widely and that they were commonly available to all – though it is hardly plausible that locals did not try using some of the more easily available substances, such as vinegar or simple herbal recipes. Lemon juice in particular seems to have been a popular remedy, as evidenced in the account of pharmacist Lubenau who went to Galata to buy fresh lemons during a plague epidemic.[71]

This, however, takes us into a second methodological question, that is, how this body of knowledge was received, circulated, and applied. It is difficult to comment on the circulation of these texts, which would involve tracing different manuscript copies in different libraries and establishing the chain of ownership.[72] The available number of manuscript copies of some of the sixteenth-century treatises, for example, those of Taşköprizade and İdris-i Bidlisi, seems considerably high. They also seem to have been widely circulated. Other works with fewer copies, such as İlyas's and Bistami's, may suggest a more limited circulation.[73] In conjunction with this, there is also the question of who read them beyond other treatise writers. Until the end of the sixteenth century, almost all Ottoman plague treatises were composed in Arabic. As such, they were scholarly texts not intended for

---

[68] Marcus Milwright, "The Balsam of Matariyya: An Exploration of a Medieval Panacea," *Bulletin of the School of Oriental and African Studies* 66, no. 2 (2003): 193–209; J. P. Griffin, "Venetian Treacle and the Foundation of Medicines Regulation," *British Journal of Clinical Pharmacology* 58, no. 3 (2004): 317–25; Belon, *Les Observations*, 51–52; Heath W. Lowry, *Fifteenth Century Ottoman Realities: Christian Peasant Life on the Aegean Island of Limnos* (Istanbul: Eren, 2002), 153–71.

[69] Jérome Maurand, *Itinéraire de Jérome Maurand d'Antibes à Constantinople* (Paris: E. Leroux, 1901), 240–41.

[70] Gerlach, *Türkiye Günlüğü*, 189, 273, 284–85, 339–40, 365, 391, 396–98, 401, 452, 668–69, 768; Busbecq, *Turkish Letters*, 416.

[71] Lubenau, *Beschreibung*, 2:25.

[72] For an example of tracing the chain of owners and the story of a seventeenth-century plague treatise, see Curry, "Scholars, Sufis, and Disease."

[73] E.g., although only a handful of copies are listed for Bistami's treatises, and even fewer copies for İlyas's work, the number of copies for İdris-i Bidlisi's and Taşköprizade's is much greater. See *Osmanlı Tıbbi Bilimler Literatürü Tarihi* [History of the literature of medical sciences during the Ottoman period], ed. Ekmeleddin İhsanoğlu, 4 vols (Istanbul: IRCICA, 2008), 1:50–53, 97–98, 101–2, 139–40.

the general readership. They stand in stark contrast, for example, with the medical compendia of the fifteenth century composed in vernacular Turkish. This may suggest that these authors wrote for other scholars, judges, and physicians, in other words, for the learned.

Nevertheless, the measures adopted by the Ottoman state to deal with plague epidemics (as discussed at length in Chapter 8) seem to suggest some basic understanding of and familiarity with this body of knowledge. Even if we cannot show how this link functioned (i.e., who read these works, who put them to use, etc.), it is difficult to ignore these connections altogether. In fact, it would be impossible to think of the Ottoman state-formation process, especially as regards its growing claims to oversee the health of the urban populace, without exploring how it might have made use of this growing body of knowledge. Recent scholarship shows that the Ottoman state machinery was one of the important foci of power in shaping the production of knowledge in the empire. For example, it has been demonstrated how the Ottoman imperial ideology shaped the content, orientation, and discourses of geographical works in the sixteenth century in a manner to support and legitimize its expansion. The Ottoman geographical corpus produced under the auspices of imperial patronage deliberately situated the empire at the center of the world. The same corpus of geographical knowledge, in turn, was utilized to expand the power of the empire and further legitimize its expansion.[74] Similarly, it should be possible to explore how the body of knowledge on plague was shaped by the rise of the Ottoman administrative measures for dealing with epidemics, especially in large urban centers like Istanbul, through the sixteenth century.

It remains to be said that the knowledge of plague stands in a complex relationship with the Ottoman imperial project. Inquiries of this relationship need to consider the transformative effects of the imperial ideology and the mechanisms through which knowledge was promoted, circulated, and canonized. Yet it should be possible to maintain that some forms of knowledge would be seen as easier to use for the purposes of developing policy and for responding to the needs of a state. For example, the diagnosis of plague, as distinct from other diseases, seems to have been used for administrative practices of counting plague deaths, keeping separate records for plague and nonplague cases during epidemics, and in legal cases that necessitated posthumous identification of plague.[75] Similarly, knowledge of plague etiology might have shaped the precautionary measures of urban cleanliness adopted in this era, aimed at eliminating observable causes of disease. Even when there was not much to be done in terms of taking precautionary measures about divine and cosmic causes, it was possible to do

---

[74] Pınar Emiralioğlu, *Geographical Knowledge and Imperial Culture in the Early Modern Ottoman Empire* (Burlington, VT: Ashgate, 2014).

[75] See Chapter 8.

something for the more tangible causes such as miasma or corruption of the air. In fact, the nature of the precautionary measures was such that they entailed an understanding of the causes and/or the mechanism of causation. A close analysis of the kinds of measures taken against epidemic outbreaks in this era suggests that dead human and animal bodies as well as garbage, seen as a source of putrefaction, needed to be removed quickly. In fact, for a society in which miasma was the main causal explanation for epidemic disease, foul smells were associated with the unclean. In other words, cleanliness was not only something that could be seen but also smelled; a place was considered clean when it was free of bad smells. This suggests that some aspects of that body of knowledge was adopted and put into use by the state as practicable knowledge. Perhaps it should not be surprising that it was the kind of knowledge that empowered the state to implement policies for transforming the environment or imposing social control that became more prevalent than others. After all, in the seventeenth century, this view seems to have become part of common wisdom, as testified in the words of Evliya Çelebi in the epigraph to this chapter.

In the light of this discussion regarding the two stages of medicalization, let us look into the third stage, that is, the changing views about claims over predicting or healing the plague in sixteenth-century Ottoman society. These claims were intimately linked to the question of causation. In the medieval Islamic plague cosmology, as we have seen, the disease was seen as divine decree, and only God had the power over it. To that end, one could pray or seek the intercession of saints for protection from it. What seems interesting is that such powers in the sixteenth century gradually moved away from the authority of the saints. The stories in the hagiographic literature may offer glimpses of this process of change.

In the Ottoman hagiographic literature, the trope of miraculous cures of plague for entire communities *gradually faded out*, if not disappearing entirely.[76] Later in the sixteenth century, the writers of hagiographic works no longer deemed it appropriate to attribute to the mystics the power to protect entire communities against plagues – even though healing the sick individual continued, as a common trope of the genre. For example, Akhisarlı Şeyh İsa (d. 1531), a mystic from Anatolia, curses a group of nomads for fleeing from an outbreak that afflicted both humans and animals and for

---

[76] According to John Curry, these claims did not disappear completely; on the contrary, cases of miraculous cures can still be found in the hagiographies composed in later centuries. E.g., the hagiographies of eighteenth-century Halveti figures like Muhammad Nasuhi Efendi (d. 1718) and Ünsi Hasan Efendi (d. 1723) made use of such tropes. However, it seems that although the supporters and followers of these figures continued to make these claims, the actual Sufi leaders themselves began to downplay miraculous occurrences in general to put the focus on other elements of the mystical path that did not involve some worldly benefit. See, e.g., Ömer el-Fuadi's reconstruction of the life of Şaban-ı Veli as discussed in Curry, *Transformation of Muslim Mystical Thought*, Part III.

leaving their dead behind, unburied. In another instance, he predicts that a plague will break out in town and kill a certain percentage of its population. Yet there is no evidence in these stories for his intercession in lifting the pestilence in either case.[77] Another example is Şaban-ı Veli (d. 1569), a sixteenth-century Sufi leader, who refused the demands of his followers to lift the catastrophes that afflicted his community.[78] This does not mean that the issue of plagues *disappeared entirely* from the narratives of Ottoman hagiographic literature. On the contrary, the trope of the Sufi master's inflicting plagues and pestilence upon the enemies of the order, a long-established motif in these narratives, continued, and even flourished.[79] To be sure, those who wrote these stories by the turn of the seventeenth century still believed in the intercessional powers of the mystics, but there was no longer any belief in the *necessity* of their intervention to relieve the populace from plagues and pestilence. Such relief was now being divorced from the order of supernatural powers. Hence, the narratives mainly retained the role of the Sufi masters as inflictors of plague, not alleviators of its suffering.

If so, then where could people turn to seek for relief from plague? Whose prerogative was healing now? One of Evliya Çelebi's stories can offer some valuable insights. According to the story, Armağani Mehemmed Efendi, a much-admired mystic in Istanbul, encounters "the soldiers of plague." In the year 1623, when the mystic left the capital with the intention of visiting his hometown, he had a miraculous vision in Üsküdar, where he stopped to pray. While praying, the mystic found himself surrounded by countless numbers of soldiers. These soldiers looked nothing like ordinary soldiers he knew. They were divided into two encampments. In one camp were those dressed in white garments, in white tents; those were the good or benevolent spirits (*ervah-ı tayyibe*). In the other camp were those dressed in black, holding spears, in black tents; those were the evil or malevolent spirits (*ervah-ı habise*). Seeing this, the mystic conversed with members of the former encampment, who told him that they were good and benevolent spirits. When they pierced someone with their spear, the wounded contracted the plague, but only to recover and ultimately to survive the disease. Pointing to the encampment of soldiers in black tents, they told the mystic that whenever those soldiers pierced someone with their spear, the wounded died of the plague – if a Muslim, then as martyr. Upon hearing this, the mystic fearfully inquired about the people of Istanbul, about whether they were going to be pierced by the soldiers of plague. The answer was yes.

---

77 This hagiography is a sixteenth-century account written by the mystic's son İbn İsa-yı Saruhani. See İbn Isa-yı Saruhanî, *Akhisarli Şeyh İsâ Menâkıbnâmesi*, ed. Sezai Küçük and Ramazan Muslu (Sakarya: Aşiyan Yayınları, 2003), 96–97, 109.

78 Curry, "Scholars, Sufis, and Disease." These requests may not have directly involved plague but rather other concerns his followers felt threatened by, such as storms at sea or business calamities.

79 Curry, "Scholars, Sufis, and Disease."

He was told that a terrible plague was about to break out in the city, in which many were to die. Then, he was presented with the names of all those who were to die of plague and those who were to survive. The mystic meticulously recorded all those names in a register. Having found out what was about to befall the city and its people, he rushed back to the capital to see the Ottoman sultan to tell him about his experience and to give him the register he had prepared. Exclaiming the good news to the sultan that the latter's life was going to be spared, he handed him the register. Sultan Murad IV (r. 1623–40) read the register and dismissed it by saying, "This is a register of a lunatic-dervish" (*bir meczub kaydıdır*). The next morning, Istanbul woke up to a terrible plague, and in forty days, three hundred thousand people had died. Everything the mystic recorded in his register came true, exactly as he had it.[80]

A close reading of this story allows glimpses of the changing Ottoman mentalities about who held the prerogative of predicting or healing plagues. As we have seen, predicting, inflicting, or healing plagues were long seen as powers of the mystics. As is suggested in the story, Mehemmed Efendi claims to maintain this long-held spiritual power to predict plagues. Interestingly enough, this prediction takes the form of a written document, a register that distinguished between those who would die from plague and those who would survive.[81] This register symbolizes not only the prerogative of predicting a plague outbreak but also an embodiment of the knowledge of the very names of people to be affected by it. What is even more interesting is that the Ottoman sultan takes a look at it and immediately dismisses it. This suggests that by the mid-seventeenth century, the Ottoman state saw itself as having taken over that power and thus in a position to discredit the claims of other parties to share it. The authority to predict or lift a plague, which was once the mystical prerogative of the saints and Sufi orders, was now transferred to the domain of the Ottoman sovereignty.

By the mid-seventeenth century, it seems that plague counting, recording, and healing had become a political power. This was indeed the ramification of a process that started in the sixteenth century. The sixteenth-century Ottoman texts clearly testify to a growing association between plague (or rather the power to lift it) and sovereignty. In the first half of the century, this power is seen as vested in the person of the Ottoman sultan – we see this clearly in the example of Süleyman (r. 1520–66). In the second half of the century, they come to be extended to the state and its growing powers or

---

[80] Evliya Çelebi, *Seyahatnâme*, 4: 319–20. In another place, he tells the same story briefly, giving different numbers: "in seven days, 70,000 people died." Evliya Çelebi, *Seyahatnâme*, 1: 178.

[81] The reference to the distinction between the benevolent and malevolent spirits in the story must symbolize basic understanding between plague morbidity vs. mortality. This is also reflected in the way the register was organized. All of these practices of counting appear to be common knowledge in the seventeenth century. See Chapter 8.

claims to oversee the health of the populace.[82] Going back to Evliya Çelebi's story, we see that the state had won – or so it triumphantly proclaims to. However, the next twist in the story challenges this view. The day after the sultan dismisses the mystic's register, plague comes to Istanbul, as had been predicted, and everything the mystic had recorded comes true. This last twist in the story can be read as the expression of a sullen resentment on the part of the Sufi orders and their supporters for losing their prerogatives over plagues.

There is further evidence for the growing claims of the state to take over this power, even in the spiritual domain. Certain religious activities were organized for supplication to God for the lifting of the plague, such as processions or communal prayers.[83] Selaniki Mustafa Efendi gives examples of such communal prayers and processions in Istanbul organized in the reign of Murad III (r. 1574–95), in which men of religion and Sufi leaders took part.[84] It is interesting to bear in mind that these activities were organized by the state, suggesting that even the communal spiritual efforts were now brought closer to the state's control. It may be worthwhile to contrast this situation to the intercession of the holy men of the previous century. Unlike the individual initiative of the holy men to lift plagues, now the holy men or the men of religion were asked to intercede by the sovereign or the state.

As a last point, it may be useful to indicate that it is difficult to know to what degree medical professionals were involved in the process. We have rather vague ideas about the extent of involvement of medical professionals in the diagnosis, prophylaxis, and treatment of plague. It appears that receiving treatment for plague from a physician was a relatively limited phenomenon in early modern Ottoman society, which may not have gone beyond the limited circles of the ruling elite and their households. There is some information that comes from the testimonies of European diplomatic missions to the Ottoman Empire, which also had physicians on board.[85] One well-known case was the physician of the Habsburg ambassador Busbecq, William Quacquelben, who himself fell prey to plague.[86] Another example is the surgeon in the retinue of Baron Wratislaw who, while kept in prison in the Rumeli fortress, was let out to treat patients in nearby villages.[87] Other

---

[82] I explore the relationship between plague and sovereignty extensively elsewhere. See my "From '*Bête Noire*' to '*le Mal de* Constantinople.'"

[83] Such processions, as sporadic efforts of communities to pray for forgiveness in the face of natural disasters (e.g., plague, drought, famine), had a long history in the medieval and early modern Muslim world. See, e.g., Dols, *Black Death*, 246–54; Dols, "Communal Responses."

[84] Selânikî, *Tarih-i Selânikî*, 285–87.

[85] E.g., see the Venetian case as discussed in Dursteler, "Bailo in Constantinople," 17.

[86] See Chapter 8.

[87] Wratislaw, *Adventures*, 162. This is also confirmed by the testimony of Friedrich Seidel, the apotheracy in the Habsburg embassy sent to Istanbul in 1591. See Friedrich Seidel,

such foreign missions, even when they had a physician on board, could still seek the advice of local physicians. For example, Gerlach sent a letter to Haim Abenxuxen, a Portuguese Jewish physician, to request advice about what to do for protection from plague, for which he received a reply in a letter that included such advice.[88] Perhaps in view of circumstances at times of plague, the process of consulting a physician and receiving advice on what to do or what not to do, via correspondence, may have been appropriate.

Changes in Attitudes toward Plague: Canonization

While the perception of plague was undergoing thorough changes and the knowledge about it was being rigorously formulated, a third significant line of change was taking place in the attitudes of sixteenth-century Ottoman society toward plague. Unlike the other two processes of naturalization and medicalization, changes in attitudes are difficult to trace by what people wrote about plague. Attitudes may or may not manifest themselves in actual or observable behavior, so they cannot always be discerned from action. Nevertheless, by studying prescriptive principles of right conduct, it may be possible to detect some tangible changes in attitudes. It may especially be important to pay attention to a set of principles, maintained and exercised by some, that comes to be sanctioned by law and approved as norm by the state. In this case, this principle not only becomes a guide for the members of a society but also turns into a tradition that is passed down to later generations. Here I argue that the principles of conduct as regarding plague underwent a process of *canonization* in this manner. First, there was a set of principles, maintained and exercised by some. In this case, this was avoiding plague-infested locations and, if necessary, leaving those areas for the purpose of preserving one's health. Then, treatise writers strove to render this principle, already practiced by some, compatible with the tenets of Islamic law. Once this was accomplished, the legal opinion by the Chief Juristconsult approved this principle and by doing so sanctioned it as approved practice by the state. It should be noted that this process of canonization does not refer to how a certain principle was held and practiced by some sections in Ottoman society; rather, it aims to explain how that certain practice becomes canonical and is passed on to the later eras as *the* right principle of conduct at times of plague.

To be sure, the issue of right conduct at times of plagues busied the minds and hearts of many people before the Ottomans.[89] The question of to flee

---

Sultanın Zindanında: Osmanlı İmparatorluğu'na Gönderilen bir Elçilik Heyetinin İbret Verici Öyküsü (1591–1596), trans. Türkis Noyan (Istanbul: Kitap Yayınevi, 2010), 56–57.

88 Gerlach, *Türkiye Günlüğü*, 427, 872. The text of the letter (in Latin) is not included in the Turkish translation.

89 For an excellent overview of flight debates both in the Muslim and Christian view, see Stearns, *Infectious Ideas*.

or not to flee, which, in some cases, could mean a choice between life and death, divided communities in the face of plague. This question, which for brevity's sake will be referred to here as the *flight dilemma*, was especially tricky for Ottoman society because of its controversial legal and religious standing in the Islamic tradition. To be clear, there had been those who were pro-flight and those who opposed the practice since early Islamic history.

People of all walks of life in the Ottoman world maintained different types of intuitions about avoiding plague, and some indeed fled from plague-infected cities, as cases from *mühimme* registers amply evince. In such cases, the refuge for the empire's urban population could be nearby villages within a reasonable distance. For example, in summer 1544, Jérôme Maurand went to the vineyards on account of the raging plague in the city. He described the vineyard as a pleasant environment, with a nicely painted house, a well, and good water, at about two miles away from Pera.[90] Eventually, the villages north of Istanbul, toward Kemer, especially the village of Belgrad (or Belgradcık), became popular destinations for the non-Muslim residents of the city at such times. In the seventeenth century, Eremya Çelebi Kömürcüyan writes that this village was particularly popular among the Greek and European residents of Istanbul who wanted to take refuge from plagues. The clean air and water of the village were much praised by its contemporaries, and it was still a popular destination for flight in the nineteenth century.[91] Similarly, Jewish residents of Thessaloniki took refuge in the surrounding villages at times of plague. Some of these nearby villages, such as Livadi, became especially popular destinations for the Jewish residents of Thessaloniki.[92] In a similar vein, the Christians in Trabzon did the same in taking refuge in the countryside.[93] French and British ambassadorial missions in Istanbul started to maintain summer residences outside the city in which they could take refuge in times of plague.[94] It has been shown that the Muslim urban classes also fled plagues, including members of the Ottoman *askeri* class.[95] The Venetian *bailo* Lorenzo Bernardo observed in the late sixteenth century the increasing popularity of flight among the Ottoman urban population, including Muslim religious scholars. British historian Rycaut makes similar

90 Maurand, *Itinéraire de Jérome Maurand*, 204–5, 224–27.

91 Eremia Kömürcüyan, *İstanbul Tarihi: XVII. Asırda İstanbul*, trans. Hrand D Andreasyan (Istanbul: Eren, 1988), 31. For evidence that the Europeans went there in the early part of the eighteenth century, see Webb and Webb, *The Earl and His Butler*, 19–26.

92 See my "Plague, Conflict, and Negotiation."

93 For the flight of Christian communities in Trabzon, see Jennings, "Plague in Trabzon," 30–32.

94 İnalcık, "Istanbul." Also, the Habsburg ambassador Busbecq took refuge in the Princes' Islands during a plague outbreak in Istanbul in 1561. Busbecq, *Turkish Letters*, 180, 182–90.

95 Miri Shefer-Mossensohn, *Ottoman Medicine: Healing and Medical Institutions, 1500–1700* (Albany: State University of New York Press, 2009), 174–75. E.g., there is evidence that the *tımar*-holder *sipahi*s fled their lands during a plague outbreak in Trabzon in 1565–66. See Jennings, "Plague in Trabzon," 31.

observations in the second half of the seventeenth century.[96] As a matter of fact, we know that Ottoman sultans themselves preferred spending time outside the capital when there was pestilence or any major natural disaster in Istanbul.[97] Examples can be multiplied to show that flight was one of the means of protection for Ottoman urban populations of the sixteenth century, though it seemed to be more or less limited to those who could afford it, that is, the elite.

Yet there was another question, at least for the Muslim population of the empire: the question of whether flight was permissible according to Islamic legal principles. So, this was a matter of whether those who were already fleeing, or pondering flight, were justified in doing so because of the religious and legal controversy on this issue. Revolving around the issue of God's will, the good or well-being of the community, and the individual's free will, this controversy was well known to Ottoman scholars, who have written extensively to resolve it. The Ottoman plague treatises written in the sixteenth century reveal a new legal perspective on proper conduct during times of plague. These treatises proposed justifications for flight from epidemic outbreaks.

The earliest examples of this voice can be found in the plague treatises composed around the turn of the sixteenth century. Sources note Muslihuddin ibn-i Evhadüddin (d. 1505–6) wrote a treatise about the permissibility of flight from plague. Katip Çelebi lists it as *Risaletü'l-veba ve cevazi'l-firari anh* (Plague and the Permissibility of Fleeing from It). Mustafa Ali concludes from this treatise, clearly written to justify fleeing from plague, that he was an erudite scholar.[98] Another treatise written slightly after that was İlyas's *Majannah*, which adamantly advocates flight from diseased areas as the first and foremost measure.[99] In its straightforward recommendation of flight and exclusive use of medicine, this treatise is different from the works produced by Ottoman religious and legal scholars. For this latter group, disease transmission and flight were not merely medical or etiological problems but rather more complex religious and legal matters. In an attempt to bring a resolution to this long-debated issue, these scholars employed theological explanations, exegetical interpretations, and methods of jurisprudence. Plague treatises written by leading Ottoman scholars of the sixteenth

---

[96] Both Lorenzo's and Rycaut's ideas with respect to flight have been extensively discussed in Chapter 2.

[97] For the flight of the Ottoman sultans from plague, see Lowry, "Pushing the Stone Uphill." However, this practice did not end in the sixteenth century, as Lowry suggests. We have many examples of Ottoman sultans spending time in Edirne or in their summer residences on the Bosporus in the sixteenth century. See, e.g., my "Conquest, Urbanization, and Plague."

[98] Mustafa Âli, *Künhü'l-ahbâr*, 157b. Katip Çelebi lists the author's name as Muslihu'd-dîn Mustafâ ibn Evhadi'd-dîn el-Yarhisarî. See Katip Çelebi, *Keşfü'z-Zunûn* (Istanbul: Tarih Vakfı Yurt Yayınları, 2007), 2:729. I could not locate the treatise itself.

[99] İlyas, *Tevfîkât*, 27–28.

century, İdris-i Bidlisi (d. 1520), Kemalpaşazade, and Taşköprizade, can be
cited in this group. All of these works demonstrate a distinct approach in
their treatment of disease transmission and the issue of flight and argue
that plague is something that should be avoided. In doing so, they diverge
from the conventionally accepted stereotype of the Muslim attitude toward
plague: *fatalism.*[100]

In the early sixteenth century, the Ottoman historian İdris-i Bidlisi wrote
Risalah al-ʿiba' ʿan mawaqiʿ al-waba' (Treatise on Avoiding Places of Infection) in response to certain religious scholars who forbade flight from plague
on the grounds that it was incompatible with belief in God's will. The background of this story merits close attention. When Bidlisi was in Syria in
1511, on his way to Mecca for pilgrimage, he heard that plague broke out
in Egypt. Upon hearing this, he wanted to return to Anatolia immediately
by way of sea, perhaps simply to avoid the contagion. However, religious
scholars of Aleppo and Damascus opposed his departure and may even have
forbidden it on the grounds that it was incompatible with a certain legal and
theological understanding of God's will. Bidlisi's work is a complex and
lengthy justification of flight. It includes theological discussions of catastrophes in the context of the delicate relationship between God's will and
human free agency. It also presents medical discussions of the etiology of
plague and other epidemic diseases, the issue of contagion and flight, and
spiritual and physical precautions to be taken against epidemic illnesses, and
even a few medical recipes. Ultimately, this work is invaluable as an indica-
tor of new approaches to contagion and the justification and preferability of
flight.[101]

It is worth mentioning that two other plague treatises composed in the
sixteenth century reach very similar conclusions and provide additional evidence of a shift in emphasis in matters pertaining to the proper response to
plague. The plague treatise written by Chief Jurisconsult Kemalpaşazade (d.
1534) concurs that it is advisable and justified to avoid plague. He favors
caution in the face of plague and advises that certain measures be taken to
prevent exposure to it. He concludes that it is very dangerous to travel to
and from plague-stricken areas.[102]

---

[100] Until recently, scholarship held that Muslim attitudes toward plague were exemplified in
the works written after the Black Death. Especially the plague treatise of Ibn Hajar al-
ʿAsqalani (d. 1449), *Badhl al-maʿun fi faḍl al-taʿun*, came to be seen as the encapsulation
of Muslim attitudes toward plague (that one should not flee from plague because it is a
mercy from God and is a means of martyrdom for the believer). See Dols, *Black Death*.
However, recent research shows that there was no single tradition in the Islamic world
universally accepted by all Muslim scholars on the issue of flight. See Stearns, *Infectious
Ideas*.

[101] İdris-i Bidlisi, *Risālah al-ʿibā' ʿan mawāqiʿ al-wabā'* [Treatise on avoiding places of infec-
tion], Süleymaniye Library, ms. Aşir Efendi 275/3. Also see Dols, *Black Death*, 332.

[102] Kemalpaşazade, *Risālah fī al-ṭāʿun*, 160–61. Also see Dols, *Black Death*, 332.

In his work on plague, *Risalah al-shifa' li-adwa' al-waba'* (Healing Treatise for the Treatment of Plague), the renowned sixteenth-century scholar Taşköprizade discusses the issue of legal authorization of whether one should flee a plague-infested place. His work can be considered as the synthesis of the contemporary legal and medical knowledge in the eastern Mediterranean in the sixteenth century. Arguably the climax of the genre in the Ottoman tradition and demonstrably the model for later treatises, this work was not only a comprehensive compendium on plague, it also became canonical within the Ottoman legal perspective on the issue. Perhaps it can be considered in conjunction with the legal opinion (*fatwa*) issued by Chief Jurisconsult Ebussuud, who legally authorized exiting a plague-stricken city in search of a safer place and for taking precautions against plague.[103]

The plague treatise of Taşköprizade is noteworthy for its representative discussion of four important problems about the plague. He emphasizes that these problems revolve around the question of trust in God, which serves as a ground for the discussion of whether one should flee a plague-stricken area. Formulating dialectical disputes, Taşköprizade weighs the pros and cons of each of the arguments for and against flight from plague. Then, using rational argumentation based on logical principles (*'aql*) as well as reports from the hadith literature (*naql*), he concludes that clean air is a cause in preserving health and bad or corrupt air is a cause of disease. Following this, he devotes seven chapters to a consideration of religious and medical characteristics of plague and the response to it, including the permissibility of prayers for deliverance from its threat and the efficacy of material and spiritual cures, even providing a list of such prayers and cures.[104]

Combining his mastery of the Islamic sciences and notions of disease transmission, Taşköprizade defended an intriguing resolution to the flight dilemma: if there is an outbreak in a certain location, there is no harm for an individual to depart, as long as that individual is seeking clean air or medical treatment, not merely fleeing from that which is sent by God. The permission to depart – rather than to flee in panic – is based on the proof that preservation of health requires sound air and that corrupted or fetid air brings forth disease. He consults the hadith literature to find evidence in support of his resolution of the flight dilemma, which assisted in establishing an applicable and sound basis for the right behavior of a believer. The novelty of Taşköprizade's work consisted not only in his bid to wed knowledge on disease transmission with the principles of Islamic law but also in his formulation of an idea that was practical in real-world scenarios and applicable in legal cases.

---

[103] Ertuğrul M. Düzdağ, *Şeyhülislam Ebussuud Efendi Fetvaları Işığında 16. Asır Türk Hayatı* (Istanbul, 1983), nos. 395, 499, 754, 888, 912, 913.
[104] Taşköprizade, *Risalah al-shifa'*.

By formulating this new legal interpretation, Taşköprizade's work was certainly speaking to an ongoing discussion of the permissibility of flight. It is worth mentioning here that, even in the absence of legal authorization, people were nevertheless fleeing from plague outbreaks. As we have seen, we have ample evidence for the practice of flight from different sections of Ottoman society during this period. Nonetheless, there was no clear guideline for conduct available to the Muslim population. It was for this purpose that Ebussuud's legal authorization of Taşköprizade's resolution of the flight dilemma provided such readily applicable guidelines.

The shift toward the authorization of flight notwithstanding, it may be more difficult to determine how this controversy or its resolution was received in Ottoman society. For example, what sections of Ottoman society found the idea of fleeing appealing or justified? What groups were opposed to the idea? It is difficult to find robust evidence to answer this question until the latter part of the sixteenth century. By the late sixteenth century, when the controversy seems to have been resolved, or rather when the prescriptive principle of flight became sanctioned, things can be better identified. The Venetian *bailo* Lorenzo Bernardo observed in 1592 that Ottoman society was moving toward favoring flight at times of epidemic, which he believed was a recent change. About three-quarters of a century later, Rycaut observed that the Ottoman religious scholars favored flight because they were learned, which he contrasted to the ignorance of the common people.[105] It is difficult to comment whether the Ottoman religious scholars did actually spearhead flight from plague or if this was highlighted because it was most shocking to a European observer who held widespread beliefs about Muslim fatalism. Perhaps a man of religion fleeing from plague would sound more scandalous to readers than the flight of an ordinary citizen. That said, there are indications that members of the Ottoman tax-exempt *askeri* class did indeed flee from plagues, despite regulations against it. This was possibly because they could afford to leave their residences to take refuge in nearby villages. Hence, it is conceivable that the tax-exempt bodies of the empire were better protected than most taxpaying subjects; especially the urban poor seem to have suffered the worst of plague.

On the whole, this new perspective and its legal ramifications not only played a key role in defining the Ottoman response to plague but also was a factor concomitant with the broader changes taking place in the Ottoman society of the sixteenth century, especially with respect to changing administrative attitudes toward epidemic diseases. To better understand the Ottoman response that emerged in the face of plague during this era, one should consider the measures and means by which the central administration tried to monitor these epidemics, as discussed in the next chapter.

---

[105] See Chapter 2.

It is therefore in this particular context that one can better evaluate the significance of this shift toward the acceptance of flight as a legitimate social practice in the Ottoman plague treatises of the sixteenth century.

The legal justification of the flight dilemma and the new administrative measures taken against plague, in the form of public health policy, stand in a rather complex relationship. What is clear and uncontroversial is that all of this took place in the sixteenth century. The precise chronology of what followed what within that century is less apparent. The most parsimonious explanation may be that the notions about plague's etiology, transmission, and effects, as implied in the legal authorization of flight under proper conditions, facilitated taking other administrative steps to handle potential outbreaks, such as organizing urban hygiene or regulating burial practices. In a sense, it does not matter whether these administrative steps followed after or were being undertaken even as the flight dilemma was being discussed and its resolution authorized legally. What may count here is that notions of health and disease opened administrative practices to a new and broader dimension of justification, such that not only flight for proper reasons but urban cleanliness and other matters could be justified and implemented as legally authorized practices of the state. In other words, the question that this matter opens is in fact whether the authorization of the resolution of the flight dilemma and the concomitant justification it offered for other "public health" practices provided (or at least represented the provision of) new powers of government in a process of early modern state formation, which is discussed in the next chapter.

Conclusion

This chapter has demonstrated that the late medieval Ottoman perceptions, knowledge, and attitudes toward plague changed dramatically in the sixteenth century. These changes are studied here in three distinct but concurrent processes: *naturalization*, *medicalization*, and *canonization*.

The discussion devoted to *naturalization* has characterized the late medieval Ottoman perception of plague as (1) divine decree, (2) portent of apocalypse, and (3) a result of social and moral transgression. Drawing from works of poetry, hagiographies, and early Ottoman chronicles, this section has illustrated this particular perception in Ottoman literary, religious, and historical imagination. In the sixteenth century, even though plague as (1) divine decree and as (3) resulting from social and moral ills was retained, (2) the apocalyptic context gradually vanished. As the apocalyptic character of plague diminished, a new perception took hold, which corresponds to the process of *naturalization*, by which plague came to be seen as a familiar presence in the social texture of urban life. A number of sources were used to demonstrate this change, especially drawing from the use of language, metaphors, and imagery in historical, hagiographic, and literary texts.

The chapter has shown how plague became naturalized in the Ottoman cultural landscape in the sixteenth century.

The process of *medicalization* was traced here in three stages: (1) the rise of a distinct body of knowledge on plague (symptoms, etiology, prognosis, prophylaxis); (2) the crystallization and adoption of this body of knowledge by the Ottoman state; and (3) the changing authority and expertise over plague from the domain of the saints and Sufis to the institutions of the state. First, late medieval knowledge of plague was presented, highlighting the nature and organization of that body of knowledge. It has been demonstrated here that this body of knowledge was imbued with supernatural elements, eclectic in nature, and did not necessarily distinguish plague from other diseases with respect to prevention and treatment purposes. Then, the rise of a new body of plague literature in the sixteenth century was discussed especially with respect to the rise of the genre of treatises. Once the body of knowledge in the treatises was surveyed, this new body of knowledge as something tangible and quantifiable, and therefore something that could be used as a basis for administrative policies of the state, was discussed. In the last stage of this transformation, it was demonstrated that the saints and Sufis gradually seemed to have lost their prerogative over predicting or healing the plague – something they claimed to have held in the late medieval era. Some of these powers were transferred to the rising Ottoman state, with its new claims to oversee the health of its urban populace starting in the sixteenth century.

While the processes by which the perception of plague became less supernatural and cataclysmic, the knowledge about it became more tangible and categorized, and the attitudes toward plague became *canonized*. Through the sixteenth century, the Ottoman treatise writers struggled to meet the tenets of Islamic religion and traditions with the acquired wisdom of plague drawn from their experience. This effort seems to have culminated after the mid-sixteenth century, when a legal orthodoxy was reached about what the right conduct ought to be at times of plague. The formulation of this orthodoxy continued into the post-1600 era as the Ottoman canon, at least in the circles that associated themselves with the imperial project. Ultimately, all of these processes of transformation can be best understood in their immediate Ottoman context (i.e., the rise of the early modern Ottoman state and the imperial project), which takes us to the next chapter.

8

The State of the Plague

Politics of Bodies in the Making of the Ottoman State

Halk içinde muteber bir nesne yok devlet gibi
Olmaya devlet cihanda bir nefes sıhhat gibi
– Muhibbî

A skilled physician is needed in every town since the Prophet said: "Do not live in a place where there is no wise sovereign, cautious governor, or skilled physician."
– Nidaî[1]

In the sixteenth century, the Ottoman central administration adopted and implemented a series of new regulations in response to plague. These ranged from monitoring daily death tolls at times of outbreak to more comprehensive and ambitious undertakings, such as ensuring cleanliness in urban areas and promoting a system of public health. Taken as a whole, this body of administrative responses to plague reverberates the popular and scholarly responses of Ottoman society to this phenomenon. In other words, both the popular beliefs about this disease and the scholarly knowledge of its signs, transmission, and treatment are key in understanding the rationale of the official administrative response. My argument here is that, in tandem with the *naturalization*, *medicalization*, and *canonization* of plague, successive and harsh outbreaks forced the Ottoman central administration to respond by developing a series of new regulations. These, in turn, paved the way for the establishment of an early modern public health administration. Stated differently, the threat of epidemics compelled the Ottoman central administration to exercise a new form of governance that manifested in the development of technologies for the surveillance of bodies, the regulation of their movement, and control of the space in which they lived, worked,

---

[1] Nidâî, *Menâfiü'n-nâs*, quoted in Nil Sarı, *Osmanlılarda Hekimlik ve Hekimlik Ahlakı* (Istanbul, 1977), 25.

248

and died. The sum of these new technologies of surveillance and governance of bodies not only left their lasting legacy in the emergence of Ottoman institutions of public health but also contributed to the making of the early modern Ottoman state.

The sixteenth century was a period of profound transformation in Ottoman history, during which the Ottoman landholdings expanded enormously. Immense changes in administration followed territorial growth. Both the central and the provincial governments expanded, and consequently new bureaucratic career paths emerged and developed during this period. New institutions were set up and gradually consolidated in this new social and administrative structure. This was also when the imperial law was codified. In brief, there was change in almost all aspects of life, most visibly in the major urban centers of the empire. In particular, this was the time when Istanbul forged a new identity as the new imperial center, but also as the center of learning and arts that flourished in this era. The multifaceted transformations of this era are discernible not only in the administrative and institutional aspects of the Ottoman state but also in the idea of the state and its expanding capabilities. The reign of Süleyman in particular was a time when the idea of the state's powers and responsibilities expanded enormously. As one axis of this redefinition, the function of the state in the sphere of health deserves a more extensive consideration, especially in the form of its increasing presence in matters related to the body of the Ottoman subjects.

The corpus of legislation that developed, especially during and after plague outbreaks, is invaluable for studying the manner in which the Ottoman administration tried to deal with such crises. As the following pages show, early measures were steered toward immediate crisis management. Later in the sixteenth century, as plagues persisted and intensified, the regulations were extended to promote hygiene and cleanliness in the capital and to ensure a healthy urban environment. Regulations to maintain urban cleanliness, control burial practices, monitor the health of the tax-exempt elites, and regulate the burgeoning medical profession all underscore the emergence of a new consciousness for the definition of the idea of state and its newly assumed roles in matters that related to the body of the individual. These efforts combined to reflect a greater visibility of the Ottoman administration in health-related issues, which parallels the great political, ideological, and social transformations of the sixteenth century.

To clarify, the purpose here is not limited to documenting the official response to plague, as imperative as that may be. It is also to contextualize that response and explore its ramifications as manifested in the growing powers of governance of the Ottoman state. As we see in the following, the institutionalization of urban health programs, the creation of a medical establishment, and the implementation of regulations governing the body of the individual were manifestations of a new consciousness largely triggered by plague epidemics. Hence, this initial response to plague as well as its long-term legacy in the formation of a public health system represents a critical turning point in Ottoman history. By the second half of the sixteenth century, some of these regulations turned into institutions and practices that would retrospectively be perceived as "classical," similar to processes that were witnessed in arts, architecture, and religious and legal life.

How the early modern Ottoman central and provincial administrations responded to plague epidemics has not been hitherto systematically surveyed. As a first attempt to reconstruct this body of response, this chapter draws extensively from *mühimme* collections. These documents are copies of orders sent by the Ottoman central administration to the provincial administrators. As such, they constitute an indispensable source of information for the student of Ottoman history by shedding light on many aspects of Ottoman political, social, economic, and, more recently, environmental life. They are also an invaluable resource to trace the Ottoman administrative efforts for healthscaping.[2]

The use of these sources presents some methodological problems that need to be addressed at the outset. First, looking at this body of legislation, we are faced with an impression of ever-expanding powers of governance as held by the Ottoman administration over the body of Ottoman subjects. Regulations oversaw the location, movement, and interaction of bodies, living and dead. As such, these orders may seem to suggest that the Ottoman state was becoming all-powerful. However, one may need to remember that a discourse of power is embedded in these very orders. Such orders were produced to project power. In studying them, we see how they *intended* to govern bodies. If they are studied in isolation, these orders may not be the most useful of sources. For example, they may state what action needs to be taken, without necessarily explaining the rationale behind the adoption of such regulations – a methodological difficulty than can partially be overcome by the integration of evidence from narrative sources (e.g., chronicles), records of social practice (e.g., court registers), and medical works. Second, these documents do not inform us regarding whether a particular order is *actually* carried out. Studying the orders in isolation, we cannot learn how the categories of power they projected were negotiated by those who executed them. All these limitations make it imperative to study these orders in context. Third, this corpus brings to mind questions about whether they really represent something new or they simply offer better documentation. It is true that there is better documentation of all things

---

[2] This term has recently been introduced to the field of urban history. One historian defines such urban efforts as "a physical, social, legal, administrative and political process of providing their environments with the means to safeguard and improve residents' wellbeing." See Guy Geltner, "Healthscaping a Medieval City: Lucca's Curia Viarum and the Future of Public Health History," *Urban History* 40, no. 3 (2013): 395–415, quotation on 396.

Ottoman starting in the sixteenth century and that the sheer availability of better documentation can lead to an assumption that things reflected in documents are new phenomena. It is also true that the lack of documents for the preceding period does not necessarily mean the complete absence of such practices. Nevertheless, the mere presence of documents, in itself, can be seen as testimony of a new consciousness. This can be taken as evidence for a new bureaucratic mechanism that systematically produced data and maintained registers, in a manner that we do not observe until that time. All in all, what better evidence can there be to trace the expanding powers of governance of the Ottoman administration than following the paper trail it produced during that process? Hence, the availability of documents showing the Ottoman administration's increasing visibility in *biopolitics* – to use a modern term – can be taken as an indication for the emergence of an early modern Ottoman state and its expanding powers of governance.[3]

It may seem controversial to situate the formation of an Ottoman public health mechanism and a system of health administration in the mid-sixteenth century. The mainstream Ottomanist scholarship seems to search for such changes in the late empire, perhaps because of the association of public health with medical sciences, on one hand, and with modernity, on the other.[4] Recent scholarship, however, has offered to disentangle the history

---

3 For notions of biopower, biopolitics, and governmentality, the classic works are Michel Foucault's. See, e.g., Foucault, *The Birth of Biopolitics: Lectures at the Collège de France, 1978–79* (New York: Palgrave Macmillan, 2008); Foucault, *The History of Sexuality* (London: Penguin, 1998). Several of Foucault's ideas were influential in the scholarship on the history of medicine, public health, and governance in the 1980s and 1990s. For a critical assessment of his influence on the social history of medicine, see, e.g., Colin Jones and Roy Porter, eds., *Reassessing Foucault: Power, Medicine, and the Body* (London: Routledge, 1994). Later scholarship raised serious criticism about some of his notions, such as governmentality, and offered new insights. See, e.g., Bruce Curtis, "Foucault on Governmentality and Population: The Impossible Discovery," *The Canadian Journal of Sociology/Cahiers Canadiens de Sociologie* 27, no. 4 (2002): 505–33; Mitchell Dean, *Governmentality: Power and Rule in Modern Society* (London: Sage, 1999). Perhaps more relevant for the discussion here is the political theorist James C. Scott's concept of "legibility." See Scott, *Seeing Like a State: How Certain Schemes to Improve the Human Condition Have Failed* (New Haven, CT: Yale University Press, 1999).

4 The scholarship on public health in the Ottoman Empire seems to consider this issue as part and parcel of the modernization scheme and thus seeks to situate it in the nineteenth century. Efforts for public health before modern medicine and its institutions are generally regarded as "folk/traditional healing." See, e.g., Özaydın and Hatemi, *Bir Bibliyografya Denemesi*, 114–42. More recently, this question was revisited by Miri Shefer Mossensohn, who, despite situating the Ottoman public health policies in the nineteenth century, acknowledged the significance of the sixteenth and seventeenth centuries. See Miri Shefer-Mossensohn, "Health as a Social Agent in Ottoman Patronage and Authority," *New Perspectives on Turkey* 37 (2007): 147–75, esp. 149–50, and the bibliography therein. There is also a prolific body of scholarship that focused on public health in the nineteenth-century Muslim Middle East. See, e.g., Nancy Gallagher, *Medicine and Power in Tunisia, 1780–1900* (Cambridge: Cambridge University Press, 1983); Gallagher, *Egypt's Other Wars: Epidemics and the Politics of Public*

of public health from medical sciences. Doing so opened the notion of public health to premodern contexts, which has been most productively used in studies of late medieval and early modern urban history.[5] Hence, efforts to improve the conditions of health and safety in a city can be viewed through that lens.

In this context, it may be useful to reconsider how health was defined in early modern Ottoman society. In the available literature, this issue is predominantly approached from the perspective of medicine, medical knowledge, and institutions.[6] In fact, reducing the understanding of health to medicine can seriously distort the picture of what constituted the well-being of the Ottoman subject and the collective to which it belonged. As this chapter shows, health was understood to be a complex equilibrium in which the individual lived and flourished. As such, bodily health could not be established in the absence of moral, spiritual, and social harmony that affected the individual's relationship to the broader world. Neither was the health and well-being of the individual independent from good governance. Hence, a holistic approach to the subject that covers various aspects of health, ranging from disease to healing, and to moral and social dimensions of health in early modern Ottoman society, promises to afford a more nuanced understanding.

As a last point, the formation of an Ottoman public health administration in the mid-sixteenth century, triggered by aggravating plagues, should not be seen as an isolated phenomenon. In fact, the adoption of urban health regulations can be seen as a larger phenomenon throughout the Mediterranean world in the late medieval and early modern eras. As such, this process can be studied in the larger post–Black Death Mediterranean context. The scholarship has fruitfully explored institutions of health in conjunction with epidemic diseases, plague in particular.[7] Nevertheless, as we saw

---

Health (Syracuse, NY: Syracuse University Press, 1990); LaVerne Kuhnke, *Lives at Risk: Public Health in Nineteenth-Century Egypt* (Berkeley: University of California Press, 1990); Hormoz Ebrahimnejad, *Medicine, Public Health, and the Qājār State: Patterns of Medical Modernization in Nineteenth-Century Iran* (Leiden: Brill, 2004).

[5] G. Geltner, "Public Health and the Pre-Modern City: A Research Agenda," *History Compass* 10, no. 3 (2012): 231–45; J. Coomans and G. Geltner, "On the Street and in the Bathhouse: Medieval Galenism in action?," *Anuario de Estudios Medievales* 43, no. 1 (2013): 53–82; Geltner, "Healthscaping a Medieval City."

[6] A quick look at a recently published collection of articles, ironically titled *Health in/among the Ottomans*, proves the point, as it does not include a single attempt to define notions of health as defined by the Ottomans; it is based on assumptions drawn from modern concepts of health. See *OS*.

[7] For the Italian context, see, e.g., Carlo Cipolla, *Cristofano and the Plague: A Study in the History of Public Health in the Age of Galileo* (Berkeley: University of California Press, 1973); Cipolla, *Public Health and the Medical Profession in the Renaissance* (Cambridge: Cambridge University Press, 1976); Ann G. Carmichael, "Plague Legislation in the Italian Renaissance," *Bulletin of the History of Medicine* 57, no. 4 (1983): 508–25; Carmichael,

in Chapter 2, the assumed differences in responses to plague have heavily revolved around religious differences. For the early modern European travelers, the lack of quarantine applications in the Ottoman Empire meant that they were *passive* in the face of plague and *fatalistic*. This vision became a staple of European thought, down to the modern era, to find itself integrated into modern scholarship. For example, William McNeill assigned a central importance to measures of quarantine in his discussion of the Christian response to plague, which differentiated it, for him, from that of the Muslims.[8] Such perceived differences have hitherto hindered the development of inquiries seeking a relationship between plague and the formation of a public health administration in early modern Ottoman society. Responding to plague meant adopting a set of new regulations and policies that redefined the role of the Ottoman state, with its increased involvement in matters pertaining to the health of individuals and the community alike.

Calculus of Bodies

As a fortunate accident, a small number of documents dating from the late fifteenth and/or early sixteenth century have survived in the Topkapı Palace Museum Archives. The earliest of these documents is a short undated petition that contains invaluable information about epidemics in Istanbul (Figure 3). Undated and unsigned, this is a brief report submitted to the sultan, probably written by the *kadı* or *subaşı*, and again probably during the reign of Bayezid II (r. 1481–1512). The document reports the number of deaths caused by the epidemic during three days, without clearly stating what disease was involved. Being the earliest of the few surviving documents of its sort, this petition reveals that the *kadı* and the *subaşı* of Istanbul were ordered to make detailed investigations in the city and find out how many dead bodies were taken out of the city gates. The report states that Muslims and Jews who fell victim to the disease were taken outside the city walls for burial, whereas the Christians were buried in the churches, presumably *intra muros* (Table 5). In addition to giving the number of deaths recorded daily, the document also makes a distinction between the kinds of diseases

---

Plague and the Poor in Renaissance Florence (Cambridge: Cambridge University Press, 1986); Samuel Kline Cohn, *Cultures of Plague: Medical Thinking at the End of the Renaissance* (Oxford: Oxford University Press, 2010). For other European contexts, see, e.g., Paul Slack, *The Impact of Plague in Tudor and Stuart England* (London: Routledge and Kegan Paul, 1985); Kinzelbach, "Infection, Contagion, and Public Health"; Alexandra Parma Cook and Noble David Cook, *The Plague Files: Crisis Management in Sixteenth-Century Seville* (Baton Rouge: LSU Press, 2009); Kristy Wilson Bowers, *Plague and Public Health in Early Modern Seville* (Rochester, NY: University Rochester Press, 2013). For the Russian context, see John T. Alexander, *Bubonic Plague in Early Modern Russia: Public Health and Urban Disaster* (Baltimore: Johns Hopkins University Press, 1980).

[8] McNeill, *Plagues and Peoples*, 271.

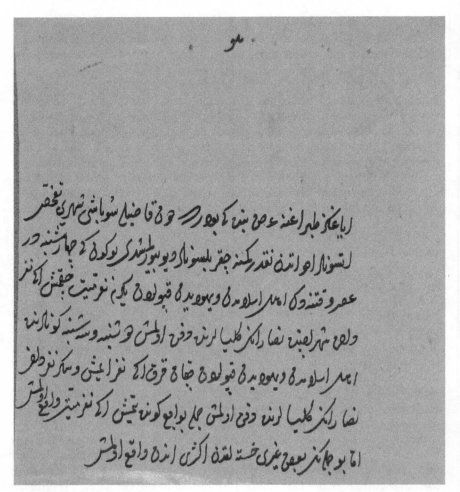

FIGURE 3. Brief note submitted to the Palace reporting the death toll during an epidemic in Istanbul. Undated. E. 10038. Document from Topkapı Palace Museum Archives.

the deaths resulted from. Of the seventy-two people who died in three days, some lost their lives because of "other diseases" (*gayrı hastalıktan*) but most died of "it" (*andan*).[9]

This document attests to a number of important practices, albeit in an embryonic form. To my knowledge, this is the earliest surviving document

---

[9] TSMA, E.10038, undated. The catalog dates it to Bayezid II's reign, which seems very likely in view of the burial practices mentioned in it: "bu üç günde 72 nefer meyyit vaki olmuş ama bu cümlenin bazısı gayrı hastalıktan ekseri andan vaki olmuş."

TABLE 5. *Burial of Plague Victims, (probably) During the Reign of Bayezid II*
(r. 1481–1512)

Day	Confession	Number of Deaths	Place of Burial
Wednesday	Muslim and Jewish	20	Buried outside city walls
	Christian	2	Buried in churches (*intra muros*)
	Total	22	
Monday and	Muslim and Jewish	42	Buried outside city walls
Tuesday	Christian	8	Buried in churches (*intra muros*)
	Total	50	
Total (in three	Muslim and Jewish	62	Buried outside city walls
days)	Christian	10	Buried in churches (*intra muros*)
	Total	72	

Source: Topkapı Palace Museum Archives, E. 10038.

issued during an epidemic outbreak in Ottoman Istanbul, and it bears a clear testimony that the daily death toll was kept during epidemics. Moreover, it suggests that a working knowledge was in place about the need to distinguish the mortality caused by diseases other than the dominant epidemic disease. In fact, even though it is not clearly stated what disease was involved, for reasons discussed earlier, we have good reason to believe this was an outbreak of plague.[10] Unfortunately, the many unknowns limit our ability to make further observations about the nature and progress of the epidemic and the rate of mortality.

Fortunately, we have two other documents dating from a slightly later date that are much more detailed. These two documents, both written on the same day during an outbreak of plague in Istanbul in May 1513, demonstrate that the daily death toll was meticulously recorded at the city gates[11] (Figures 4 and 5). One document is written by İlyas, Chief of Janissaries (*Yeniçeriler Ağası*), and the other, by Hamza, *kadı* of Istanbul, who made inspections at the gates to determine the death toll.[12] An important difference from the earlier document is that now all dead bodies seem to be taken outside of city gates during epidemics, as there is no longer a reference to *intra muros* burials

[10] The fact that the disease is simply referred to as "it" reveals more than it conceals. In the light of the discussions of Chapter 7, this manner of referencing plague (as a *black hole* or *bête noire*) suits well to the mentalities of that period. For plague in Bayezid II's reign, see Chapter 4.

[11] TSMA, E.6155, E.2544. (The full text of E.6155 has been published in *OS*, 2:35 (doc 49).

[12] E. 6155, signed as "Efkaru'l-verâ Hamza el-müvellâ be-Mahrûse-i Kostantiniye," was probably Karasili Nureddin b. Yusuf (Sarı Gürz or Görez). See Aḥmad ibn Muṣṭafa Ṭāshkubrīzādah, *al-Shaqā'iq al-nu'māniyah fī 'ulamā' al-Dawlat al-'Uthmāniyah* (Istanbul, 1985), 298–99. I am grateful to Abdurrahman Atcıl for his help in establishing the identity of this figure.

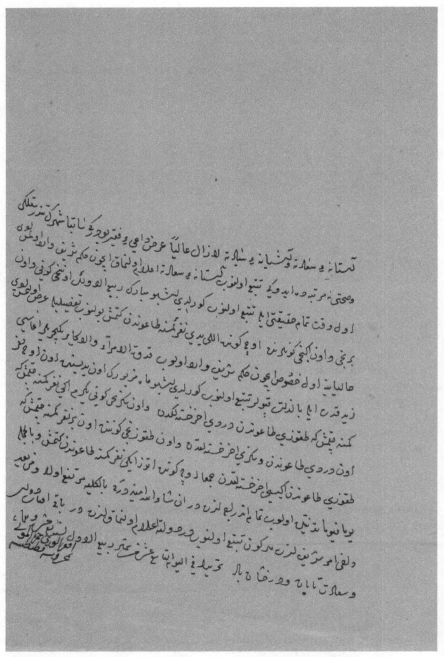

FIGURE 4. Report by the *kadı* of Istanbul submitted to the Palace during a plague epidemic. May 1513. E. 6155. Document from Topkapı Palace Museum Archives.

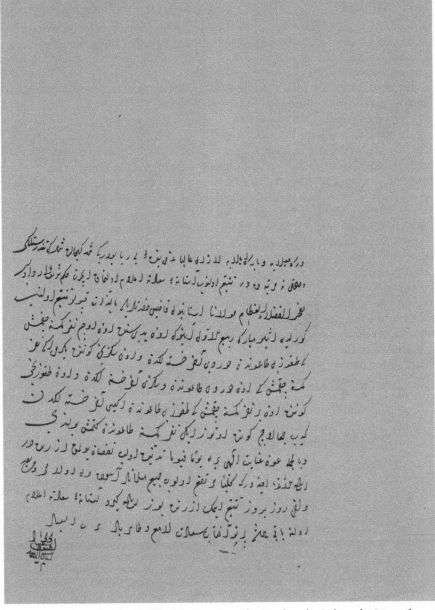

FIGURE 5. Report by the Chief of Janissaries submitted to the Palace during a plague epidemic. May 1513. E. 2544. Document from Topkapı Palace Museum Archives.

in churches. Similarly, there is no reference to which confessional community plague victims belonged, suggesting all were taken outside the walls for burial. Another difference is the care given to distinguish the number of deaths caused by plague (now clearly stated as such) as opposed to deaths caused by other diseases (Tables 3 and 4). In these reports, the daily number of deaths from plague was recorded separately from those who died from other diseases. One of these documents clearly states that the number of deaths is reported to the Ottoman palace daily.

Taken together, these documents indicate a systematic record keeping of daily mortality in Istanbul (and perhaps in other cities) at times of plague.[13] Until now, we did not have access to known collections of registers containing daily mortality records at times of plague dating from this era, but we find evidence for the practice of counting in the narrative accounts. The piecemeal information that has survived in the narrative accounts suggests that such records were kept at city gates. One eyewitness account testifies to this practice in Aleppo, in the mid-sixteenth century, by calling it "real science." According to this, before the dead bodies were taken outside the city gates for burial, they were counted by officials who reported these figures to the authorities on a daily basis.[14] Another eyewitness testimony comes from the late sixteenth century. Pharmacist Reinhold Lubenau, who witnessed a plague outbreak in Istanbul in winter 1587, wrote that during this outbreak, the number of dead bodies taken outside the gates was diligently recorded. It was found that the daily mortality was eight hundred for that outbreak, which lasted three months.[15] A later source offers a different method instead. In a letter dated November 23, 1751, Mordach Mackenzie, the physician of the Levant Company in Istanbul, claims that "the Turks have no bills of mortality," but they allegedly reckoned mortality figures on the basis of bread consumption. He explained, "One killow makes bread enough for 50 persons per day; but the consumption of bread in the months of July, August, and September, was 3000 killows short: from which it is concluded,

---

[13] Despite many efforts, I have not been able to locate such mortality registers at the Topkapı Palace Museum Archives (TSMA) or the Prime Ministry Ottoman Archives (BOA) in Istanbul. I remain convinced that these registers, if they survived, will be discovered some day. Nevertheless, such recording may have been limited to the walled city. Semavi Eyice notes that not all of the dead were taken outside Istanbul in the sixteenth century; some must be buried in the three main graveyards of Istanbul (based on personal communication with Semavi Eyice, March 24, 2006). For Istanbul's graveyards, also see Hans-Peter Laqueur, *Hüve'l-Baki: İstanbul'da Osmanlı Mezarlıkları ve Mezar Taşları* (Istanbul: Tarih Vakfı Yurt Yayınları, 1997), 7–62; Eldem, *Death in Istanbul.*

[14] *Albèri*, 1:219–20.

[15] Lubenau also notes that after the outbreak, the Sultan ordered the counting of males over the age of twenty in the city, which revealed a total of 180,000. See Lubenau, *Beschreibung*, 1:140.

that $3000 \times 50 = 150000$ must have died of the plague."[16] We do not know whether this was a commonly used method, at least as far as the sixteenth century is concerned. Perhaps this was what common wisdom prescribed for the Istanbuliotes. Regardless of whether mortality figures were kept, such estimates – accurate or not – seem to have circulated beyond Ottoman administrative circles. The population of the city was most likely aware of the fluctuations in those figures and perhaps used it as a measure to decide whether it would be better to leave the city.

The figures we encounter in narrative accounts tend to be much larger. For Istanbul, we have figures before, during, and after the sixteenth century, which may admit grounds for some comparison. For example, Kritovoulos mentioned a daily death toll of more than six hundred for the plague of 1467.[17] According to Busbecq, the daily toll at the height of the outbreak in summer 1561 was around one thousand to twelve hundred. He found out that when five hundred died per day, the people of Istanbul thought that plague was lessening.[18] An early-seventeenth-century eyewitness account further clarified the meaning of daily mortality figures. It was common to have two hundred to three hundred deaths a day, according to this account, and not at all uncommon for daily mortality figures to reach a thousand a day, or as many as twelve hundred to fifteen hundred in very violent outbreaks, which would continue for three to four months. When such was the case, the sultan did not leave the palace, according to this testimony.[19] In the mid-seventeenth century, Evliya Çelebi recounts that a great plague epidemic broke out in Istanbul during the reign of Selim II (r. 1566–74), during which every day three thousand corpses were carried out of the twenty-seven gates of the city.[20]

Even though most information is about Istanbul, there are somewhat comparable figures for other cities. For example, during the outbreak of 1548 in Thessaloniki, which was described by eyewitness testimonies as an especially devastating one, it was said that one could count up to ten deaths in one single household and 314 victims in a single day. The Jewish residents of Thessaloniki claimed to have lost seven thousand to that outbreak alone.[21] There is also some scattered evidence about mortality in

---

[16] Mordach Mackenzie, "Extracts of Several Letters of Mordach Mackenzie, M. D. Concerning the Plague at Constantinople," *Philosophical Transactions (1683–1775)* 47 (1752): 389–90.

[17] Kritovoulos, *History of Mehmed the Conqueror*, 220.

[18] Busbecq, *Turkish Letters*, 180, 182–90.

[19] Üçel-Aybet, *Avrupalı Seyyahların Gözünden*, 371–72.

[20] Evliya Çelebi, *Seyahatnâme*, 1:56.

[21] I. S. Emmanuel, *Histoire des Israélites de Salonique* (Paris: Librairie Lipschutz, 1936), 156. This figure seems to be too high, as it would imply an approximately 50 percent mortality rate within the Jewish population of the town. For figures of the Jewish population of

other provincial settings. For example, around mid-century, Salona, a market town in southern Thessaly, reported the loss of two thousand souls to plague, which must have been detrimental to a town that size. In fact, the local market stopped being held in the wake of the outbreak owing to soaring mortality.[22] Shortly thereafter, Hoybersin, a town on the Transylvanian border, reported a loss of about eight thousand people to plague.[23] We do not know anything about how mortality registers were kept in provincial towns – if they were at all – but we do come across figures that were reported to the center.

Elsewhere in the Mediterranean world, mortality registers were kept during plague epidemics of the late medieval and early modern eras. For example, several Italian cities adopted this practice from very early on.[24] We also hear of such practices in late medieval Cairo, as reported by Mamluk chroniclers.[25] It seems that the Ottomans knew about such record keeping practices elsewhere. Rumors about particularly high figures of plague mortality seem to have circulated across the Mediterranean, as suggested by the accounts of Ottoman historians. For example, Oruç mentions the case of the Mamluk Egypt while narrating the plague raging there in late fifteenth century.[26]

The calculus of bodies was not at all foreign to the Ottomans in this era. After all, they were already experts in counting bodies; tax registers constitute the ultimate evidence for this familiarity. Even though these registers included data for tax collection purposes, they nevertheless translated taxable sources of income into countable units and numbers; they counted individual bodies in the case of single males and households in the case of families. The oldest surviving examples of such registers come from the early fifteenth century, with indications that the practice probably started earlier.[27] At any rate, it may be useful to remember that the first decades of the sixteenth century witnessed the rise of a new Ottoman bureaucracy,

Thessaloniki in 1567–68, see *Melek Delilbaşı*, "The Via Egnatia and Selanik (Thessalonica) in the 16th century," in Zachariadou, *Via Egnatia under Ottoman Rule*, 67–84.

[22] MD 4, 192/2009 (29 Cemaziyelahir 968 H./March 17, 1561). See Chapter 5 for this outbreak. An early-nineteenth-century visitor to Salona reported the presence of more than eight hundred households, which in comparison may suggest that the mid-sixteenth century outbreak had been a detrimental blow to the town's population. See Sir Henry Holland, *Travels in the Ionian Isles, Albania, Thessaly, Macedonia, &c. during the Years 1812 and 1813* (printed for Longman, Hurst, Rees, Orme, and Brown, 1819), 2:153.

[23] MD 28, 334/843 (13 Şaban 984 H./November 4, 1576). For this outbreak, see Chapter 6.

[24] For such record keeping practices in late medieval Florence, see Carmichael, *Plague and the Poor in Renaissance Florence*.

[25] For discussion of urban mortality during and after the Black Death and the practices of recording plague deaths in the Mamluk case, see Dols, *Black Death*, 169–85.

[26] Oruç, *Tarih*, 153.

[27] Halil İnalcık, "Ottoman Methods of Conquest," *Studia Islamica* 2 (1954): 109–10.

which heavily made use of new technologies of record keeping. Among the most important agents of using these new practices, the Ottoman scribes actively experimented with techniques of keeping, storing, and retrieving records.[28] Yet all these registers recorded information about the living bodies, which may leave us wondering: why count the dead bodies? Can this be seen as an attempt to monitor the changing rhythm of an epidemic or to keep the pulse of the plague as an urban health problem? What was the nature of the information these numbers revealed to those in the administration? These questions are difficult to answer with the narrative accounts we have at hand, though it is possible to offer some preliminary observations. Even on the basis of a small sample of documents, it can be argued that the numbers were the result of a conscious effort at measuring the epidemic and translating mortality into numbers, precisely because it meant something to its contemporaries about the intensity of the epidemic. For example, the document composed on May 25, 1513, may have been written when plague was thought to be lessening. The fact that the number of plague deaths was decreasing was taken as an indication that the outbreak was abating, followed by a statement of wish and prayer for its complete disappearance.[29] It may be helpful to remember that human mortality during plague epidemics typically followed a recognizable bell curve, with a gradual increase, peak, and gradual decrease. This pattern should have been familiar to those who experienced the outbreaks repeatedly.

It is also equally significant that this recording process distinguished plague deaths from deaths caused by other diseases. Even though we do not hear what other diseases were involved, this practice is worthy of consideration. First of all, it tells us something about the presence of a working knowledge of plague diagnosis in Ottoman society. There is no reason to doubt that plague, with its gruesome manifestations and capacity to kill fast, was familiar to early-sixteenth-century Ottoman society. At this stage, we do not have evidence about who was making plague diagnoses, but it is most likely that no medical professional was involved. Second, this also informs us about the familiarity with the prevalence of multiple diseases during epidemics – a well-known epidemiological phenomenon. The practice of recording plague deaths separately from deaths caused by other diseases demonstrates an awareness of this epidemiological phenomenon and

[28] Fleischer, *Bureaucrat and Intellectual in the Ottoman Empire*, 214–24; Cornell H. Fleischer, "Preliminaries to the Study of the Ottoman Bureaucracy," *Journal of Turkish Studies* 10 (1986): 135–41; Kaya Şahin, *Empire and Power in the Reign of Süleyman: Narrating the Sixteenth-Century Ottoman World* (Cambridge: Cambridge University Press, 2013), 215–20.

[29] TSMA, E.6155, E.2544. If this statement is not a completely empty statement of wishful thinking or a formulaic phrase, then it may be that there was already some understanding of the patterns of mortality in a plague outbreak and its relation to changes of season.

plague's potential power of masking mortality caused by other diseases.[30] Third, this practice can be evaluated with respect to its immediate practical value to the Ottoman authorities. Even though the earlier document made a vague distinction between deaths from plague and those caused by other diseases, it was a general observation, not one expressed in a conscious effort of counting. However, the documents dating from 1513 did show separate numbers of plague and nonplague deaths, a significant change in itself for the diagnosis and counting of the plague victims.

Unfortunately, we know very little about how these registers were kept, if at all. Were the names of individuals or, for that matter, any other personal information recorded? Or was it only the numbers? As we shall see, more detailed registers were kept when the tax-exempt Ottoman elite (*askeri*) died of plague. Regardless, if such registers did exist – and there is good reason to believe they did – an organized attempt to count the dead and record this information can be taken as evidence for the beginning of a new consciousness on the part of the Ottoman administration. Perhaps this may be seen as an attempt to monitor the course of epidemics and to collect information, for possible uses of controlling and taking precautions against it. What we do know is that those who were in charge of counting the dead, recording the information, and reporting the figures represented the Ottoman state. Hence, the calculus of bodies can be seen as the initial stage of a process that contributed to the "making" of the early modern Ottoman state, by rendering the state of the bodies more "legible" to the mechanisms of control.[31] Once the state of the bodies was transformed into a form of quantifiable data, then the next stage followed in the form of regulating the logistics for the disposal of plagued bodies. As we shall see, regulations developed as to where, when, how, and whom to bury.

Disposal of Bodies

During epidemics, the quick burial of victims was a major source of concern, especially when mortality was high. Unfortunately, we do not have clear evidence about how plague victims were buried. Yet, it can be assumed that funeral rites could diverge from the norm, at times when the fast burial of the victims became a pressing problem. In the second half of the fifteenth century, Kritovoulos's account suggests that burial rites were not fully observed for victims of plague in Istanbul because the mortality was too high. He wrote, "More than six hundred deaths a day occurred, a multitude greater than men could bury, for there were not men enough." It is true that *the dead outnumbering the living* was a known trope in the

---

[30] Compare with Renaissance Florence as discussed in Carmichael, *Plague and the Poor in Renaissance Florence.*

[31] Scott, *Seeing Like a State.*

Byzantine chronicle-writing tradition, used to emphasize high mortality.[32] Yet, Kritovoulos accounts for the shortage of men of religion and workers to bury the dead, as well as the lack of coffins. He wrote, "There were often two or three dead, or even more, buried in a single coffin, the only one available.... There were not enough ... priests for the funerals and burials or the funeral chants and prayers, nor could the dead be properly interred, for the workers gave out in the process. They had to go through the long summer days without eating or drinking, and they simply could not stand it."[33] Such difficulties are not unheard of in cases of high mortailty. In fact, Byzantine Constantinople had seen worse during the Plague of Justinian, when corpses had to be thrown in the sea, inside the towers, or in pits dug for mass burial purposes.[34]

Writing not too long after the Ottoman conquest of the city, Kritovoulos described the burial customs of what appears to be a heavily Christian population. Interestingly enough, we do not hear of mass burial practices in Ottoman society in times of plague. Other situations of high mortality, such as soldiers fallen dead on the battlefield, may have at times necessitated deviating from funerary rites in Ottoman society.[35] However, nowhere in the sources is there mention of mass burials or throwing corpses in large pits or elsewhere at times of plague. On the contrary, the testimonies of travelers' accounts confirm that funeral customs and practices were kept even in time of plague. The burial customs of Muslims as well as Jews and Christians have been a source of interest for foreign observers. Many left detailed descriptions of such practices in Ottoman society. For example, Stephan Gerlach, the Lutheran chaplain of the Habsburg ambassadorial mission to the Porte between 1573 and 1578, recorded in his memoirs detailed accounts of funeral rites and customs for Muslim, Jewish, and Christian burials, though he did not openly mention the plague in the city.[36]

There is no doubt that the members of the Ottoman imperial family and the high-ranking elite, whose funerals have been better recorded in the sources, enjoyed more elaborate funeral processions. Even though most

32 Stathakopoulos, *Famine and Pestilence*, 141.
33 Kritovoulos, *History of Mehmed the Conqueror*, 220.
34 Paul Magdalino, "The Maritime Neighborhoods of Constantinople: Commercial and Residential Functions, Sixth to Twelfth Centuries," *Dumbarton Oaks Papers* 54 (2000): 218–19.
35 Vatin and Yerasimos suggest that funeral rituals may not have been fully observed for soldiers who died on the battlefield or people who died elsewhere. This may have also been the case at times of epidemics, when exceptionally high mortality occurred. Nicolas Vatin and Stephane Yerasimos, *Les Cimetières dans la ville: status, choix et organisation des lieux d'inhumation dans Istanbul intra muros* (Istanbul: Institut français d'études anatoliennes Georges Dumézil, 2001), 26.
36 Gerlach, *Türkiye Günlüğü*, 330, 431. Gerlach also described the funerals of the Greek Orthodox community of Istanbul, which he found very interesting, especially the loud weeping of the hired mourners, 680–81. He noted that the Jews also had particular funerary customs, 681.

funerals have been described in the sources as solemn and inconspicuous occasions, some, such as Süleyman's, are remembered to have been quite ostentatious.[37] This, however, does not necessarily inform us about how the ordinary Ottoman subjects were interred, especially those who died during epidemics. In such cases, it can be presumed that funerals took place without big processions, at best with a small gathering of closest family members undertaking their final duty for their loved ones. Despite the challenge posed by epidemics and the high mortality that ensued at those times, some customary burial practices seem to be in place for the Muslim community. For example, all bodies, including those that fell victim to plague, seem to have been washed, shrouded, and prepared according to Muslim customs of burial.[38] A *mühimme* order from 1576 suggests that washing the body of the deceased, even for those who died of plague, would have been considered customary. In this case, a death that was registered as caused by plague was later suspected to have been a case of murder and was ordered to be inspected on the basis of the testimonies of those who washed and buried the body.[39] There are also testimonies of foreign observers about this practice, which they commented on with some apprehension. For example, Baron Wratislaw, who witnessed a plague epidemic in Istanbul in the 1590s, mentioned with great astonishment that the dead bodies were washed before burial, even at times of serious plague.[40] This may not have been standard practice everywhere, as suggested by the experience of Evliya Çelebi during his visit of Fener-abadan, a small fortress in Thessaly. The traveler wrote that the locals there flee plagues and leave their houses and belongings behind unattended and their sick untended. Upon seeing an abandoned man who died of hunger, Evliya Çelebi takes upon himself to wash the body of the dead man with the help of his servants, perform the funeral prayer, and bury him. The same evening, much to his surprise, their host family fled from them saying that they handled and washed a plagued body.[41] This incident is at least some evidence that washing plague victims cannot be accepted as standard

---

37 Zeynep Tarım Ertuğ, *XVI. Yüzyıl Osmanlı Devletinde Cülûs ve Cenaze Törenleri* (Ankara: Kültür Bakanlığı, 1999).

38 For death rites in early Islam, see Leor Halevi, *Muhammad's Grave: Death Rites and the Making of Islamic Society* (New York: Columbia University Press, 2007). The Ottomans followed the Muslim burial tradition with slight local variations. Washing the body of the deceased, placing it in a seamless shroud, and carrying the shrouded body in a coffin to a mosque was standard funerary custom. After the funeral prayer at the mosque, the body was carried to the grave and interred facing the direction of Mecca without the coffin. See Edhem Eldem, "Death and Funerary Culture," in Ágoston and Bruce Alan Masters, *Encyclopedia of the Ottoman Empire*, 177–80; Eldem, *Death in Istanbul*.

39 MD 27, 261/612 (12 Zilkade 983 H./February 12, 1576).

40 Wratislaw, *Adventures*, 107. Compare with Reinhold Lubenau's description of the burial of plague victims from the Habsburg ambassadorial residence. Lubenau, *Beschreibung*, 2:25.

41 Evliya Çelebi, *Seyahatnâme*, 8:91: "halkı Urûmşa olup dağ âdemîsi olmak ile tâ'ûndan firâr edüp niçe hânedânların cümle bakır avânîleri durup hâneleri berbâd oluyor." "Bunlar tâ'ûnlu ölü yanına varup ölü yaykadılar."

practice everywhere. In another instance, when an adolescent slave of our traveler died, he washed the body and buried it, for which he was accused by Albanians of handling the deceased's body. He convinced them with great difficulty that the slave had died from diarrhea and not from plague.[42] Another case of a plague victim who was prepared for burial in Istanbul suggests that full funerary rites were performed even for plague deaths, not only in the Muslim community, but also among the Christians. In this particular instance, when the fourteen-year-old Constantine of Moldavia died of plague in Istanbul, his body was prepared for burial, first according to the customs of the Orthodox creed (confession, consecration with bread and wine). Then, when the Muslims found out about this, they performed Muslim rites, whereupon they circumcised the deceased, had testimonies heard by witnesses that the deceased wanted to convert to Islam before he died, and carried him to the burial ground in a coffin with a Muslim headgear placed on top, according to custom.[43] Even though these examples suggest that full funerary rites were performed even for plague deaths, further research about religious and social norms of burial of plague victims in Ottoman society is necessary.

After the body was prepared for burial according to custom, it had to be carried to the burial site on top of the shoulders of those who bid farewell to the deceased. Even though wooden coffins were normally used for transporting the dead, it is plausible to surmise that coffins could become expensive or scarce in times of high mortality. At such times, corpses were most likely placed directly on wooden biers or anything that would serve that purpose. The woodcut by the Flemish artist Pieter Coecke van Aelst depicts a scene of burial just outside of Edirne in 1533. In this scene, the dead body is placed on a wooden bier, carried on the shoulders of a small number of men, as the grave was being prepared for interment[44] (Figure 6). Visually speaking, this is presumably as close as we can get to the funeral of an ordinary

---

42 Evliya Çelebi, *Seyahatnâme*, 8:281: "bu hakîrin bir nâ-resîde gulâmı merhûm olup kendim gasl edüp bu haremde defn etdim. Hattâ cümle Arnavud halkı, 'Sen meyyit yaykadın' deyü hakîrden nefret etdiler. 'Bire vallâhi tâ'ûnlu değil idi, ishâlden merhûm oldu' deyü niçe bin yemîn-i muğallazalar edüp gücile halkı i'timâd etdirdim."

43 Dernschwam, *İstanbul ve Anadolu'ya Seyahat Günlüğü*, 104–5. According to the order of events in his narrative, Constantine seems to have died on March 26, 1554.

44 Alexandrine N. St Clair, *The Image of the Turk in Europe* (New York: Metropolitan Museum of Art, 1973), 27, illustration 4: woodcut after Pieter Coecke van Aelst from *Ces Moeurs et fachons de faire de Turcz...*, [Antwerp], 1553. Also see Pieter Coecke van Aelst, *The Turks in MDXXXIII: A Series of Drawings Made in That Year at Constantinople* (London: privately printed for W. S. M., 1873). It may be worthy of note that a horse (presumably of the deceased) is depicted here to follow the procession. Bringing the horse of the deceased to the funeral (usually with its tail cut) was a custom that continued until the sixteenth century and even longer in some places. See Eldem, "Death and Funerary Culture." Another interesting detail is the depiction of people carrying decorated saplings walking along the procession, apparently used as *nahıl* (decorated trees or poles more commonly utilized in wedding and circumcision processions). See Özdemir Nutku, "Nahil,"

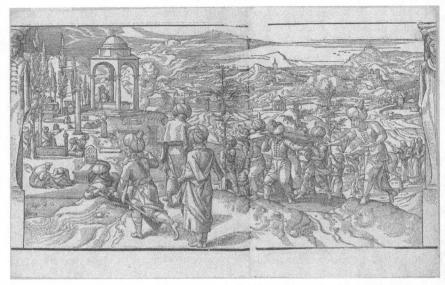

FIGURE 6. Pieter Coecke van Aelst, *A Turkish Funeral* from the frieze *Ces Moeurs et fachons de faire de Turcz* (Customs and Fashions of the Turks), 1553. The Metropolitan Museum of Art, Harris Brisbane Dick Fund, 1928, www.metmuseum.org.

Ottoman subject in the early sixteenth century. Other visual representations from the sixteenth century also testify to the material aspects of funerary practices among the Christian, Jewish, and Muslim members of Ottoman society (Figures 7–9).[45] Yet we do not know whether this scene comes from a time of plague. We do not have evidence as to whether there were practices that distinguished plague burials from those of others,[46] except for an

TDVİA; Mehmet Arslan, "Osmanlı Dönemi Düğün ve Şenliklerinde Nahıl Geleneği, 1675 Edirne Şenliği ve Bu Şenlikte Nahıllar," in *Osmanlı Edebiyat, Tarih, Kültür Makaleleri* (Istanbul 2000), 593–617. In the Ottomanist literature, *nahıl* is generally associated with fertility because of its symbolism. See, e.g., Babak Rahimi, "*Nahıl*s, Circumcision Rituals and the Theatre State," in Sajdi, *Ottoman Tulips*, 90–116. If this depiction was not entirely a product of the artist's imagination, then, the use of *nahıl* in funeral processions may have had other associations, such as symbolizing life and longevity, in a meaning similar to the common custom of planting cypress trees by the tombs. See F. W. Hasluck, *Christianity and Islam under the Sultans* (Oxford: Clarendon Press, 1929). On the depiction of a man climbing the cypress tree by the grave, see Godfrey Goodwin, "Gardens of the Dead in Ottoman Times," *Muqarnas* 5 (January 1, 1988): 62.

45 E.g., see *Bartholomäus Schachman (1559–1614): The Art of Travel* (Milan: Skira, 2012), 111, 155, 313.

46 Archeological research could provide such evidence. Compare with comparative study of plague burials in rural and urban Europe during and after the Black Death on the basis of archeological evidence in Sacha Kacki and Dominique Castex, "Réflexions sur la variété des modalités funéraires en temps d'épidémie. L'exemple de la peste noire en contextes urbain et rural," *Archéologie Médiévale* 42 (2012): 1–21.

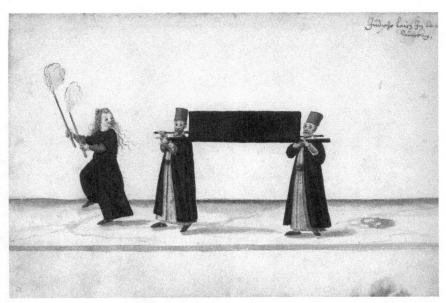

FIGURE 7. *Jewish Burial in Turkey*, from the *Travel Album of Bartholomäus Schachman* (17r), 1590. Orientalist Museum, Doha, OM. 749.

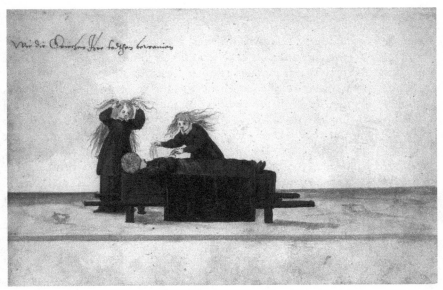

FIGURE 8. *Christians Lamenting Their Dead*, from the *Travel Album of Bartholomäus Schachman* (86v), 1590. Orientalist Museum, Doha, OM. 749.

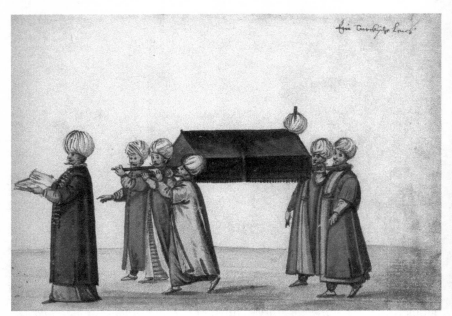

FIGURE 9. *Turkish Burial*, from the *Travel Album of Bartholomäus Schachman* (3v), 1590. Orientalist Museum, Doha, OM. 749.

early-nineteenth-century testimony that referred to "the customary sign or token of a red cloth thrown over the bier, and enveloping the dead body" for plague victims. But after the body was taken to the cemetery, they were buried in exactly the same manner as others were.[47]

Similarly, the presence of men of religion for performing funerary rites could be surmised even in the smallest of the funerals. This was indeed crucial to Muslim burials so much so that the absence of men of religion to undertake this duty could cause delays in burials. For example, a document from 1566 reported the unavailability of men of religion to perform this duty in some Muslim villages near Roda on the Lim River (probably Brodarevo in Serbia), which caused delays in the interment of the dead for several days.[48] Even though there is no direct reference to the conditions of an epidemic in this document, it is clear that such cases of high mortality would make things all the more difficult. As with other members of society, high mortality left

[47] William Wittman, *Travels in Turkey, Asia Minor, Syria, and across the Desert into Egypt* (Philadelphia: printed and sold by James Humphreys, 1804), 76–77. Compare with Figures 7, 8, and 9. Only in the scene depicting a Muslim funeral (Figure 9) the coffin is covered in red cloth, whereas the other two are not.

[48] *5 Numaralı Mühimme Defteri (973/1565–1566): özet ve indeks*, ed. Hacı Osman Yıldırım et al. (Ankara: T. C. Başbakanlık Devlet Arşivleri Genel Müdürlüğü, 1994), 1235.

men of religion in reduced numbers, which may have caused interruption in the burials of plague victims.

All of these steps – from washing, shrouding, and preparing the body for burial to the manufacture and acquisition of a coffin or bier for the transportation of the deceased to the grave, from the actual process of digging graves, interring the dead, and preparing tombstones to praying for the eternal peace of the soul of the deceased – must have created a certain demand for a funeral industry. Although there is no clear indication as to when the goods and services of this industry became widely available to the ever-growing population of Istanbul, the number of professionals offering them seems to have gradually increased. For example, Evliya Çelebi mentions gravediggers (*esnaf-ı mezar-kazan* or *gur kazan*) and gives their number as 2,008 but mentions exclusively their services at times of war. However, one wonders whether those gravediggers or others who could perform such tasks were utilized in Istanbul at times of high mortality, when they did not serve on military campaign. In a similar vein, he mentions professional corpse washers (*esnaf-ı mürde-şuyan*), whose number he gives as four thousand. Again, it seems these are exclusively in charge of serving at times of war for the purpose of washing the bodies of deceased soldiers in military campaigns. In addition to this, other professionals, such as coffin makers (*esnaf-ı tabutcıyan*), tombstone carvers, and funeral witnesses (*cenaze şahidleri*), seem to have served the funeral industry in Istanbul. Furthermore, a special group of porters in Istanbul who carried sick people could have also been involved in providing their services in the transportation of plague victims.[49]

The variety of goods and services, however, was no guarantee of their availability at times of crises and heavy mortality. For example, it is conceivable that plagues would reduce the number of those laborers and artisans, as they fell prey to the disease like everybody else, and perhaps even more so because of the very nature of their profession. It is also equally conceivable that they would flee plagues or simply refuse to perform such risky jobs. At least in one case, we see the intervention of the state in assigning the duty of burying plague victims to the local gypsy population. This is attested by a *mühimme* order of 1572, which commanded that non-Muslim plague victims be buried by the gypsies of Kırkkilise (Kırklareli).[50] Even though gypsy communities were traditionally associated with certain professions, such as blacksmiths, palm reading, and entertainers, in Ottoman society,

---

49 Evliya Çelebi, *Seyahatnâme*, 1:241–42, 246, 321–22, 10:183. About the grazing of animals and begging in cemeteries, see *7 Numaralı Mühimme Defteri (975–976/1567–1569)*, 162. For porters, see Evliya Çelebi, *Seyahatnâme*, 1:281, 315; Nejdet Ertuğ, *Osmanlı Döneminde İstanbul Hammalları* (Istanbul: Timaş Yayınları, 2008), 47, 218–19, 266; Seidel, *Sultanın zindanında*, 39.

50 KK 67, 241/480, no. 1698, cited in Rıfat Günalan, "XVI. Yüzyılda Bab-ı Defteri Teşkilatı ve Maliye Ahkam Defterleri," PhD diss., Marmara University, Istanbul, 2005.

gravedigging and burial does not seem to appear among these.[51] Their admittedly low ranking in this society may have caused the assignment of such tasks to this community.

Even when such goods and services were to be available, this did not guarantee that all members of Ottoman society could use them equally. At times of plague, having access to the goods and services of the funeral and burial industry may have become too difficult or expensive, especially for Ottoman subjects of modest income. Even though there is some evidence for the regulation of prices for funerary services, only an extensive consideration of the prices at different years, especially epidemic and nonepidemic years, can better shed light to this issue.[52] Guild organizations or pious foundations may have provided assistance to those in need in such cases.[53]

Almost all of these practices presume a certain degree of public order to be executed. However, it is difficult to comment on the extent to which that order was possible to maintain, especially in cases of heavy mortality. Drawing analogies from other cases of crises in Istanbul, such as in great fires, enforcing public order must have been challenging, especially in view of escalating crime.[54] Similar problems would likely arise in urban areas at times of plague, the significance of which might even be partly obscured by heavy plague mortality. Crime could also surface in rural areas, especially along the highways. Archival documents attest to the increased presence of highway robberies at times of plague, even on the main highways of the empire, such as that connecting Istanbul to Edirne and the Balkans.[55]

Reduced numbers in the workforce would have to struggle for burials. The burial of those plague victims who did not have family members or had family also carried off by the plague must have been particularly worrisome. There is also the problem of the availability of men of religion

[51] Elena Marushiakova and Vesselin Popov, *Gypsies in the Ottoman Empire: A Contribution to the History of the Balkans* (Hatfield: University of Hertfordshire Press, 2001), 41–44. On the status of gypsies in Ottoman society, Eyal Ginio, "Neither Muslims nor Zimmis: The Gypsies (Roma) in the Ottoman State," *Romani Studies* 14, no. 2 (2004): 117–44.

[52] Vatin and Yerasimos present a good selection of cases from the early modern era. See Nicolas Vatin and Stefanos Yerasimos, *Les cimetières dans la ville: statut, choix et organisation des lieux d'inhumation dans Istanbul intra muros* (Istanbul: Institut français d'études anatoliennes Georges Dumézil, 2001), 25–38.

[53] Vatin and Yerasimos noted that pious foundations must have supported funerary services, though there is no direct evidence that shows the employment of personnel for carrying out such tasks by *waqfs*. See ibid., 2, 8–9.

[54] For a treatment of such crises in Istanbul based on primary sources of this era, see Boyar and Fleet, *A Social History of Ottoman Istanbul*, 72–128. For crimes in Istanbul, see Fariba Zarinebaf, *Crime and Punishment in Istanbul 1700/1800* (Berkeley: University of California Press, 2010).

[55] MD 22, 38/82 (23 Muharrem 981 H./May 25, 1573); MD 22, 164/344 (28 Receb 981 H./November 23, 1573); MD 27, 300/721 (26 Zilkade 983 H./February 26, 1576). For a discussion of these cases in context, see Chapter 6.

to perform religious rites of burial and gravediggers to dig graves. Were individuals responsible for arranging and executing these duties entirely on their own? Were there any charitable organizations they could turn to for help at such times? Did the state organize or offer any of those services for plague victims? Again, we have limited information to adequately address these questions. It seems that pious foundations (*waqf*) offered some of these services, as implied in the account of Evliya Çelebi in Buda. According to his account, there were people appointed by pious foundations for washing the dead. For example, the locals of Buda used the waters of thermal springs for this purpose.[56] Another piece of evidence comes from a seventeenth-century payroll register of the hospital in Bursa in which a corpse washer (*gassal*) by the name of Hacı Ebubekir was listed to have received a daily stipend of two aspers.[57] Sources indicate the presence of similar organizations among the Jewish population of Thessaloniki around this time, established to help alleviate the troubles caused by disasters. These brotherhood organizations helped their community in difficult times by assisting with burials and performing burial rites, as they faced an especially challenging task during epidemic outbreaks. They also tended for the sick and helped the poor and orphans in the aftermath of such crises.[58]

Given the frailty of public order in times of epidemics, there is more reason to construe that the state would be involved in regulating burials. This manifested most importantly in the organization of burial space. At least in the case of Istanbul, the rise of the first communal graveyards, just outside of the city walls, dates back to major outbreaks of plagues. In the first decades after the conquest, there was no organized space entirely dedicated to burials. Around this time, it appears that while the Muslims were buried *intra muros* around mosques, the non-Muslims could be buried *intra muros* or elsewhere. However, as the city's population increased, and the number of plague victims increased in proportion with this, it became necessary to establish graveyards outside the walled area of the city. As a result, communal graveyards started to appear encircling the city walls, stretching from the shores of the Marmara Sea to the Golden Horn. During the reign of Bayezid II, the first communal graveyards of Istanbul arose, organized exclusively on the basis of confessional communities. While the first Muslim graveyards began to form in the area outside of the Edirnekapı, Yenikapı, and Topkapı gates, those reserved for the Orthodox were located in the area that extended from the Topkapı to the Silivrikapı gates, and the

56 Evliya Çelebi, *Seyahatnâme*, 6:139.
57 Osman Çetin, "Bursa Şeriyye Sicilleri Işığında Osmanlılarda İlk Tıp Fakültesi: Bursa Darüşşifası ve Tıbbi Faaliyetler," *Osmanlı Tarihi Araştırma ve Uygulama Merkezi Dergisi (OTAM)* 4 (Ankara, 1993), 128.
58 I. S. Emmanuel, *Histoire des Israélites de Salonique* (Paris: Librairie Lipschutz, 1936), 68, 220, 222.

Jewish graveyards were located in the area that stretched from the Eğrikapı gate to the Golden Horn.[59] We do not know to what extent burial in these graveyards was enforced, but if we were to rely on the testimony of Evliya Çelebi, the Jews seem to have been required to bring their dead to the Jewish cemetery, even when this meant bringing their dead from areas outside the walled city – a practice that seems to have continued up to the seventeenth century.[60]

It seems likely that starting in the sixteenth century, most of Istanbul's dead were buried outside of the city, which is also evidenced in the earlier mentioned documents relating to plague burials. The Ottoman central administration started to mandate the taking of the dead outside of the city, even when there was no plague going on. It seems that the taking of the dead outside the city walls, at least for *intra muros* Istanbul, became standard practice that continued into the seventeenth century.[61]

However, the communal graveyards outside of the walls of the historical peninsula were not the only burial grounds that served the greater Istanbul area (i.e., including Galata, Hasköy/Eyüp, and Üsküdar); there were cemeteries in Pera and Üsküdar.[62] A big graveyard – Grand champs des mort – was located on the northern end of Pera, over the hill from modern-day Taksim to Fındıklı. On the western end of Pera lay another graveyard – Petit champs – on the hills of modern-day Tepebaşı and Kasımpaşa.[63] A panoramic representation of Istanbul dating back to 1533 produced by Pieter Coecke van Aelst shows Muslim and Jewish graveyards on the hills of Galata, behind the fortress (Figure 10). By the late sixteenth century, the Europeans who lived in Pera must have been buried in these cemeteries. For example, this was where Busbecq's physician William Quacquelben was buried when he fell victim to plague in 1561.[64] Stephan Gerlach, who visited this graveyard more than a decade later, confirms this, as he mentions a physician being buried there. Gerlach's testimony is important because he wrote that this graveyard, beyond the neighborhoods of Galata and Pera, was reserved for ambassadors of German and Hungarian origin. He also

---

[59] Vatin and Yerasimos, *Les cimetières*, 2.

[60] After the Jewish cemetery in Kasımpaşa was moved to Hasköy in the late sixteenth century, it seems that the Jews were required to bury their dead only there. Evliya Çelebi writes that the Jews brought their dead even from Üsküdar and Galata, as they were not allowed to bury elsewhere. See Evliya Çelebi, *Seyahatnâme*, 1:193. Also see Abraham Galante, *Histoire des juifs de Turquie* (Istanbul: Isis, 1985), 1:299–306.

[61] Vatin and Yerasimos, *Les cimetières*, 19–22.

[62] Evliya Celebi, *Seyahatnâme*, 1:194, 197–99, 222.

[63] Laqueur, *Hüve'l-Baki*, 7–9.

[64] Hans-Peter Laqueur suggests that this cemetery was where plague victims were buried, but he only mentions the case of Quacquelben. He claims that the latter's tomb is currently in Feriköy cemetery and that his tombstone still stands. See Laqueur, *Hüve'l-Baki*, 8n4. For Quacquelben, see Chapter 5.

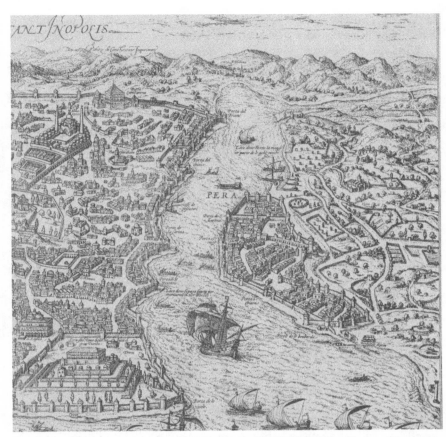

FIGURE 10. Pieter Coecke van Aelst, *The Turks in MDXXXIII: A Series of Drawings Made in That Year at Constantinople*. London: privately printed, 1873, Ott 3100.1, Houghton Library, Harvard University.

recorded that the clockmaker who had fallen ill on the way to Istanbul with thirteen others in their retinue died and was buried in this graveyard.[65]

In the seventeenth century, the burial grounds seem to have further expanded, as suggested by the testimony of Eremya Çelebi, who noted the areas reserved for the Muslim, Greek, European, and Armenian graves.[66] It appears that burial space was organized according to confessional, ethnic, and social differences. Writing in the early seventeenth century, Ottaviano Bon observed that whereas higher-rank state administrators could be buried

[65] Gerlach, *Türkiye Günlüğü*, 99.
[66] Eremya Çelebi Kömürciyan, *İstanbul Tarihi: XVII. Asırda İstanbul*, trans. Hrand D Andreasyan (Istanbul: Eren, 1988), 34, 38.

in the city, common people were carried out of the city gates for interment.[67] Evliya Çelebi mentions a graveyard reserved for gypsies outside of the gate of Eğrikapi.[68] The quality, shape, and design of tombstones as well as their epitaphs also suggest that such differences were to be found even within a single graveyard.

It is more difficult to comment on the rise of communal graveyards in other Ottoman cities mainly because of the fragmentary nature of the evidence. For example, it has been suggested that there were no communal graveyards in Thessaloniki before 1492.[69] Travelers' accounts sometimes note the location of cemeteries in Anatolia and the Balkans. For example, traveling along the main caravan route of the Balkans in the mid-sixteenth century, Dernschwam noted the presence of Muslim graveyards outside of the cities he passed.[70] Yet, it is difficult to comment on the development of cemeteries. A snapshot image of a burial area outside of Edirne, which comes from the Flemish artist Pieter Coecke van Aelst's depiction of a burial site in 1533 (see Figure 6), bears testimony to the gradual nature of the development of these cemeteries. In this scene, burial takes place on top of a hill, outside of residential areas. The other graves that can be seen in the background are not very regular. In addition to clearly identifiable Muslim graves, Christian (and possibly Jewish) graves can be seen scattered in the surrounding areas. Cypress trees, a picturesque marker of Ottoman cemeteries, are also visible.

How exactly burial space was organized in Istanbul and in other Ottoman urban centers is not clear. Policies that oversaw and regulated burial seems to have developed gradually, and mostly on an ad hoc basis. Istanbul's increasing exposure to epidemics and high levels of mortality that ensued appears to have contributed to the development of such policies. What remains to be addressed is the rationale behind the adoption of such policies and how they related to plague. Was there a link between plague and the emergence of communal graveyards outside the city walls, at least in the example of Istanbul? To better understand the rationale behind these policies, it is important to consider ideas of miasma. Dead bodies and the effluvia believed to arise from them were associated with miasma, the prevalent epidemiological paradigm. The motivation behind taking plague victims outside the city walls may have been to ensure health in the city and to protect the healthy from the miasma of the dead. If so, graveyards were to be regulated as areas that could be potentially hazardous to the air. Once the air was

---

[67] Bon, *Sultan's Seraglio*, 142–43.
[68] Evliya Çelebi, *Seyahatnâme*, 8:35.
[69] Joseph Nehama, *Histoire des Israélites de Salonique* (Salonique: Librairie Molho, 1935), 4:147.
[70] To name but a few examples, he notes Muslim graveyards just outside of Belgrade, Smederevo, Sofia, and Edirne along the way. See Dernschwam, *İstanbul ve Anadolu'ya Seyahat Günlüğü*, 21, 22, 36–37, 45.

contaminated with miasma, then the health of the rest of the population was to be endangered. Hence, the state would remove the plagued bodies outside the walls to a controlled area. Yet, the designation of burial areas outside of the city walls was not the only regulation. There seems to be additional measures to ensure a "healthy air," free from bad air or miasma. These included proper digging of the graves and possibly using lime scattered on top. Some Western travelers claimed that the Ottomans did not dig their graves deep enough. This, they thought, was the origin of miasma, which resulted in plagues in the city. How deep the grave was dug varied according to local practices. For example, in Bursa in 1502, the grave of a man had to be dug as deep as a man's chest, while that of woman had to be up to her shoulders. In the same year, in Istanbul, it had to be deep enough for a man's waist and a woman's chest.[71] When the graves were close to houses, like those of *intra muros* Istanbul, they were surrounded by walls.[72] Such efforts aimed to reduce the contamination of the air from miasmas.

The state's involvement was not only limited to counting the dead and deciding where bodies had to be buried. It also extended over controling which bodies had to be buried in those designated places as well as who was to bury whom in times of plague. These initial efforts that addressed the immediate needs of a time of crisis gradually turned into a growing concern to maintain hygiene in the cities and laid the basis for the development of a mechanism to ensure urban cleanliness and health.

Regulating Bodies in Urban Space

The Ottoman central administration was of course not only trying to regulate the dead bodies. Its growing control extended to the world of its living population. This can be seen most clearly in the efforts for regulating the hygiene, cleaning, and planning in Istanbul. Chronologically speaking, these measures seem to have followed the crisis-management regulations that started in the first half of the sixteenth century. Hence, it can be suggested that the latter were born out of the set of embryonic regulations that aimed to preserve health in the city. However, before trying to associate the regulations pertaining to dead bodies to those that aimed to regulate the living, a word of caution is in order. Here my goal is not to suggest that the latter was born out of the former just because of the chronological order. Instead, it is about the rationale of the two, which were drawn from the very same body of knowledge. It is important to pay attention not only to what the regulations aimed to do but also to why they were adopted in the first place.

---

[71] Vatin and Yerasimos, *Les cimetières*, 29. Goodwin notes that the grave of a man needed to be as deep as his height, while that of women needed to be breast high. See Goodwin, "Gardens of the Dead in Ottoman Times," 62.

[72] They had windows that made the onlookers see the tombstones. Eldem, "Death and Funerary Culture."

In turning our attention from dead bodies to those of the living, it is imperative to explore the locus of the regulations and the sites that brought the living bodies under the growing powers of governance, by means of imposing those regulations. In particular, these regulations focused in three critical components of health, as understood in the early modern Ottoman society: air, water, and morals. Health was something that could be attained by living in a place that had clean air, clean water, and inhabited by people with clean souls. In other words, the health of the body (*microcosmos*) was conceived broadly within the general environment (*macrocosmos*). This notion, which was informed by the Galenic-Avicennan model of disease etiology, dictated that the miasma that caused disease was a product of the environment. Swamps and marshy lands, dead bodies, and corrupting matter could release miasma into the air. For this purpose, the regulations first targeted urban filth and the perceived sources of miasma. Most visibly, they aimed at cleaning and paving the streets, banning sources of bad smells and fetid air, improving the nature of the construction of the houses, and maintaining a clean water supply for urban population. Nevertheless, the conception of health and well-being (*ten-dürüstlük*) was not limited to clean air and clean water; it also had a spiritual dimension. The individual could only attain a desired state of health and flourish while living in a clean soul. Behaving morally, following the right path of the *sharia*, and avoiding sinful and immoral behavior were also considered to be critical components of ensuring health and wellbeing. Eliminating any such behavior deemed contrary to the moral values of the community would help improve the health, well-being, and tranquility of the community. These regulations were fully visible in sixteenth-century Istanbul, in particular in thee loci: streets, houses, and morals.

While considering the regulations aimed at improving the conditions of the streets, the goal is not to determine whether the streets of sixteenth-century Istanbul were clean or filthy, especially with modern criteria in mind.[73] Nor is it to assess the efficacy of the adopted measures in curtailing the ravages of the plague. Perhaps more important, it is to explore the roots of a new consciousness for the exercise of a new form of control over the subjects by regulating the natural and the built environment in which they lived for the purpose of ensuring their health, a newly assumed role on the part of the Ottoman administration.

Descriptive accounts on the streets of early modern Istanbul mostly come from foreign observers. European travelers commented on the streets of Istanbul, typically describing them as notoriously filthy, dark, and unpaved. Many travelers have observed that the streets were narrow and crooked and commented on the mud and dirt. Some have commented on the accumulated

---

[73] For the streets of one neighborhood in sixteenth-century Istanbul, see Cem Behar, *A Neighborhood in Ottoman Istanbul: Fruit Vendors and Civil Servants in the Kasap İlyas Mahalle* (Albany: SUNY Press, 2003), 44–49.

garbage and animal carcasses, all contributing to the heavy stench of the city, only to be deteriorated at times of plague.[74] Such descriptions in travelogues continued more or less unchanged until the nineteenth century, which may easily create a vision of Istanbul, or other Ottoman cities for that matter, as unchanging entities. Was this another trope of the genre – a locus in reference to which the foreign observer could pass judgment about the Ottoman society, especially in comparison with an idealized Western model in mind? As such, the streets of Istanbul could turn into a rhetorical tool used as a marker of "uncivilized" Ottoman society.

Despite this seemingly unchanging image, a careful consideration of Ottoman sources suggests that there were important changes about the maintenance of the streets of Istanbul starting in the second half of the sixteenth century. These changes appeared in the form of sporadic inspections and regulations adopted for their cleanliness and maintenance. At first glance, they may not seem a systematic body of regulations aimed at keeping the urban space clean, and probably were not so at that early point. However, as a whole, they seem to represent a significant change in the growing presence of the state in the urban texture of Istanbul in the second half of the sixteenth century. It should be possible to situate this body of legislation in a continuum reflecting the growing powers of governance; it grew out of the control of bodies and expanded into spaces where bodies occupied. In other words, the locus of the control has now extended from the bodies (dead or alive) to the urban space of the city, a space where bodies walked, worked, or watched. As with other forms of regulations, these developed gradually, in ad hoc manner, mostly in response to urban disasters.

An age-old maxim dictated that the cleaning of streets was the responsibility of property or shop owners facing the street: "If every household cleaned in front of their house, the streets would be all clean." This principle must have continued over time, though gradually came to be limited to the side streets and alleys, whereas the central administration operated military units for the cleaning and maintenance of main thoroughfares,[75] which suggests a gradual encroachment of the state in this area. It is not exactly clear when the state took upon the task of dictating and overseeing the cleaning of the streets. Over the course of the sixteenth century, perhaps in conjunction with the increasing visibility of the state in other realms of life, urban cleanliness came to be associated with good governance, at least in the case of Istanbul.

Paving was a critical component of the maintenance of streets, as unpaved streets could easily be covered in mud and waste carried by rainwater. The Jewish rabbi Moses ben Baruch Almosnino noted in 1567 that "all the

---

[74] İnalcık, "Istanbul"; Robert Mantran, *Istanbul au siècle de Soliman le Magnifique* (Paris: Hachette, 1994), 105–8; Mehmet Mazak, *Orijinal Belge ve Fotoğraflar Işığında Osmanlı'da Sokak ve Çevre Temizliği* (Istanbul: İSTAÇ, 2001).

[75] İnalcık, "Istanbul."

streets in Istanbul were paved with stone." He wrote that the rainwater washed all waste accumulated in the streets and courtyards streaming to the sea, cleaning the streets, but that in heavy rains it became impossible to walk because of water and mud.[76] One of the early examples of such practices can be found in a *mühimme* order from 1556. This order comments that the marketplace and the streets of Galata were found to be filthy after an inspection. A certain Mustafa was given the task of cleaning the neighborhood of Galata.[77] Whether this attempt made any difference on the overall condition of the neighborhood is difficult to determine, but this order appears to be significant enough to be an early example of a series of such attempts to maintain the streets of Istanbul. In the early 1570s, there seems to be an official to oversee the repairs and maintenance of the pavements in Istanbul who worked like a contractor; if the pavement were to break within a given time (three years, in this case), he was to be responsible for finding cobblestones to replace broken ones. The repair of broken pavements in front of *waqf*-owned shops was to be undertaken by the trustees of the endowment under the supervision of an appointed official. Efforts to regulate and maintain the pavement of the streets of Istanbul is testified by repeated *mühimme* orders in the last decades of the century.[78] Taken as a whole, these orders reveal the process of emergence of institutions for the care of pavements.[79] Regardless, most visual depictions of Istanbul from late sixteenth century show the ground as being unpaved.[80]

For a society in which miasma was the main causal explanation for disease, foul smells were associated with the unclean. In other words, cleanliness was not only something that could be seen but also, and perhaps even more so, smelled. A place was considered clean when it was free of bad smells.[81]

---

[76] Almosnino, *Extremos y grandezas de Constantinopla*, 6–7.

[77] MD 2, 73/667 (29 Cemaziyelahir 963 H./May 10, 1556).

[78] İnalcık, "Istanbul"; Ahmet Refik, *İstanbul Hayatı 1553–1591*. Also see various *mühimme* orders, e.g., MD 21, 126/304 (20 Şevval 980 H./Feburary 23, 1573); MD 21, 131/318 (20 Şevval 980 H./February 23, 1573); MD 21, 202/482 (21 Zilkade 980 H./March 25, 1573); MD 21, 285/677 (23 Zilhicce 980 H./April 26, 1573); MD 23, 340/760 (23 Zilkade 981 H./March 16, 1574); MD 53, 154/450 (2 Ramazan 992 H./September 7, 1584); MD 64, 217/556 (20 Safer 997 H./January 8, 1589); MD 73, 133/313 (21 Şaban 1003 H./May 1, 1595); MD 73, 239/557 (18 Ramazan 1003 H./May 27, 1595).

[79] Evliya Çelebi notes that there were eight hundred artisans of pavements (*esnâf-ı kaldırımcıyân, neferât 800*). See Evliya Çelebi, *Seyahatnâme*, 1:321. Even though these orders most prominently addressed the case of Istanbul, there is evidence that streets were paved in other cities as well. See, e.g., the case of Edirne, MD 26, 178/485 (10 Cemaziyelevvel 982 H./August 28, 1574).

[80] E.g., few of the Istanbul depictions included in Salomon Schweigger's account show the ground as paved. See Schweigger, *Sultanlar Kentine Yolculuk*.

[81] The classic study on the subject is Alain Corbin, *The Foul and the Fragrant: Odor and the French Social Imagination* (Cambridge, MA: Harvard University Press, 1986). Recently, smell and other aspects of sensory history started to receive scholarly attention in Middle Eastern studies. See, e.g., Khaled Fahmy, "An Olfactory Tale of Two Cities: Cairo in the Nineteenth Century," in *Historians in Cairo: Essays in Honor of George Scanlon*, ed.

In discussing the qualities of clean air, fifteenth-century physician İbn Şerif remarked that it should be free of smells, and added, "It should not smell like the streets of the city of Bursa."[82] Anything that caused stench was considered a source of filth and thus required cleaning, such as garbage on the streets. There are *mühimme* orders that aimed to regulate the disposing of such substances on the streets or in places that could offend the senses of others. By the same token, littering the streets and breaking the paving was prohibited, and slaughterhouses or other sources of stench were to be removed outside the city.[83] As much as a Galenic model of disease etiology informed these regulations and hygiene was defined along the lines of miasma, it had some practical implications for prevention from plague epidemics that may not meet the eye at first glance. Even though it is difficult to comment on the degree of their efficacy, we know today that paving streets can limit the movement of rat colonies. Similarly, moving slaughterhouses or other potential food sources attractive to rats, such as accumulated garbage on the streets, could have curtailed the growth of their numbers to a certain extent. Overall, these embryonic efforts within the walled area of Istanbul can be seen as an expression of the desire to regulate urban space and to demonstrate good governance.

Similarly, a series of measures were adopted to regulate the construction of houses in Istanbul in the second half of the sixteenth century. Generally speaking, these regulations dictated where houses could be built, the distance between them as well as from shops and walls, and how high they could be built.[84] The nature of the regulations suggests that they had been developed primarily with the threat of fires in mind – a perfectly legitimate source of fear when the frequent and destructive fires were considered.[85] To a lesser extent, though, concerns of hygiene and fear of epidemics also seem to have informed decisions about where to build houses. This partly factored in the building of residences outside the walled area of Istanbul, especially on the northern side of the Golden Horn and along the shores of the Bosphorus.[86] This was perhaps most pronounced in the efforts of European embassies

J. Edwards, 155–87 (Cairo: American University in Cairo Press, 2002); Ziad Fahmy, "Coming to Our Senses: Historicizing Sound and Noise in the Middle East," *History Compass* 11, no. 4 (2013): 305–15; Nina Ergin, "The Soundscape of Sixteenth-Century Istanbul Mosques: Architecture and Qur'an Recital," *Journal of the Society of Architectural Historians* 6, no. 2 (2008): 204–21.

82   İbn-i Şerîf, *Yâdigâr*, 1:36.
83   İnalcık, "Istanbul"; Ahmet Refik, *İstanbul Hayatı 1553–1591*. See, e.g., MD 26, 49/128 (5 Rebiülevvel 982 H./June 25, 1574); MD 58, 9/29 (8 Rebiülahir 993 H./April 9, 1585); MD 58, 212/551 (17 Şaban 993 H./August 13, 1585); MD 58, 350/897 (8 Şevval 993 H./October 3, 1585).
84   İnalcık, "Istanbul." Ahmet Refik, *İstanbul Hayatı 1553–1591*. See, e.g., MD 9, 75/201 (Şevval 977 H./March–April 1570).
85   Boyar and Fleet, *A Social History of Ottoman Istanbul*, 77–89.
86   İnalcık, "Istanbul." A similar point has been made about the effects of fires and the dislocation of non-Muslim populations. For a recent discussion of the issue, see Marc David

moving to Pera; first the French and then the British embassies moved there in the mid-sixteenth century on account of frequent plagues in the city.[87] This trend soon caught up with the Ottoman elite, as we see the building of imperial residences and gardens outside the walled area of Istanbul and along the Bosphorus. While the Ottoman sultans left Istanbul at times of plague for Edirne and its environs in the fifteenth century, they started to retreat to these new residences at the end of the sixteenth. For example, during a violent episode of plague in Istanbul, Mehmed III (r. 1595–1603) took refuge in his Bosphorus retreat in Küçüksu until the outbreak receded.[88] Seventeenth-century English ambassadors built a residence in the village of Belgradcık, which eventually became a favorite location to take refuge from plague.[89]

These basic measures can also be seen in water policies that developed in the same era. Efforts to bring large quantities of clean water supplies to Istanbul, regulations for the distribution and use of clean water, maintenance and inspection of waterways, and prohibition of contamination correspond to the very same vision of urban hygiene and cleanliness. Taken as a whole these regulations represent yet another aspect of healthscaping in sixteenth-century Istanbul. Under the reign of Süleyman, the water problem of the city was seriously reconsidered. Water channels were improved and measures were taken to regulate water distribution.[90] There was a great effort to properly maintain clean water resources. To prevent the contamination of water, any buildings reported to contaminate the water channels were carefully inspected and banned. For instance, an order dated January 26, 1583, ordered the inspection of all water channels and removal of houses that could contaminate the water supply of the city.[91] Similarly, it was also prohibited to dispose of garbage at locations that could potentially contaminate water supplies. For instance, in a *mühimme* order sent to the *kadı* of Istanbul and the chief architect, the inhabitants of two neighborhoods were forbidden to dispose of their waste on the streets, which was reported to have contaminated the water of the fountains.[92]

Baer, "The Great Fire of 1660 and the Islamization of Christian and Jewish Space in Istanbul," *IJMES* 36 (2004): 159–81. Also see Halil İnalcık, "Ottoman Galata, 1453–1553," in *Essays in Ottoman History* (Istanbul: Eren, 1998), 275–376. On the dislocation of the Jews, see Uriel Heyd, "The Jewish Community of Istanbul in the Seventeenth Century," *Oriens* 6 (1953): 311–13; Avram Galante, *Histoire des juifs d'Istanbul* (Istanbul: Imprimerie Hüsnütabiat, 1941), 15, 53; Yerasimos, "La Communauté juive d'Istanbul à la fin du XVIe siècle," *Turcica* 27 (1995): 108.

[87] Louis Mitler, "The Genoese in Galata: 1453–1682," *IJMES* 10, no. 1 (1979): 71–91.
[88] Selânikî, *Tarih-i Selânikî*, 759–68.
[89] For Belgradcık Village, see Chapter 7.
[90] "Su," *Dünden Bugüne İstanbul Ansiklopedisi*, 7:47–49.
[91] MD 48, 272/780 (2 Muharrem 991 H./January 26, 1583).
[92] MD 58, 324/828 (17 Ramazan 993 H./September 11, 1585). Also see MD 68, 41/86 (21 Ramazan 999 H./July 13, 1591).

Even though Istanbul was the prime locus for the experimentation where the boundaries of governance expanded, such regulations were not limited to the capital. Outside of Istanbul, regulations were issued to maintain urban hygiene, though perhaps less forcefully. The question of ensuring clean air and water was especially sensitive in the case of the holy cities of Mecca and Medina, but also in other major cities such as Thessaloniki, Edirne, Aleppo, and Damascus. There are examples for similar policies in the same era in the form of relocating slaughterhouses away from towns, paving and maintaining streets, keeping water channels free of contamination, and cleaning of ditches so as to preserve clean air.[93] In rural areas, local communities were held responsible for cleaning riverbeds and drying out marshlands and swamps.[94]

Notwithstanding the emphasis placed on clean air and water, the urban environment was not the exclusive focus. For a society that envisioned health not only in a clean environment but also as moral conduct, the leap from ensuring urban hygiene to moral hygiene was perhaps not a big one. By extension, one can envision the efforts for ensuring moral purity. Here, the association between plague and morals may be less visible than efforts for controlling the built environment of the city. Nevertheless, in early modern Ottoman society, health was not conceived independently from moral behavior and just governance. There was a belief that a special bond existed between a city and its citizens; a city could only be healthy when it was inhabited by moral people. By association, this could lead to the purging of unwanted elements from cities to assure the moral purification and cleanliness of cities. Clean souls would be maintained in clean bodies, so they would live in "pure" cities, clean in morals, piety, justice, and good governance. Morals and government, on one hand, and the healthy living a place offered, on the other, were two sides of a coin: the place is blessed with health, which encourages morality; and the morality practiced is rewarded with a flourishing healthscape. The efforts of moving the unclean outside of the walled area of a city can be seen as an effort to purge the town of its unwanted elements. In line with a definition of health and well-being

93 See, e.g., MD 9, 90/234 (22 Şevval 977 H./March 30, 1570); MD 21, 56/138 (24 Ramazan 980 H./January 28, 1573); MD 26, 140/364 (19 Rebiülahir 982 H./August 8, 1574); MD 26, 178/485 (10 Cemaziyelevvel 982 H./August 28, 1574); MD 27, 55/140 (25 Receb 983 H./November 1, 1575); MD 28, 51/123 (25 Receb 984 H./October 18, 1576); MD 30, 46/114 (28 Muharrem 985 H./April 17, 1577); MD 31, 334/744 (23 Receb 985 H./October 6, 1577); MD 31, 386/858 (1 Şaban 985 H./October 14, 1577); MD 43, 68/138 (5 Cemaziyelevvel 988 H./June 18, 1580); MD 67, 133/256 (1 Ramazan 999 H./June 23, 1591).

94 See, e.g., MD 23, 235/497 (13 Ramazan 981 H./January 6, 1574); MD 35, 258/654 (27 Receb 986 H./September 29, 1578); MD 35, 286/725 (27 Receb 986 H./September 29, 1578); MD 43, 9/16 (18 Rebiülevvel 988 H./May 3, 1580); MD 43, 25/51 (18 Rebiülevvel 988 H./May 3, 1580); MD 43, 223/405 (24 Receb 988 H./September 4, 1580).

of an individual or community defined in a social and spiritual context, clean bodies were imagined to flourish in clean conscience. Just in the same way, the slaughterhouses, waste, and plague miasma were purged; neighborhoods were cleansed of unwanted elements, such as prostitutes, beggars, bachelors, illegal immigrants, criminals, and other such unwanted elements. It is interesting to observe the parallels between the state's growing control of the human body, and by association, its struggle to assert right and moral conduct.

A number of *mühimme* documents testify that such action was taken. For example, in February 1576, an order stated that drinking houses and prostitutes that had recently appeared in an area called *Taş Merdiven*, close to the mosque in Galata, had to be removed.[95] This was probably neither the first nor the last attempt to control prostitution in Istanbul, as orders for the banishment and exile of prostitutes occurred repeatedly throughout the early modern era.[96] Soon after this, for instance, we hear of another scrutiny for women of "lax morals" in Galata. This time, we find out from the account of Stephan Gerlach that the *kadı* and *sipahi ağası*, on the sultan's order, searched houses in Galata in June 1577 and found married women who did not "lead a moral life with their husbands." These women were exiled to Cyprus and to other islands. According to Gerlach, the investigation was carried out by questioning women as they entered or exited through the city gates. They were asked who they were, whether they were married or not, and where they lived. Then the administration acquired documents from the local *imam* about where their husbands were. It appears that this had a precedent in Süleyman's reign, which was still fresh in the memory of the city's population. It was said that the latter had exiled nine galleys filled with prostitutes to overseas locations, but the women later returned. Gerlach's account makes clear that such investigations continued and more women were found guilty of leading "immoral lives," outside of wedlock. In September 1577, it was reported that 250 more such women were identified.[97]

As it were, these were heavy plague years not only in Istanbul but everywhere else in the empire.[98] At first glance, how the concerted efforts to purge anxieties concerning plague were channeled toward social control may not meet the eye. However, a closer look into the rationale of such efforts can give us glimpses of that process. Islamic wisdom dictated that moral decay was one of the causes of plagues. Adultery and fornication, morally unacceptable behaviors according to Islamic religious principles, have often been

---

[95]   MD 27, 302/725 (29 Zilkade 983 H./February 29, 1576).
[96]   Dror Ze'evi, *Producing Desire: Changing Sexual Discourse in the Ottoman Middle East, 1500–1900* (Berkeley: University of California Press, 2006), 147.
[97]   Gerlach, *Türkiye Günlüğü*, 600, 640.
[98]   See Chapter 6.

mentioned in association with plague in the hadith literature. Basing themselves on an Islamic tradition of social and moral associations of plagues, Ottoman authors did not fall short of formulating such visions.[99] It is difficult to determine to what extent this line of thinking informed the adoption of such measures for purging those who were perceived to be immoral in Ottoman society. Seeking a direct causal link might be tricky or even misleading. Nevertheless, it is unmistakable that the powers of governance now went beyond regulating bodies and sought to infiltrate on moral conduct and lifestyle. Perhaps it should not come as a surprise that these regulations especially targeted perceived danger zones, where disordered interactions were imagined to take place. For example, an order issued in May 1571 forbade laundresses from working in shops in Istanbul on account of rumors about their promiscuous conduct.[100] Similarly, the backrooms of barbershops in Istanbul were flagged as places where immoral behavior was said to have been taking place; an order dated October 1579 ordered them to be destroyed.[101] As these examples suggest, these regulations sought to bring order as they redefined the proper moral conduct and its loci. Istanbul was the prime site of this experimentation of increasingly regulated social and moral life, but not the only one. There were similar measures in other cities of the empire that mimicked them.[102]

Economy of Bodies

This body of legislation also gives us glimpses of the kinds of policies enforced by the Ottoman central administration during and after plague outbreaks outside of Istanbul. Sometimes communities requested relief measures from the central administration. At other times, there was a process of negotiation between them. These requests and negotiations left behind paper trails that can be traced in the Ottoman *mühimme* collections of the sixteenth century. Generally speaking, these documents inform us about the development of technologies used by the Ottoman central administration in dealing with postmortality crises. This is most straightforward in cases of demographic interventions, such as recalling dispersed populations back to their place in the wake of a plague or replenishing the population lost due to an outbreak by resettling others in that area. For example, after residents deserted the villages between Edirne and Hasköy on account of plague, the central administration called them back because of the escalating

---

[99] For the association between plague and adultery, see Chapter 7.

[100] MD 10, 332/543 (4 Muharrem 979 H./May 28, 1571).

[101] MD 40, 183/405 (20 Şaban 987 H./October 11, 1579).

[102] See, e.g., MD 22, 81/169 (20 Safer 981 H./June 21, 1573); MD 29, 167/402 (25 Zilkade 984 H./February 13, 1577); MD 30, 160/378 (18 Safer 985 H./May 7, 1577); MD 30, 256/600 (27 Rebiülevvel 985 H./June 14, 1577); MD 30, 271/629 (28 Rebiülevvel 985 H./June 15, 1577); MD 36, 42/129 (28 Zilkade 986 H./January 26, 1579).

threat of banditry.[103] Equally common were requests from provincial communities for tax relief or reassessment of their tax rates following heavy plague mortality. The central administration sometimes postponed taxes for a certain time on account of plague or carried out investigations for fair taxation.[104] In these cases, it is possible to see how provincial communities would petition the center, what legal idioms they use in reference to plague and plague mortality, and how the central administration responds to them. As much as they document the communications regarding crisis management between provincial and central authorities, these *mühimme* orders also enable us to envision the context in which such communications took place. A careful study of these orders illustrates the processes of information flow, decision making, and technologies of communication in this era. Quite significantly, they underscore the fast flow of information in and out of Istanbul, the prompt decision-making process, and the efficacy of crisis-management communications. Hence, as a body of regulations, they help illustrate that the growing powers of governance were not only exercised in the urban space of Istanbul but also extended to the provinces as well.

Nevertheless, one must not assume that such efforts went uncontested. Looking at the reception of this power at the local level can sometimes shed light on the conflicting interests of the provincial communities that are affected by plagues and those of the center. One of the best examples for this sort of conflicting interests and the process of negotiation that ensued is the case of the Jewish broadcloth weavers of Thessaloniki. A careful examination of the repeated orders in this collection about the effects of plagues on the Jewish weavers and Istanbul's insistence on the preparation of broadcloth on schedule regardless of the effects of the plague, illustrates the multiple layers of mediation and negotiations involved in the process.[105]

Regardless, these documents enable us to comment at the level of communities and not of individuals. At best, they yield information about how plague mortality affected market conditions, how prices and wages fluctuated at times of plague or in their wake. For example, it is stated that plague took so many lives in Thessaloniki that there was a scarcity of weavers there in summer 1577 – a labor shortage severe enough to cause a dramatic increase in the price of broadcloth.[106] Be that as it may, many questions remain as to what kinds of measures were taken to support those who lost their sustenance as a result of plague mortality. For example, were there measures to help women who lost their husbands to plague? Was there a

---

[103]   MD 22, 38/82 (23 Muharrem 981 H./May 25, 1573).
[104]   See, e.g., MD 33, 177/352 (17 Şevval 985 H./December 28, 1577); MD 40, 135/296 (20 Şaban 987 H./October 12, 1579).
[105]   Varlık, "Plague, Conflict, and Negotiation."
[106]   MD 31, 48/124 (4 Cemaziyelevvel 985 H./July 20, 1577).

kind of practice for providing pensions for widows of plague victims? What happened to the children who were left orphan in the wake of an outbreak? Further research in *waqf* documents and Islamic court registers is needed to answer these questions.

Overall, plague mortality posed a variety of challenges to the central administration, including difficulty of calculating, registrating, and collecting taxes or raising other revenues and services from the empire's taxpaying population. Concern for the loss of public order and escalating crime often exacerbated these problems. The manner in which the Ottoman central administration responded to these challenges was similar to the governance of bodies in Istanbul in that it represented a concern to monitor, count, and regulate the movement of the bodies.

Elite Bodies

The bodies of the military, administrative, and religious elite who enjoyed a tax-exempt status in the empire (*askeri*) were monitored more closely than the rest of the taxpaying population (*reaya*). The members of the elite were subjected to close surveillance at every stage of their professional careers, at times of peace or war. Their lives and the state of their bodies are therefore better documented. The corpus of documentation enables us to see how their bodies were governed in health and in sickness by the Ottoman administration. For example, a description of physical appearance (including height, eye and skin color, and notable marks on body) accompanied the registration of military personnel as a marker of their identity. This enables the historian to acquire a kind of visual evidence about these bodies that cannot be gathered for the taxpaying subjects of the empire. The surveillance over their bodies and the documentation that ensued at times of military campaigns was certainly greater. For example, there were separate registers prepared for those who fell dead during military undertakings.[107]

The armed bodies were not only regulated at times of military campaigns but at other times as well. We are much better informed about how their bodies were governed even when they were not in military campaigns. This also includes some glimmerings of evidence about the armed bodies at times of plague. Even though it is difficult to find supporting evidence for their professional dispositions, it is not unrealistic to assume that plague was an important threat for the janissaries who lived in close proximity of each other in their military barracks. Yet most of the evidence comes from those who were given to the protection of Muslim families before serving in the Janissary corps. The death of such novice janissary boys (*acemi yeniçeri*) had to be registered at the court of the *kadı*. When a boy died while in the host family, it was the family's responsibility to report his death and register it

---

[107] For an example of such death registers, see KK 332 (996 H./1587–88).

because the novice boy, as slave, would be legally considered the property of the Ottoman sultan. When such boys died, their death had to be registered in the presence of witnesses, including the name, origin, identifying brief physical description, and the cause of death. We have many extant examples in court registers in which death as a result of plague is noted.[108] Similarly, *mühimme* registers have countless cases that refer to health-related issues of armed bodies and their interaction with authorities for that purpose. To clarify, the goal here is not to assess the health of the *askeri* per se, as reflected in these documents. It is rather to trace the processes that ruled their bodies, with respect to reporting, registering, authenticating, and negotiating their problems with the Ottoman powers of governance. A systematic study of those cases promises to yield invaluable evidence regarding the governance of armed bodies, even at times of peace.

Documents make it clear that the *askeri* were responsible for reporting their health-related circumstances to the authorities, especially when this affected their ability to go on military campaigns. It is clear that they had greater liability for their bodies than the *reaya*. It is not uncommon to find cases in these registers where *timar* holders reported their health problems to the central administration for various reasons. If illness or other health-related circumstances prevented a member of the military class from going on an expedition, this needed to be demonstrated. For instance, a certain Mahmud Çavuş sent a letter to his local *kadı* reporting that he was unable to join the campaign due to his illness, which was approved by the *kadı* and reported to the central administration.[109] In another instance, Nail, a *timar* holder from Çorum, requested that his *timar* not be given away. Others testified at court to his illness so that he could keep his *timar*.[110] When the ill recovered, this was also reported so they could be dispatched to join the army. This was the case of Çorum Alaybeyi İsa, who was ordered to join defense troops after he reported that he had recovered from his condition.[111]

If a disease went unreported, this could result in the loss of *timar*. This was why Musa, a *timar* holder from the town of Ladik in Amasya, reported his illness and requested that his *timar* be given to his son. In accordance with an order sent to the governor of Rumeli, his *timar* was granted to his son İsa upon his request.[112] Musa's appeal seems prudent when we consider the case of Korkmaz, whose *timar* was given away to someone else because he was sick and failed to register it. The latter had to appeal to the governor of Aleppo as an intermediary for the granting of another *timar*.[113]

---

[108] See e.g., Ali Haydar Bayat, "Şer'iye Sicilleri ve Tıp Tarihimiz I: Rıza Senetleri," *Türk Dünyası Araştırmaları* 79 (1992): 9–19.

[109] MD 1, 194/111 (24 Zilhicce 961 H./November 20, 1554).

[110] MD 4, 4/24 (25 Rebiülahir 967 H./January 24, 1560).

[111] MD 22, 281/555 (26 Rebiülahir 981 H./August 24, 1573).

[112] MD 1, 29/107 (7 Şevval 961 H./September 5, 1554).

[113] MD 1, 218/1363 (21 Muharrem 962 H./December 16, 1554).

If the health of the *tımar* holder was affected by a permanent condition, this could cause even bigger problems. For instance, the *tımar* of Karagöz, from Birecik, was assigned to someone else because of a seizure he had.[114] In cases of permanent health issues, old age, or disability, retirement could be requested. For instance, a soldier was granted pension because he was old and blind.[115]

It also becomes clear in these examples that the *kadı* played a key role in this process, as the intermediary between the armed bodies and the central administration. *Kadı*s were responsible for reporting the health-related problems of *tımar* holders to the central administration and executing the orders sent by the center. However, they performed more than this role of intermediaries. At the same time they were the decision-making unit for advising the central administration, which at times entailed their acting as authority and experts in health-related issues. Whenever necessary, they inspected the situation, collected evidence, listened to witnesses, and decided on how to advise the center. In fact, as the following pages show, these duties of the *kadı* were not limited to elite bodies alone. It appears that the taxpaying Ottoman population also went through similar procedures when their health-related problems involved legal issues.

The Body as Site of Governance: The State of the Bodies

As we have seen so far, the governance of bodies assumed different forms, ranging from counting them to registering their features and the surveillance of their movement to regulating the space in which they lived, worked, and died. Even though the elite bodies were more closely regulated, the taxpaying bodies were also subjected to surveillance. This control became most visible at times that marked important moments of transition of those bodies, such as birth, marriage, divorce, illness, medical treatment, and death. These moments of transition not only involved changes in the physical state of the bodies but also marked significant changes in their social status. Those moments of transition, especially when they involved legal problems that affected others, came under the scrutiny of the state. Whenever the state was involved, we have a paper trail that enables us to trace those interactions. Hence, the bodies function as sites where we can trace the changing powers of the state – a change that typically manifested itself in an increasing force throughout the sixteenth century. Looking at documented cases of interaction between the state and the taxpaying bodies, one can gain valuable insight into the manners in which these bodies were governed, how the technologies of governance were operationalized, and how the Ottoman officials were involved in them.

---

[114] MD 1, 34/137 (18 Şevval 961 H./September 16, 1554).
[115] MD 4, 14/121 (17 Rebiülahir 967 H./January 16, 1560).

As the representative of the state's authority, the *kadı* oversaw the physical and social transitions of taxpaying bodies. He recorded deaths, decided on causes of death, and, whenever this involved a legal dispute, solved health-related legal problems both among individuals and between patients and medical professionals. He also recorded and approved the consent of individuals before undergoing medical treatment or surgery. Islamic court registers present invaluable data about various types of health-related issues among individuals as well as controversies between individuals and health professionals. In these cases, we see the role of the *kadı* as judge for solving legal disputes among individuals, as notary public for registering contracts between parties, and, whenever necessary, as decision maker in matters related to bodies. At times, this task required expertise in matters related to diagnosis, prognosis, and treatment of health problems. In such cases, the *kadı* mostly relied on the testimony of witnesses.

Deaths could be registered at the office of the *kadı*, though not all deaths were registered at the court. When the taxpaying bodies were involved, deaths were not regularly registered unless they caused legal disputes. In some cases, a death could even be registered years later, in the event that a legal problem arose. In a sixteenth-century case from the court of Konya, the death of Hacı Ali is registered in the court by his wife Kerime and in the presence of two witnesses three years after his death.[116] Even when death was registered at the court, the cause of death is not always mentioned in the register.[117]

Occasionally, the cause of the death is openly mentioned in the court records. A case of accidental death due to drowning in water is mentioned in a sixteenth-century court register from Konya. In another instance from the same register, the death of a certain Fatima was registered by her parents on grounds that she was previously sick and died as a result of her illness, which was testified by their neighbors at court.[118] Sometimes, registering a death as caused by plague could cause further problems. For instance, the death of a certain Akkoca was known to be from plague. But, according to the petition given to the court by a certain Budak, the death was claimed to be because of physical aggression, in which case the court appointed

---

[116] Yılmaz Ceylan, "Konya Şeriyye Sicillerinden ikinci defterde kayıtlı olaylar ve hükümleri," MA thesis, Selçuk University, Konya, 1991, 48.

[117] In her study of the Üsküdar estates, Yvonne Seng puts forward that, out of the eighty-nine registered deaths between March 1521 and May 1524 in the Üsküdar courts, one was the result of murder and another of an accident. See Seng, "The Üsküdar Estates," 284. Seng therefore assumes that the rest died either in their sleep or of other natural causes. This leaves us with "health" as the main factor determining death. The concentration of deaths in summer months suggested that plague outbreaks might have been a factor contributing to deaths, 43–44. She concluded that the concentration of deaths in summer 1522 was the result of such an outbreak, 45.

[118] Ceylan, "Konya Şeriyye Sicillerinden," 42–44.

Abdi Çavuş to investigate the issue.[119] As this case clearly illustrates, even after the death of a person, the governance of bodies manifested itself in posthumous investigation for determining the cause of death. Similarly, in cases where the cause of death was unclear, death was registered on the basis of the testimony of witnesses. For instance, in a case from the court registers of Konya in the year 1570, the death of Ali Çelebi was considered suspicious and the registry of the court was needed, whereupon two witnesses testified to his death in Istanbul and to his burial.[120]

In addition to these cases, there are myriad others whereby a contract of consent was signed between a patient and a surgeon, before the *kadı* and witnesses. Such contracts were needed for healers who did not want to be liable for the failure of their treatment. In such cases, the patient and his or her relatives or future inheritors gave their consent for not holding the healer responsible in case of death as a result of the treatment.[121] As understood from these cases, the healer administering treatment could be held responsible for lack of success. Because oral consent was not enough, unless such a contract was signed between the parties, the patient or his or her relatives could take the healer to court. These contracts protected the healers from charges of malpractice and causing death.[122] For instance, a certain Dimitri Nikola was suffering from a bladder stone in sixteenth-century Bursa. He came to terms with surgeon Seyyid Ali for surgery. The surgeon agreed to carry out the operation in return for three hundred aspers. Yet he wanted to sign a contract in the presence of the *kadı* and the witnesses that the aforesaid Dimitri would not hold him responsible for any undesired outcome, including death. Witnesses testified to his consent.[123] In some cases, the consent of the patient was given when a serious intervention involved his or her bodily integrity. For instance, in a late-fifteenth-century case from the court of Bursa, it is recorded that a certain Hamza, Ahmed Çelebi's slave, had fallen off a horse and broken his leg. When the possibility of gangrene appeared, the surgeon offered the option of amputating the leg. Ahmed gave his consent at court for the amputation and agreed that he would not hold the surgeon responsible for failed treatment.[124] When such

---

[119] Budak's son Himmet and the aforementioned Akkoca had some problems nine months before this court case. It is understood that Akkoca's cause of death was important for inheritance problems. See Halit Ongan, ed., *Ankara'nın 1 Numaralı Şeriye Sicili* (Ankara, 1958), 115.

[120] Ceylan, "Konya Şeriyye Sicillerinden," 45.

[121] Bayat, "Şer'iye Sicilleri."

[122] For legal responsibilities of Ottoman physicians, see Nil Sarı (Akdeniz), *Osmanlılarda Hekim ve Hekimlik Ahlakı* (Istanbul, 1977); Nil Sarı, "Osmanlı Hekimliğinde Tıp Ahlâkı," *OS*, 1:207–35.

[123] Bayat, "Şer'iye Sicilleri," 14.

[124] In this case, we see that such consent was given by the owner of the slave. Çetin, "Bursa Şeriyye Sicilleri Işığında," 136.

a contract of consent was not signed between the parties, the patient or his or her relatives could sue the healer if the treatment were to fail. The case of a certain Veli who lived in Bursa in the late fifteenth century is an example of such failed treatment. The aforesaid Veli allegedly suffered from scrofula and had tumors around his neck. Physician Rıdvan promised to treat him by removing the tumors. But the treatment failed and Veli died. His three brothers Alemşah, Ali, and Salim brought the matter to court.[125]

Taken as a whole, cases such as these afford us glimpses of an emerging body politics in an early modern empire. Many factors along the way have clearly contributed to the adoption and implementation of the particular set of policies in the management of bodies. Technologies used by the Ottoman state to gather, record, classify, and interpret information developed into means for surveillance and social control in times of plague and nonplague alike. The challenge of plague, in particular, prompted the development of techniques for maintaining social order through increased regulation over the individual's life and body. The legacy of plague in shaping the policies of surveillance remains persuasive.

Conclusion

New administrative responses to plague developed in the sixteenth-century Ottoman Empire. This body of response entailed new forms of surveillance technologies over bodies, regulating their movement and the space in which they lived, worked, and died. These regulations can be better understood in conjunction with the changes in popular and scholarly perceptions of plague, as plague was being *naturalized, medicalized,* and *canonized.* Taken as a whole, this body of administrative effort represents the core of a new public health consciousness.

Regulations came during and in the wake of crises. For example, in the late-fifteenth- and early-sixteenth-century plagues in Istanbul, there is evidence of a growing concern to monitor daily mortality and prompt removal of dead bodies outside the city walls. Evidence also suggests that these policies were informed by a basic working knowledge of plague diagnosis and patterns of epidemic mortality. Such record-keeping practices were products of efforts to translate plague mortality into quantifiable information to make epidemics "legible" to the Ottoman central administration. In return, it was these figures that prompted the development of practices for dealing with immediate and long-term consequences of mortality. The more immediate efforts focused on the removal of plague deaths and the regulation of burial practices. We see efforts to regulate burial space, to make goods and

---

[125] However, we find out in the records that the brothers withdrew their claim. Çetin, "Bursa Şeriyye Sicilleri Işığında," 136.

services available for the funeral industry, and to ensure a certain level of public order at such times.

The immediate efforts gradually developed into attempts to maintain a basic level of cleanliness and hygiene in the urban space of the cities, most prominently in the case of Istanbul. Regulations mainly targeted improving three essential components of health, as defined by the Ottomans in this era: air, water, and morals. To this end, measures were implemented for improving the quality of the air by freeing it from stench and causes of corruption (e.g., regulating garbage disposal and slaughterhouses, cleaning and paving the streets), providing and maintaining clean water, and purging the cities of unwanted elements that were imagined to disturb the moral well-being of the community (e.g., prostitutes, bachelors, illegal immigrants).

Alongside these efforts, the Ottoman central administration also kept in close contact with provincial administrators to oversee and intervene in postmortality crises in the provinces. These responses ranged from regulating the movement of people to postponing some taxes or offering temporary tax relief. Taken as a whole, the body of response generated enables us to evaluate the development of technologies for communicating, controlling, and handling such crises outside of the capital as well.

Generally speaking, we are better informed about plague mortality among the religious, administrative, and military elite of the empire, that is, the tax-exempt class. It has been demonstrated here that the policies adopted to respond to plague mortality came to be expanded to overseeing the elite bodies and their health-related problems. Though to a lesser extent, the Ottoman state became increasingly visible in governing the bodies of the taxpaying population of the empire. This mostly focused on the critical turning points of their lives, such as birth, marriage, divorce, illness, medical treatment, and death. Taken as a whole, such efforts for regulating bodies can be seen as the legacy of policies that were aimed at plague management.

Epilogue

> During the twenty long years I have lived in this country, here and at Smyrna, there has scarcely been a year, excepting three, in which the plague did not threaten more or less.

These were the words of Mordach Mackenzie, the physician of the Levant Company in Istanbul, from a letter he wrote in Istanbul on November 23, 1751.[1] This persistence had a backstory – the story we tried to follow in this book. Our chronological framework covered the outbreaks between 1347 and 1600. But this is by no means a break in the history of Ottoman plagues. On the contrary, plague continued to recur along the lines of activity of the third phase (as traced in Chapter 6). It established itself securely in the natural and built environment of the Ottoman Empire and followed the same mobilities of exchange to distribute itself. In the early years of the seventeenth century, plague recurred almost every year; throughout the century, it peaked in 1603, 1611–13, 1620–24, 1627, 1636–37, 1647–49, 1653–56, 1659–66, 1671–80, 1685–95, and from 1697 until the early years of the eighteenth century. It peaked again in 1713, 1719, 1728–29, 1739–43, 1759–65, 1784–86, and 1791–92 in the eighteenth century as well as in 1812–19 and 1835–38 in the nineteenth century.[2]

The story of the plague as outlined in this book is hardly the end of the inquiry. On the contrary, it invites a whole host of new questions to consider and areas of research to pursue. I shall highlight them briefly here, starting with research in Ottomanist studies. First, the history of Ottoman plagues of the seventeenth century is yet to be written. Given the patterns and loci of persistence that manifested in the last decades of the sixteenth century, the seventeenth-century plagues can be studied in that framework. The

---

[1] Mordach Mackenzie, "Extracts of Several Letters of Mordach Mackenzie, M. D. Concerning the Plague at Constantinople," *Philosophical Transactions (1683–1775)* 47 (1752): 388.
[2] İnalcık, "Istanbul"; Panzac, *La peste*.

Ottoman chronicle writing tradition of the seventeenth century acknowledged plague as a legitimate topos and produced some substantial evidence.
Such an inquiry would bridge the plagues studied here to those carefully
examined in the study of the late Daniel Panzac and produce a full temporal
and spatial spectrum of Ottoman plague histories. After having sketched the
general contours of the epidemiological experience, it would be possible to
identify the areas that need further research.

Second, future research is needed to explore the different local contexts
of Ottoman plagues so as to reveal how different regions yield different epidemiological outcomes. Both historical and epidemiological evidence point
out that the patterns of persistence, areas of coverage, and rates of mortality
of plague vary from region to region, and even within a given region over
time. Future research will need to take into consideration the differentials
of plague activity in different urban and rural contexts of the Ottoman
Empire. When and where did the enzootic plague foci form in Ottoman
areas? How long did those foci exist? What was instrumental in transmitting sylvatic plagues into Ottoman urban areas? Did urban areas themselves
sustain the disease as a result of the presence of commensal rodents? What
species of rodents and other mammals served as permanent and temporary
hosts to plagues in the Ottoman fauna? What species of arthropod vectors were instrumental in transmitting it? How did the environment (flora,
fauna, climate, altitude, etc.) affect the etiology and epidemiology of plague
in the diverse Ottoman landscape? How are we to explain the disappearance of plague from this area, which long sustained it? Did enzootic foci
disappear? If so, why? Addressing these questions and such others clearly
goes beyond the boundaries of any single discipline. Thus, third, interdisciplinary studies are sorely needed to further investigate this subject.
For example, research in archeology, bioarcheology, zooarcheology, and
archeoentomology of medieval and early modern Ottoman plagues would
be invaluable in contributing to historical studies, especially to shed light
on the burial practices of plague victims, to identify rodents and arthropod vectors in Ottoman urban and rural contexts and determine their
prevalence and distribution, not to mention to recover aDNA specimens of
Y. pestis.

This research also has implications for non-Ottomanist plague studies.
First, the applicability of the model proposed here linking imperial growth to
epidemic expansion would have to be tested with other historical examples.
At first glance, it may appear that other early modern empires, such as the
Mughals, Safavids, or Habsburgs, may stand as comparable examples to
the Ottoman case. Nevertheless, it is important to keep in mind that the
nature of communication that tied these empires both within themselves
and to the world around them may need to be carefully investigated. For
example, the maritime links of the Ottomans were mostly carried out in
the Mediterranean, where coastal shipping was the norm. How the longer

ocean trips may have helped or hindered the spread of plague in the early modern era remains to be investigated.

Second, the Ottoman experience during the Second Pandemic promises to offer some insights that may challenge some of the core conventions of the field at large. Current studies of the post–Black Death Mediterranean suffer from a Eurocentric approach to plagues. For example, the periodization of plague pandemics, which purports to be global, is in fact little more than Eurocentric. It is a system of periodization that situates Europe at the center and, as such, offers few insights for understanding the ebb and flow of plague waves in other areas, especially with regard to the "in-between" outbreaks. Studying the Ottoman plagues seems to complicate this periodization, as it blurs the boundaries between the end of the Second Pandemic and the beginning of the Third. Long after plague receded from Europe, outbreaks continued in Ottoman areas – a persistence that lasted into the mid- to late nineteenth century, when the Third Pandemic was about to spread globally. Another example is the problem of plague's focalization, in other words, the process by which the disease forms urban or natural foci to perpetuate itself independently of incoming infection. Such processes may be helpful in studying the plague experience of even those areas that are historically imagined to have received the infection from outside, for example, Europe. And as a last point, the Ottoman experience urges the elimination of old models of epidemiological boundaries that are built on flawed historical constructs. Instead, it highlights the importance of adopting more unified epidemiological perspectives for studying larger disease zones. The Ottoman epidemiological experience is not only eminently comparable to those other contemporaneous experiences but also indispensable for a full understanding of the post–Black Death Mediterranean plagues.

Bibliography

Archival and Manuscript Sources

Başbakanlık Osmanlı Arşivi (BOA, Prime Ministry Ottoman Archive, Istanbul)
    Kamil Kepeci (KK)
    Mühimme Defteri (MD)
Topkapı Sarayı Müzesi Arşivi (TSMA, Topkapı Palace Museum Archives,
    Istanbul)

Manuscripts

Atufi. *Defter-i Kütüb*. Ms. Hungarian National Library, Török F. 59.
Abdurrahman Bistami. *Wasf al-dawā' fī kashf āfāt al-wabā'*. Ms. Süleymaniye
    Library, Şehid Ali Paşa 2811/44.
_____. *al-Adʿiyyah al-muntakhabah fī al-adwiyyah al-mujarrabah*. Ms. Süley-
    maniye Library, Hacı Mahmud Efendi 4228/1.
İdris-i Bidlisi. *Risālah al-'ibā' 'an mawāqiʿ al-wabā'*. Ms. Süleymaniye Library, Aşir
    Efendi 275/3.
İlyas bin İbrahim (Eliahu ben Avraham). *Majannah al-ṭāʿūn wa al-wabā'*.
    Süleymaniye Library, ms. Esad Efendi 2484/3, 28–42ff.
_____. *Tevfikātü'l-hamidiyye fī defʿi'l-emrāzi'l-vebā'iyye*. Translated by Ahmedü'ş-
    Şami Ömeri. Ms. Istanbul University Cerrahpaşa History of Medicine Library,
    105.
Kemalpaşazade. *Risālah fī al-ṭāʿūn*. Ms. Süleymaniye Library, Aşir Efendi 430/
    36.
Tabib Ramazan. *Al-Risālah al-fathiyyah al-ungurusiyyah al-sulaymaniyyah*. Ms.
    Topkapı Palace Museum Library, Revan 1279.
Taşköprizade, Ahmed. *Risālah al-shifā' li-adwā' al-wabā'*. Ms. Süleymaniye Library,
    Aşir Efendi 275.
_____. *Bezlü'l-māʿūn fī cevāzi'l-ḫurūc 'ani't-ṭāʿūn*. Translated by Ahmed Tevhid.
    Ms. Istanbul University, Cerrahpaşa History of Medicine Library, 225.
Ünver, Süheyl. *Notlar*. Ms. Süleymaniye Library, 662.

Published Primary Sources

5 Numaralı Mühimme Defteri (973/1565–1566): özet ve indeks. Edited by Hacı Osman Yıldırım et al. Ankara: T.C. Başbakanlık Devlet Arşivleri Genel Müdürlüğü, 1994.

7 Numaralı Mühimme Defteri (975–976/1567–1569): özet-transkripsiyon-indeks. Edited by Hacı Osman Yıldırım et al. Ankara: T.C. Başbakanlık Devlet Arşivleri Genel Müdürlüğü, 1998.

Abdal Mûsa. *Abdal Mûsâ Velâyetnâmesi.* Edited by Abdurrahman Güzel. Ankara: TTK, 1999.

Ahmed Bî-cân (Yazıcıoğlu). *Dürr-i Meknun: kritische Edition mit Kommentar.* Edited by Laban Kaptein, Tom Seidel, Wouter van der Land et al. Asch: [Laban Kaptein], 2007.

_____. *Dürr-i Meknun: Saklı İnciler.* Istanbul: Tarih Vakfı Yurt Yayınları, 1999.

Ahmedî. *Dîvân.* Edited by Yaşar Akdoğan. [Ankara]: T.C. Kültür ve Turizm Bakanlığı Yayınları, 1988.

_____. *History of the Kings of the Ottoman Lineage and Their Holy Raids against the Infidels.* Edited by Kemal Sılay. Cambridge, MA: Department of Near Eastern Languages and Literatures, Harvard University, 2004.

Ahmet Refik. *On Altıncı Asırda İstanbul Hayatı (1553–1591).* Istanbul: Enderun Kitabevi, 1988.

Al-Ahrī, Abū Bakr al-Quṭbī. *Ta'rikh-i Shaikh Uwais (A History of Shaikh Uwais): An Important Source for the History of Ādharbaijān in the Fourteenth Century.* Translated by J. B. Van Loon. The Hague: Mouton, 1954.

Albèri, Eugenio, ed. *Relazioni degli Ambasciatori Veneti al Senato.* Series III. 3 vols. Florence: Società editrice fiorentina, 1840–55.

Alberti, Tommaso. *Viaggio a Costantinopoli (1609–1621).* Bologna: Romagnoli, 1889.

Almosnino, Mosé ben Baruj. *Extremos y grandezas de Constantinopla.* Madrid: Francisco Martinez, 1638.

Altuntaş, İsmail Hakkı. *Niyâzî-i Mısrî. Divan-ı İlâhiyyat ve Açıklaması.* N.p., 2010.

Aşık Paşazade. *Osmanoğulları'nın Tarihi.* Edited by Kemal Yavuz and Yekta Saraç. Istanbul: Koç Kültür Sanat Tanıtım, 2003.

Atsız, Nihal. "Fatih Sultan Mehmed'e Sunulmuş Tarihi bir Takvim." *İstanbul Enstitüsü Dergisi* 3, no. 1 (1957): 17–23.

Aydın, Mehmet Âkif, Rıfat Günalan, and Coşkun Yılmaz. *İstanbul Kadı Sicilleri.* Istanbul: İslâm Araştırmaları Merkezi (İSAM), 2010. http://www.kadisicilleri.org/.

Barkan, Ömer Lütfi. "Edirne Askerî Kassamı'na Âit Tereke Defterleri (1545–1659)." *Türk Tarih Belgeleri Dergisi* 3, nos. 5–6 (1966): 1–479.

Belon, Pierre. *Les Observations de plusieurs singularitez et choses memorables, trouvees en Grece, Asie, Judée, Egypte, Arabie & autres pays estranges.* Paris: Chez Hierosme de Marnef, 1588.

Blackburn, Richard, ed. and trans. *Journey to the Sublime Porte: The Arabic Memoir of a Sharifian Agent's Diplomatic Mission to the Ottoman Imperial Court in the Era of Suleyman the Magnificent.* Beirut: Orient-Institut, 2005.

Bon, Ottaviano. *The Sultan's Seraglio: An Intimate Portrait of Life at the Ottoman Court (from the Seventeenth-Century Edition of John Withers).* London: Saqi, 1996.

Brayer, A. *Neuf années à Constantinople, observations sur la topographie de cette capitale, l'hygiène et les mœurs de ses habitants, l'islamisme et son influence: la peste . . . les quarantaines et les lazarets.* Paris: Bellizard, 1836.

de Busbecq, Ogier Ghiselin. *The Turkish Letters of Ogier Ghiselin de Busbecq. Imperial Ambassador at Constantinople, 1554–1562. Translated from the Latin of the Elzevir Edition of 1663* by Edward Seymour Forster. Baton Rouge: Louisiana State University Press, 2005.

Celâlüddin Hızır (Hacı Paşa). *Müntahab-ı Şifâ.* Edited by Zafer Önler. Ankara: Türk Dil Kurumu, 1990.

Chesneau, Jean. *Le Voyage de Monsieur d'Aramon ambassadeur pour le Roy en Levant escript par noble homme Jean Chesneau l'un des secrétaires dudict seigneur ambassadeur.* Paris: E. Leroux, 1887.

de Clavijo, Ruy González. *Narrative of the Embassy of Ruy Gonzalez de Clavijo to the Court of Timour at Samarcand, AD 1403–6.* London: Hakluyt Society, 1859.

Coecke van Aelst, Pieter. *The Turks in MDXXXIII: A Series of Drawings Made in That Year at Constantinople.* London: privately printed for W. S. M., 1873.

Davis, James Cushman. *Pursuit of Power: Venetian Ambassador's Reports on Spain, Turkey and France in the Age of Phillip II: 1560–1600.* New York: Harper and Row, 1970.

Defoe, Daniel. *A Journal of the Plague Year.* New York: W. W. Norton, 1992.

Dei, Benedetto. *La cronica dall'anno 1400 all'anno 1500.* Edited by Roberto Barducci. Florence: F. Papafava, 1984.

Dernschwam, Hans. *İstanbul ve Anadolu'ya Seyahat Günlüğü.* Ankara: Kültür ve Turizm Bakanlığı, 1987.

Dols, Michael W. "Ibn al-Wardī's *Risālah al-Naba' 'an al-Waba':* A Translation of a Major Source for the History of the Black Death in the Middle East." In *Near Eastern Numismatics, Iconography, Epigraphy and History, Studies in Honor of George C. Miles,* edited by Dickron K. Kouymjian, 443–55. Beirut: American University of Beirut, 1974.

Doukas. *Decline and Fall of Byzantium to the Ottoman Turks.* Detroit, MI: Wayne State University Press, 1975.

Düzdağ, Ertuğrul M. *Şeyhülislam Ebussuud Efendi Fetvaları Işığında 16. Asır Türk Hayatı.* Istanbul, 1983.

Evliya Çelebi. *Evliyâ Çelebi Seyahatnâmesi.* Istanbul: Yapı Kredi Yayınları, 1996.

Gerlach, Stephan. *Türkiye Günlüğü: 1573–1576.* 2 vols. Istanbul: Kitap Yayınevi, 2007.

Giovio, Paolo. *A shorte treatise vpon the Turkes chronicles.* London: Edvvarde VVhitchurche, 1546.

Hacı Bektaş Veli. *Manakıb-ı Hacı Bektâş-ı Velî "Vilâyetnâme."* Istanbul: İnkılap Kitabevi, 1995.

Ḥāfiẓ Abrū. *Ẕayl-i Jāmi' al-Tavārīkh.* Edited by Khānbābā Bayānī. Tehran: 'Ilmī, 1317 [1939].

Hasan Rumlu. *A Chronicle of the Early Ṣafavīs.* Edited and translated by C. N. Seddon. Baroda: Oriental Institute, 1931–34.

Heberer, Johann Michael. *Aegyptiaca servitus.* Graz: Akademische Druck und Verlagsanstalt, 1967.

Hoca Saadettin Efendi. *Tacü't-tevarih.* Istanbul: Milli Eğitim Basımevi, 1979.

Holland, Sir Henry. *Travels in the Ionian Isles, Albania, Thessaly, Macedonia, &c. during the Years 1812 and 1813*. Printed for Longman, Hurst, Rees, Orme, and Brown, 1819.

Horrox, Rosemary, trans. and ed. *The Black Death*. Manchester: Manchester University Press, 1994.

Ibn Battuta. *Travels in Asia and Africa, 1325–1354*. Translated by H. A. R. Gibb. London: Routledge, 1929.

İbn Isa-yı Saruhanî. *Akhisarlı Şeyh Îsâ Menâkıbnâmesi (XVI. yüzyıl)*. Edited by Sezai Küçük and Ramazan Muslu. Sakarya: Aşiyan Yayınları, 2003.

İbn-i Şerîf. *Yâdigâr: 15. Yüzyıl Türkçe Tıp Kitabı*. Edited by Ayten Altıntaş et al., 2 vols. Istanbul: Merkez Efendi ve Halk Hekimliği Derneği, 2003–4.

de Jaucourt, Louis. "Peste." In *Encyclopédie, ou dictionnaire raisonné des sciences, des arts et des métiers*, edited by Denis Diderot and Jean le Rond d'Alembert, 12: 452–58. Paris: Sociétés Typographiques, 1751–72.

————. "Turquie." In *Encyclopédie, ou dictionnaire raisonné des sciences, des arts et des métiers*, edited by Denis Diderot and Jean le Rond d'Alembert, 16: 755–59. Paris: Sociétés Typographiques, 1751–72.

Katip Çelebi. *Keşfü'z-Zunûn*. Istanbul: Tarih Vakfı Yurt Yayınları, 2007.

Kaygusuz Abdal. *Kaygusuz Abdal (Alâeddin Gaybî) Menâkıbnamesi*. Edited by Abdurrahman Güzel. Ankara: TTK, 1999.

Kemal. *Selâtîn-Nâme (1299–1490)*. Ankara: TTK, 2001.

Kinglake, Alexander William. *Kinglake's Eothen*. London: Henry Frowde, 1906.

Klarwill, Victor, ed. *Fugger-Zeitungen; ungedruckte Briefe an das Haus Fugger aus den Jahren 1568–1605*. Vienna: Rikola, 1923.

Kömürcüyan, Eremia. *İstanbul Tarihi: XVII. Asırda İstanbul*. Translated by Hrand D Andreasyan. Istanbul: Eren, 1988.

Kritovoulos. *History of Mehmed the Conqueror*. Translated by Charles T. Riggs. Princeton, NJ: Princeton University Press, 1954.

La Brocquière, Bertrandon de. *The Voyage D'Outremer*. New York: Peter Lang, 1988.

Lubenau, Reinhold. *Beschreibung der Reisen des Reinhold Lubenau*. Edited by W. Sahm, 2 vols. Königsberg: Beyer (Thomas and Oppermann), 1914–15.

el-Mârdânî, Abdülvehhâb bin Yûsuf ibn-i Ahmed. *Kitâbu'l-Müntehab fî't-Tıb: inceleme, metin, dizin, sadeleştirme, tıpkıbasım*. Edited by Ali Haydar Bayat. Istanbul: Merkezefendi Geleneksel Tıp Derneği, 2005.

Manuel II Palaeologus. *The Letters*. Edited and translated by George T. Dennis. Washington, DC: Dumbarton Oaks Center for Byzantine Studies, 1977.

Maurand, Jérome. *Itinéraire de Jérome Maurand d'Antibes à Constantinople (1544)*. Paris: E. Leroux, 1901.

Moltke, Helmuth Karl Bernhard von. *Türkiye'deki Durum ve Olaylar Üzerine Mektuplar (1835–1839)*. Translated by Hayrullah Örs. Ankara: TTK Basımevi, 1960.

Müneccimbaşı Ahmed bin Lütfullah. *Müneccimbaşı Tarihi*. Translated by İsmail Erünsal. [Istanbul]: Tercüman, [197–].

Mustafa Âli. *Câmi'u'l-Buhûr Der Mecâlis-i Sûr*. Edited by Ali Öztekin. Ankara: TTK, 1996.

————. *Künhü'l-ahbâr: dördüncü rükn, Osmanlı tarihi*. Ankara: TTK, 2009.

————. *Mustafā Ali's Counsel for Sultans of 1581*. Edited by Andreas Tietze. Vienna: Österreichischen Akademie der Wissenschaften, 1979.

Muṣṭawfī, Zayn al-Dīn b. Ḥamd Allāh Qazvīnī. *Zayl-i Tārīkh-i Guzīda*. Edited by İraj Afshār. Tehran: Naqsh-i Jahān, 1372 [1993].

Neşrî. *Kitâb-ı Cihan-Nümâ = Neşrî Tarihi*. Edited by Faik Reşit Unat and Mehmed A. Köymen. 2 vols. Ankara: TTK, 1995.

Ongan, Halit, ed. *Ankara'nın 1 Numaralı Şeriye Sicili*. Ankara: TTK, 1958.

Oruç Beğ. *Oruç Beğ Tarihi: Giriş, Metin, Kronoloji, Dizin, Tıpkıbasım*. Edited by Necdet Öztürk. Istanbul: Çamlıca Basım Yayın, 2007.

Pouqueville, François-Charles-Hugues-Laurent. *Voyage en Morée, à Constantinople, en Albanie, et dans plusieurs autres parties de l'empire othoman, pendant les années 1798, 1799, 1800 et 1801*. Gabon (Paris), 1805.

Russell, Alexander, and Patrick Russell. *The Natural History of Aleppo: Containing a Description of the City, and the Principal Natural Productions in Its Neighbourhood: Together with an Account of the Climate, Inhabitants, and Diseases, Particularly of the Plague*. London: printed for G. G. and J. Robinson, 1794.

Rycaut, Paul. *The Present State of the Ottoman Empire*. London: John Starkey and Henry Brome, 1670.

Sabuncuoğlu, Şerefeddin. *Cerrāḥiyyetü'l-Ḫāniyye*. Edited by İlter Uzel. 2 vols. Ankara: TTK, 1992.

Sahillioğlu, Halil, ed. *Topkapı Sarayı Arşivi, H. 951–952 Tarihli ve E-12321 Numaralı Mühimme Defteri*. Istanbul: IRCICA, 2002.

Şahin, İlhan, ed. *II. Bâyezid Dönemine Ait 906/1501 Tarihli Ahkâm Defteri*. Istanbul: Türk Dünyası Araştırmaları Vakfı, 1994.

Sanjian, Avedis K. *Colophons of Armenian Manuscripts, 1301–1480: A Source for Middle Eastern History*. Cambridge, MA: Harvard University Press, 1969.

Sanudo, Marino. *I diarii di Marino Sanuto (MCCCXCVI-MDXXXIII) dall' autografo Marciano ital. cl. VII codd. CDXIX-CDLXXVII*. 58 vols. Venice: F. Visentini, 1879–1903.

Schachman, Bartholomäus. *Bartholomäus Schachman (1559–1614): The Art of Travel*. Milan: Skira, 2012.

Schiltberger, Johann. *The Bondage and Travels of Johann Schiltberger*. New York: Burt Franklin, 1879.

Schreiner, Peter. *Die byzantinischen Kleinchroniken*. Vienna: Verlag der Österreichischen Akademie der Wissenschaften, 1975–79.

Schweigger, Salomon. *Sultanlar Kentine Yolculuk, 1578–1581*. Translated by S. Türkis Noyan. Istanbul: Kitap Yayınevi, 2004.

Seidel, Friedrich. *Sultanın Zindanında: Osmanlı İmparatorluğu'na Gönderilen bir Elçilik Heyetinin İbret Verici Öyküsü (1591–1596)*. Translated by Türkis Noyan. Istanbul: Kitap Yayınevi, 2010.

Selânikî Mustafa Efendi. *Tarih-i Selânikî*. Edited by Mehmet İpşirli. Ankara: TTK, 1999.

Şeyyad Hamza. *The Story of Joseph: A Fourteenth-Century Turkish Morality Play*. Translated by Bill Hickman. Syracuse, NY: Syracuse University Press, 2014.

Solakzâde Mehmet Hemdemi Çelebi. *Solakzâde Tarihi*. Istanbul, 1880.

Spandouginos, Theodōros. *Theodore Spandounes: On the Origins of the Ottoman Emperors*. Translated and edited by Donald M. Nicol. Cambridge: Cambridge University Press, 1997.

Sphrantzes, George. *The Fall of the Byzantine Empire: A Chronicle by George Sphrantzes, 1401–1477.* Translated by Marios Philippides. Amherst: University of Massachusetts Press, 1980.

Tafur, Pero. *Travels and Adventures, 1435–1439.* Edited by Malcolm Letts. New York: Harper, 1926.

Taşköprizade, Ahmed ibn Mustafa. *al-Shaqā'iq al-nu'māniyya fī 'ulamā' al-Dawla al-'Uthmānīyya.* Istanbul: Edebiyat Fakültesi Basımevi, 1985.

———. *Risālah al-shifā' li-adwā' al-wabā'* [Cairo]: al-Matba'ah al-Wahbiyah, 1875.

Toulon, Father Maurice de. *Le Capucin charitable, enseignant la méthode pour remédier aux grandes misères que la peste a coûtume de causer parmi les peuples.* Paris, 1662.

Turan, Osman. *İstanbul'un Fethinden Önce Yazılmış Tarihî Takvimler.* Ankara: TTK Basımevi, 2007.

Tursun Bey. *Târîh-i Ebü'l-feth.* Edited by Mertol Tulum. Istanbul: Baha Matbaası, 1977.

Wiet, Gaston. "La grande peste noire en Syrie et en Égypt." In *Études d'Orientalisme dédiées à la mémoire de Lévi-Provençal* 1: 367–84. Paris: G.-P. Maisonneuve et Larose, 1962.

Wittman, William. *Travels in Turkey, Asia Minor, Syria, and across the Desert into Egypt during the Years 1799, 1800, and 1801, in Company with the Turkish Army, and the British Military Mission. To Which Are Annexed, Observations on the Plague, and on the Diseases Prevalent in Turkey, and a Meteorological Journal.* Philadelphia: printed and sold by James Humphreys, 1804.

Wratislaw, Wenceslas. *Adventures of Baron Wenceslas Wratislaw of Mitrowitz: What He Saw in the Turkish Metropolis, Constantinople; Experienced in His Captivity; and After His Happy Return to His Country, Committed to Writing in the Year of Our Lord 1599.* Translated by A. H. Wratislaw. London: Bell and Daldy, 1862.

Published Secondary Sources

Aberth, John, ed. *The Black Death: The Great Mortality of 1348–1350: A Brief History with Documents.* Boston: Bedford/St. Martin's, 2005.

Abu-Lughod, Janet. *Before European Hegemony: The World System AD 1250–1350.* New York: Oxford University Press, 1989.

Achtman, Mark, Giovanna Morelli, Peixuan Zhu, Thierry Wirth, Ines Diehl, Barica Kusecek, Amy J. Vogler, et al. "Microevolution and History of the Plague Bacillus, *Yersinia pestis.*" *PNAS* 101, no. 51 (2004): 17837–42.

Achtman, Mark, Kerstin Zurth, Giovanna Morelli, Gabriela Torrea, Annie Guiyoule, and Elisabeth Carniel. "*Yersinia pestis,* the Cause of Plague, Is a Recently Emerged Clone of *Yersinia pseudotuberculosis.*" *PNAS* 96, no. 24 (1999): 14043–48.

Ágoston, Gábor. "A Flexible Empire: Authority and Its Limits on the Ottoman Frontiers." *International Journal of Turkish Studies* 9, nos. 1–2 (2003): 15–31.

———. "Where Environmental and Frontier Studies Meet: Rivers, Forests, Marshes and Forts along the Ottoman – Hapsburg Frontier in Hungary." In *The Frontiers of the Ottoman World,* edited by A. C. S. Peacock, 57–79. Oxford: Oxford University Press, 2009.

Aharoni, Bathscheba. *Die Muriden von Palästina und Syrien.* Lucka (Bez. Leipzig): Druck von Reinhold Berger, 1932.

Akar, Metin. "Şeyyad Hamza Hakkında Yeni Bilgiler." *Türklük Araştırmaları Dergisi* 2 (1987): 1–14.

Akasoy, Anna. "Islamic Attitudes to Disasters in the Middle Ages." *The Medieval History Journal* 10, nos. 1–2 (2007): 387–410.

Akıncı, Sırrı. "*Osmanlı İmparatorluğunda Veba (Taun) Salgınları ve Yorumlanması.*" PhD diss., Istanbul University, 1969.

———. "Tarih Boyunca Veba." *Tarih Mecmuası* 6 (1973): 32–37.

Alexander, John T. *Bubonic Plague in Early Modern Russia: Public Health and Urban Disaster.* Baltimore: Johns Hopkins University Press, 1980.

Altun, Kudret. *Gelibolulu Mustafa Âli ve Divânı (Vâridâtü'l-Enîkâ).* Niğde: Özlem Kitabevi, 1999.

And, Metin. *16. Yüzyılda İstanbul: Kent, Saray, Günlük Yaşam.* Istanbul: Yapı Kredi Yayınları, 2009.

Anderson, Sonia P. *An English Consul in Turkey: Paul Rycaut at Smyrna, 1667–1678.* Oxford: Oxford University Press, 1989.

Andrews, Walter G. *The Age of Beloveds: Love and the Beloved in Early-Modern Ottoman and European Culture and Society.* Durham, NC: Duke University Press, 2005.

Andrianaivoarimanana, Voahangy, et al., "Understanding the Persistence of Plague Foci in Madagascar." *PLoS Neglected Tropical Diseases* 7, no. 11 (2013): e2382.

Anisimov, Andrey P., Luther E. Lindler, and Gerald B. Pier. "Intraspecific Diversity of *Yersinia pestis.*" *Clinical Microbiology Reviews* 17, no. 2 (2004): 434–64.

Ansari, B. M. "An Account of Bubonic Plague in Seventeenth Century India in an Autobiography of a Mughal Emperor." *Journal of Infection* 29, no. 3 (1994): 351–52.

Aplin, Ken P., Terry Chesser, and Jose ten Have. "Evolutionary Biology of the Genus *Rattus*: Profile of an Archetypal Rodent Pest." In *Rats, Mice, and People: Rodent Biology and Management*, edited by Grant R. Singleton, Lyn A. Hinds, Charles J. Krebs, and Dave M. Spratt, 487–98. Canberra: Australian Centre for International Agricultural Research, 2003.

Aplin, Ken P., Hitoshi Suzuki, Alejandro A. Chinen, R. Terry Chesser, José ten Have, Stephen C. Donnellan, Jeremy Austin, et al. "Multiple Geographic Origins of Commensalism and Complex Dispersal History of Black Rats." *PLoS ONE* 6, no. 11 (2011): e26357.

Arık, Feda Şamil. "Selçuklular Zamanında Anadolu'da Veba Salgınları." *Tarih Araştırmaları Dergisi* 15, no. 26 (1991): 27–57.

Armağan, A. Latif. "XVII. Yüzyılın Sonu ile XVIII. Yüzyılın Başlarında Batı Anadolu ve Balkanlarda Görülen Veba Salgınlarının Sosyo-Ekonomik Etkileri Üzerine Bir Araştırma." In *Proceedings of the 38th International Congress on the History of Medicine, 1–6 September 2002*, edited by Nil Sarı et al., 3: 907–14. Ankara: TTK, 2005.

Armitage, Philip L. "Unwelcome Companions: Ancient Rats Reviewed." *Antiquity* 68, no. 259 (1994): 231–40.

Arslan, Mehmet. "Osmanlı Dönemi Düğün ve Şenliklerinde Nahıl Geleneği, 1675 Edirne Şenliği ve Bu Şenlikte Nahıllar." In *Osmanlı Edebiyat, Tarih, Kültür Makaleleri*, 593–617. Istanbul: Kitabevi, 2000.

Ata (Ataç), Galib. "İstanbul'da veba salgınları." *Tıp Fakültesi Mecmuası* 3 (1918): 189.

Audoin-Rouzeau, Frédérique. "Le rat noir (Rattus rattus) et la peste dans l'occident antique et médieval." *Bulletin de la Société de Pathologie Exotique* 92, no. 5 (1999): 422–26.

———. *Les chemins de la peste: le rat, la puce et l'homme*. Rennes: Presses universitaires de Rennes, 2003.

Ayalon, Yaron. "Plagues, Famines, Earthquakes: The Jews of Ottoman Syria and Natural Disasters." PhD diss., Princeton University, 2009.

———. "When Nomads Meet Urbanites: The Outskirts of Ottoman Cities as a Venue for the Spread of Epidemic Diseases." In *Plagues in Nomadic Contexts: Historical Impact, Medical Responses, and Cultural Adaptations in Ancient to Mediaeval Eurasia*, edited by Kurt Franz et al. Leiden: Brill, forthcoming.

Aynur, Hatice. "Kurgusu ve Vurgusuyla Kendi Kaleminden Âşık Çelebi'nin Yaşamöyküsü." In *Âşık Çelebi ve Şairler Tezkiresi Üzerine Yazılar*, edited by Hatice Aynur and Aslı Niyazioğlu, 19–55. Istanbul: Koç Üniversitesi Yayınları, 2011.

Ayyadurai, Saravanan, Linda Houhamdi, Hubert Lepidi, Claude Nappez, Didier Raoult, and Michel Drancourt. "Long-Term Persistence of Virulent *Yersinia pestis* in Soil." *Microbiology* 154, no. 9 (2008): 2865–71.

Ayyadurai, Saravanan, Florent Sebbane, Didier Raoult, and Michel Drancourt. "Body Lice, *Yersinia pestis* Orientalis, and Black Death." *Emerging Infectious Diseases* 16, no. 5 (2010): 892–93.

Babinger, Franz. *Mehmet the Conqueror and His Time*. Princeton, NJ: Princeton University Press, 1978.

Babinger, Franz, and C. E. Bosworth. "Raghusa." *EI²*.

Bacot, A. W., and C. J. Martin. "Observations on the Mechanism of the Transmission of Plague by Fleas." *Journal of Hygiene* 13 (Suppl. III) (1914): 423–39.

Badiaga, S., and P. Brouqui. "Human Louse-Transmitted Infectious Diseases." *Clinical Microbiology and Infection* 18, no. 4 (2012): 332–37.

Baer, Marc David. "The Great Fire of 1660 and the Islamization of Christian and Jewish Space in Istanbul." *IJMES* 36 (2004): 159–81.

Baltazard, M. "New Data in the Interhuman Transmission of Plague." *Bulletin de l'Académie nationale de médecine* 143 (1959): 517–22.

Bang, Peter F., and C. A. Bayly. *Tributary Empires in Global History*. New York: Palgrave Macmillan, 2011.

Barkai, Ron. "Between East and West: A Jewish Doctor from Spain." In *Intercultural Contacts in the Medieval Mediterranean*, edited by Benjamin Arbel, 49–63. London: Frank Cass, 1996.

Barker, John W. "Late Byzantine Thessalonike: A Second City's Challenges and Responses." *Dumbarton Oaks Papers* 57 (2003): 5–33.

Barry, Stephane, and Norbert Gualde. "La peste noire dans l'Occident chrétien et musulman, 1347–1353." *Canadian Bulletin of Medical History/Bulletin canadien d'histoire de la médecine* 25, no. 2 (2008): 461–98.

Bartsocas, Christos S. "Two Fourteenth Century Greek Descriptions of the 'Black Death.'" *JHMAS* 21, no. 4 (1966): 394–400.

Bayat, Ali Haydar. "Şer'iye Sicilleri ve Tıp Tarihimiz I: Rıza Senetleri." *Türk Dünyası Araştırmaları* 79 (1992): 9–19.

Bayraktar, M. Sami. "Bafra ve Çarşamba'da Beylikler Döneminden Kalan Tarihi Yapılar." *Uluslararası Sosyal Araştırmalar Dergisi* 6, no. 25 (2013): 111–39.

Baytop, Turhan. "Aktarlar." *Dünden Bugüne İstanbul Ansiklopedisi*, 8 vols. (Istanbul: Türkiye Ekonomik ve Toplumsal Tarih Vakfı, 1993–95), 1:172–74.

Behar, Cem. *A Neighborhood in Ottoman Istanbul: Fruit Vendors and Civil Servants in the Kasap İlyas Mahalle*. Albany: State University of New York Press, 2003.

Ben Néfissa, Kmar, and Anne Marie Moulin. "La peste nord-africaine et la théorie de Charles Nicolle sur les maladies infectieuses." *Gesnerus–Swiss Journal of the History of Medicine and Sciences* 67, no. 1 (2010): 30–56.

Benedictow, Ole Jørgen. *The Black Death, 1346–1353: The Complete History*. Woodbridge, UK: Boydell Press, 2004.

———. *What Disease Was Plague? On the Controversy over the Microbiological Identity of Plague Epidemics of the Past*. Leiden: Brill, 2010.

Ben-Zaken, Avner. *Cross-Cultural Scientific Exchanges in the Eastern Mediterranean, 1560–1660*. Baltimore: Johns Hopkins University Press, 2010.

Beyhan, Mehmet Ali. "1811–1812 İstanbul Veba Salgını, Etkileri ve Alınan Tedbirler." In *1. Uluslararası Türk Tıp Tarihi Kongresi / 10. Ulusal Türk Tıp Tarihi Kongresi Bildiri Kitabı (20–24 May 2008)*, vol. 2, edited by Ayşegül Demirhan Erdemir et al., 1029–36. Konya: Türk Tıp Tarihi Kurumu, 2008.

Biraben, Jean-Noël. *Les hommes et la peste en France et dans les pays européens et méditerranéens*. 2 vols. Paris: Mouton, 1975.

Bitam, Idir, Saravanan Ayyadurai, Tahar Kernif, Mohammed Chetta, Nabil Boulaghman, Didier Raoult, and Michel Drancourt. "New Rural Focus of Plague, Algeria." *Emerging Infectious Diseases* 16, no. 10 (2010): 1639–40.

Blanc, G., and M. Baltazard. "Rôle des ectoparasites humains dans la transmission de la peste." *Bulletin de l'Académie nationale de médecine* 126 (1942): 446–48.

Bleukx, Koenraad. "Was the Black Death (1348–1349) a Real Plague Epidemic? England as a Case Study." In *Serta Devota in Memoriam Guillelmi Lourdaux, 2: Cultura Medievalis*, edited by Werner Verbeke, Marcel Haverals, Rafaël De Keyser, and Jean Goossens, 65–113. Leuven: Leuven University Press, 1995.

Boeckl, Christine M. *Images of Plague and Pestilence: Iconography and Iconology*. Kirksville, MO: Truman State University Press, 2000.

Bolton, James L. "Looking for *Yersinia pestis*: Scientists, Historians, and the Black Death." In *Society in an Age of Plague (The Fifteenth Century, XII)*, edited by Linda Clark and Carole Rawcliffe, 15–38. Woodbridge, UK: Boydell Press, 2013.

Boogert, Maurits van den. *Aleppo Observed: Ottoman Syria through the Eyes of Two Scottish Doctors, Alexander and Patrick Russell*. Oxford: Oxford University Press, 2010.

Borah, Woodrow W., and Sherburne F. Cook. *The Aboriginal Population of Central Mexico on the Eve of the Spanish Conquest*. Berkeley: University of California Press, 1963.

———. "Conquest and Population: A Demographic Approach to Mexican History." *Proceedings of the American Philosophical Society* 113, no. 2 (1969): 177–83.

———. *The Population of Central Mexico in 1548*. Berkeley: University of California Press, 1960.

Borsch, Stuart J. *The Black Death in Egypt and England: A Comparative Study*. Austin: University of Texas Press, 2005.

Borsook, Eve. "The Travels of Bernardo Michelozzi and Bonsignore Bonsignori in the Levant (1497–98)." *Journal of the Warburg and Courtauld Institutes* 36 (1973): 145–97.

Bos, Kirsten I., Verena J. Schuenemann, G. Brian Golding, Hernán A. Burbano, Nicholas Waglechner, Brian K. Coombes, Joseph B. McPhee et al. "A Draft Genome of *Yersinia pestis* from Victims of the Black Death." *Nature* 478, no. 7370 (2011): 506–10.

Boubaker, Sadok. "La peste dans les pays du Maghreb: attitudes face au fléau et impacts sur les activités commerciales (XVIe-XVIIIe siècles)." *Revue d'Histoire maghrébine* 79–80 (1995): 311–41.

Bowers, Kristy Wilson. *Plague and Public Health in Early Modern Seville*. Rochester, NY: University Rochester Press, 2013.

Boyar, Ebru, and Kate Fleet. *A Social History of Ottoman Istanbul*. Cambridge: Cambridge University Press, 2010.

Braude, Benjamin. "The Rise and Fall of Salonica Woollens, 1500–1650: Technology Transfer and Western Competition." *Mediterranean Historical Review* 6, no. 2 (1991): 216–36.

Braudel, Fernand. *The Mediterranean and the Mediterranean World in the Age of Philip II*. Berkeley: University of California Press, 1995.

Brentjes, Sonja. *Travellers from Europe in the Ottoman and Safavid Empires, 16th–17th Centuries: Seeking, Transforming, Discarding Knowledge*. Burlington, VT: Ashgate/Variorum, 2010.

Brockliss, L. W. B., and Colin Jones. *The Medical World of Early Modern France*. Oxford: Clarendon Press, 1997.

Brooks, J. E., and F. P. Rowe. *Commensal Rodent Control*. [Geneva]: WHO, Vector Biology and Control Division, 1987.

Buckland, Paul C., and Jon P. Sadler. "A Biogeography of the Human Flea, *Pulex irritans* L. (Siphonaptera: Pulicidae)." *Journal of Biogeography* 16, no. 2 (1989): 115–20.

Buell, Paul D. "Qubilai and the Rats." *Sudhoffs Archiv* 96, no. 2 (2012): 127–44.

Bulliet, Richard. "The Camel and the Watermill." *IJMES* 42, no. 4 (2010): 666–68.

Bulmuş, Birsen. *Plague, Quarantines, and Geopolitics in the Ottoman Empire*. Edinburgh: Edinburgh University Press, 2012.

Burbank, Jane, and Frederick Cooper. *Empires in World History: Power and the Politics of Difference*. Princeton, NJ: Princeton University Press, 2010.

Burke, Edmund. "Pastoralism and the Mediterranean Environment." *IJMES* 42, no. 4 (2010): 663–65.

Campbell, Bruce M. S. "Physical Shocks, Biological Hazards, and Human Impacts: The Crisis of the Fourteenth Century Revisited." In *Le Interazioni Fra Economia E Ambiente Biologico nell'Europa Preindustriale. Secc. XIII–XVIII (Economic and Biological Interactions in Pre-Industrial Europe from the 13th to the 18th Centuries)*, edited by Simonetta Cavaciocchi, 13–32. Florence: Firenze University Press, 2010.

Çankaya, Nurten. "Taşköprülüzade Ahmet İsameddin Efendi'nin *Risaletü'ş-şifa li-edva'il-vebâ* adlı Risalesi Üzerine bir Değerlendirme." In *VIII. Türk Tıp Tarihi Kongresi: Kongreye Sunulan Bildiriler*, 313–22. Istanbul: Türk Tıp Tarihi Kurumu, 2006.

Carmichael, Ann G. "Infectious Disease and Human Agency: An Historical Overview." In *Interactions between Global Change and Human Health: Working Group, 31 October–2 November 2004*, 3–46. Vatican City: Pontificia Academia Scientiarum, 2006.

———. *Plague and the Poor in Renaissance Florence.* Cambridge: Cambridge University Press, 1986.

———. "Plague, Historical." In *Encyclopedia of Microbiology*, edited by Moselio Schaechter, 58–72. Oxford: Elsevier, 2009.

———. "Plague Legislation in the Italian Renaissance." *Bulletin of the History of Medicine* 57, no. 4 (1983): 508–25.

———. "Plague Persistence in Western Europe: A Hypothesis." *The Medieval Globe* 1 (2014): 157–191.

———. "Universal and Particular: The Language of Plague, 1348–1500." In *Pestilential Complexities: Understanding Medieval Plague*, edited by Vivian Nutton, 17–52. London: Wellcome Trust for the History of Medicine at UCL, 2008.

Carniel, Elisabeth. "Plague Today." In *Pestilential Complexities: Understanding Medieval Plague*, edited by Vivian Nutton, 115–22. London: Wellcome Trust for the History of Medicine at UCL, 2008.

Casale, Giancarlo. "The 'Environmental Turn': A Teaching Perspective." *IJMES* 42, no. 4 (2010): 669–71.

———. *The Ottoman Age of Exploration.* Oxford: Oxford University Press, 2010.

Çetin, Osman. "Bursa Şeriyye Sicilleri Işığında Osmanlılarda İlk Tıp Fakültesi: Bursa Darüşşifası ve Tıbbi Faaliyetler." *Osmanlı Tarihi Araştırma ve Uygulama Merkezi Dergisi* 4 (1993): 121–49.

Ceylan, Ömür. "Ölümün unutulan adı: veba." *Dergâh* 15, no. 182 (2005): 20–21.

Ceylan, Yılmaz. "Konya Şeriyye Sicillerinden ikinci defterde kayıtlı olaylar ve hükümleri." MA thesis, Selçuk University, Konya, 1991.

Christie, A. B., T. H. Chen, and Sanford S. Elberg. "Plague in Camels and Goats: Their Role in Human Epidemics." *Journal of Infectious Diseases* 141, no. 6 (1980): 724–26.

Cipolla, Carlo M. *Cristofano and the Plague: A Study in the History of Public Health in the Age of Galileo.* Berkeley: University of California Press, [1973].

———. *Faith, Reason, and the Plague in Seventeenth-Century Tuscany.* Ithaca, NY: Cornell University Press, 1979.

———. *Public Health and the Medical Profession in the Renaissance.* Cambridge: Cambridge University Press, 1976.

Clair, Alexandrine N. St. *The Image of the Turk in Europe.* New York: Metropolitan Museum of Art, 1973.

Cohn, Samuel Kline. "The Black Death: End of a Paradigm." *The American Historical Review* 107, no. 3 (2002): 703–38.

———. *The Black Death Transformed: Disease and Culture in Early Renaissance Europe.* London: Arnold/Oxford University Press, 2002.

———. *Cultures of Plague: Medical Thinking at the End of the Renaissance.* Oxford: Oxford University Press, 2010.

Congourdeau, Marie-Hélène. "La peste noire à Constantinople de 1348 à 1466." *Medicina nei secoli* 11, no. 2 (1999): 377–90.

Congourdeau, Marie-Hélène, and Mohammed Melhaoui. "La perception de la peste en pays chrétien byzantin et musulman." *Revue des Études Byzantines* 59 (2001): 95–124.

Conrad, Lawrence. "The Plague in the Early Medieval Near East." PhD diss., Princeton University, 1981.

———. "*Ṭā ʿūn* and *Wabāʾ*: Conceptions of Plague and Pestilence in Early Islam." *JESHO* 25, no. 3 (1982): 268–307.

Cook, Alexandra Parma, and Noble David Cook. *The Plague Files: Crisis Management in Sixteenth-Century Seville*. Baton Rouge: Louisiana State University Press, 2009.

Cook, Michael A. *Population Pressure in Rural Anatolia 1450–1600*. London: Oxford University Press, 1972.

Cook, Sherburne Friend, and Woodrow W. Borah. *The Indian Population of Central Mexico, 1531–1610*. Berkeley: University of California Press, 1960.

Coomans, J., and G. Geltner. "On the Street and in the Bathhouse: Medieval Galenism in Action?" *Anuario de Estudios Medievales* 43, no. 1 (2013): 53–82.

Corbin, Alain. *The Foul and the Fragrant: Odor and the French Social Imagination*. Cambridge, MA: Harvard University Press, 1986.

Crawshaw, Jane L. Stevens. *Plague Hospitals: Public Health for the City in Early Modern Venice*. Burlington, VT: Ashgate, 2012.

Crespo, Fabian, and Matthew B. Lawrenz, "Heterogeneous Immunological Landscapes and Medieval Plague: An Invitation to a New Dialogue between Historians and Immunologists." *The Medieval Globe* 1 (2014): 229–57.

Crosby, Alfred W. *The Columbian Exchange: Biological and Cultural Consequences of 1492*. Westport, CT: Greenwood Press, 1972.

Cui, Yujun, Chang Yu, Yanfeng Yan, Dongfang Li, Yanjun Li, Thibaut Jombart, Lucy A. Weinert et al. "Historical Variations in Mutation Rate in an Epidemic Pathogen, *Yersinia pestis*." *PNAS* 110, no. 2 (2013): 577–82.

Cummins, Neil, Morgan Kelly, and Cormac O'Grada. "Living Standards and Plague in London, 1560–1665." SSRN Scholarly Paper. Rochester, NY: Social Science Research Network, July 3, 2013. http://papers.ssrn.com/abstract=2289094.

Curry, John J. "Scholars, Sufis, and Disease: Can Muslim Religious Works Offer Us Novel Insights on Plagues and Epidemics in the Medieval and Early Modern World?" In *Plague and Contagion in the Islamic Mediterranean*, edited by Nükhet Varlık. Burlington, VT: Ashgate, forthcoming.

———. *The Transformation of Muslim Mystical Thought in the Ottoman Empire: The Rise of the Halveti Order, 1350–1750*. Edinburgh: Edinburgh University Press, 2010.

Curtis, Bruce. "Foucault on Governmentality and Population: The Impossible Discovery." *The Canadian Journal of Sociology/Cahiers Canadiens de Sociologie* 27, no. 4 (2002): 505–33.

Dağlar, Oya. *War, Epidemics and Medicine in the Late Ottoman Empire (1912–1918)*. Haarlem: Stichting Onderzoekscentrum Turkestan en Azerbaidzjan, 2008.

Danışman, Günhan H. "Emirza Bey Türbesi, Bafra." *Anadolu Araştırmaları* 10 (1986): 543–46.

Darling, Linda T. "Ottoman Politics through British Eyes: Paul Rycaut's *The Present State of the Ottoman Empire*." *Journal of World History* 5, no. 1 (1994): 71–97.

Davis, Diana K. "Introduction: Imperialism, Orientalism, and the Environment in the Middle East: History, Policy, Power, and Practice." In *Environmental Imaginaries of the Middle East and North Africa*, edited by Diana K. Davis and Edmund Burke, 1–22. Athens: Ohio University Press, 2011.

———. "Power, Knowledge, and Environmental History in the Middle East and North Africa." *IJMES* 42, no. 4 (2010): 657–59.

Dean, Mitchell. *Governmentality: Power and Rule in Modern Society*. London: Sage, 1999.

de Groot, A. H. "Kubrus." *EI²*.

Delilbaşı, Melek. "The Via Egnatia and Selanik (Thessalonica) in the 16th Century." In *The Via Egnatia under Ottoman Rule (1380–1699)*, edited by Elizabeth Zachariadou, 67–84. Rethymnon: Crete University Press, 1996.

Devignat, R. "Variétés de l'espèce *Pasteurella pestis*: nouvelle hypothèse." *Bulletin of the WHO* 4, no. 2 (1951): 247–63.

Di Cosmo, Nicola. "Black Sea Emporia and the Mongol Empire: A Reassessment of the Pax Mongolica." *JESHO* 53, nos. 1–2 (2010): 83–108.

Dincer, Aysu. "Disease in a Sunny Climate: Effects of the Plague on Family and Wealth in Cyprus in the 1360s." In *Economic and Biological Interactions in Pre-industrial Europe, from the 13th to the 18th Century*, 531–40. Florence: Firenze University Press, 2010.

Dols, Michael W. *The Black Death in the Middle East*. Princeton, NJ: Princeton University Press, 1977.

———. "The Comparative Communal Responses to the Black Death in Muslim and Christian Societies." *Viator* 5 (1974): 269–87.

———. "Geographical Origin of the Black Death." *Bulletin of the History of Medicine* 52, no. 1 (1978): 112–13.

———. "Plague in Early Islamic History." *Journal of the American Oriental Society* 94, no. 3 (1974): 371–83.

———. "The Second Plague Pandemic and Its Recurrences in the Middle East: 1347–1894." *JESHO* 22, no. 2 (1979): 162–89.

Drancourt, Michel, Linda Houhamdi, and Didier Raoult. "*Yersinia pestis* as a Telluric, Human Ectoparasite-Borne Organism." *The Lancet Infectious Diseases* 6, no. 4 (2006): 234–41.

Drancourt, Michel, Véronique Roux, La Vu Dang, Lam Tran-Hung, Dominique Castex, Viviane Chenal-Francisque, Hiroyuki Ogata et al. "Genotyping, Orientalis-like *Yersinia pestis*, and Plague Pandemics." *Emerging Infectious Diseases* 10, no. 9 (2004): 1585–92.

Drancourt, Michel, Michel Signoli, La Vu Dang, Bruno Bizot, Véronique Roux, Stéfan Tzortzis, and Didier Raoult. "*Yersinia pestis* Orientalis in Remains of Ancient Plague Patients." *Emerging Infectious Diseases* 13, no. 2 (2007): 332–33.

Dunn, Ross E. *The Adventures of Ibn Battuta, a Muslim Traveler of the Fourteenth Century*. Berkeley: University of California Press, 1986.

Dursteler, Eric R. "The Bailo in Constantinople: Crisis and Career in Venice's Early Modern Diplomatic Corps." *Mediterranean Historical Review* 16, no. 2 (2001): 1–30.

Easterday, W. Ryan, Kyrre L. Kausrud, Bastiaan Star, Lise Heier, Bradd J. Haley, Vladimir Ageyev, Rita R. Colwell, and Nils Chr Stenseth. "An Additional Step in the Transmission of *Yersinia pestis*?" *The ISME Journal* 6, no. 2 (2012): 231–36.

Ebrahimnejad, Hormoz. *Medicine, Public Health, and the Qājār State: Patterns of Medical Modernization in Nineteenth-Century Iran.* Leiden: Brill, 2004.

Eisen, Rebecca J., Lars Eisen, and Kenneth L. Gage. "Studies of Vector Competency and Efficiency of North American Fleas for *Yersinia pestis*: State of the Field and Future Research Needs." *Journal of Medical Entomology* 46, no. 4 (2009): 737–44.

Eisen, Rebecca J., and Kenneth L. Gage. "Transmission of Flea-Borne Zoonotic Agents." *Annual Review of Entomology* 57, no. 1 (2012): 61–82.

Eisen, Rebecca J., Jeannine M. Petersen, Charles L. Higgins, David Wong, Craig E. Levy, Paul S. Mead, Martin E. Schriefer et al. "Persistence of *Yersinia pestis* in Soil under Natural Conditions." *Emerging Infectious Diseases* 14, no. 6 (2008): 941–43.

Eldem, Edhem. "Death and Funerary Culture." In Ágoston and Masters, ed., *Encyclopedia of the Ottoman Empire*, 177–80.

―――. *Death in Istanbul: Death and Its Rituals in Ottoman-Islamic Culture.* Istanbul: Ottoman Bank Archives and Research Centre, 2005.

Ell, Stephen R. "Immunity as a Factor in the Epidemiology of Medieval Plague." *Review of Infectious Diseases* 6, no. 6 (1984): 866–79.

―――. "Some Evidence for Interhuman Transmission of Medieval Plague." *Review of Infectious Diseases* 1, no. 3 (1979): 563–66.

Ellerman, John Reeves, and Terence Charles Stuart Morrison-Scott. *Checklist of Palaearctic and Indian Mammals, 1758–1946.* London: printed by order of the Trustees of the British Museum, 1951.

Emecen, Feridun M. *İlk Osmanlılar ve Batı Anadolu Beylikler Dünyası.* Istanbul: Kitabevi, 2001.

Emiralioğlu, Pınar. *Geographical Knowledge and Imperial Culture in the Early Modern Ottoman Empire.* Burlington, VT: Ashgate, 2014.

Emmanuel, I. S. *Histoire des Israélites de Salonique.* Paris: Librairie Lipschutz, 1936.

Erder, Leila. "The Measurement of Preindustrial Population Changes: The Ottoman Empire from the 15th to the 17th Century." *Middle Eastern Studies* 11, no. 3 (1975): 284–301.

Ergin, Nina. "The Soundscape of Sixteenth-Century Istanbul Mosques: Architecture and Qur'an Recital." *Journal of the Society of Architectural Historians* 6, no. 2 (2008): 204–21.

Erickson, David L., Nicholas R. Waterfield, Viveka Vadyvaloo, Daniel Long, Elizabeth R. Fischer, Richard ffrench-Constant, and B. Joseph Hinnebusch. "Acute Oral Toxicity of *Yersinia pseudotuberculosis* to Fleas: Implications for the Evolution of Vector-Borne Transmission of Plague." *Cellular Microbiology* 9, no. 11 (2007): 2658–66.

Erler, Mehmet. *Osmanlı Devleti'nde Kuraklık, 1800–1880.* Istanbul: Libra Kitap, 2010.

Ertuğ, Nejdet. *Osmanlı Döneminde İstanbul Hammalları.* Istanbul: Timaş Yayınları, 2008.

Ertuğ, Zeynep Tarım. *XVI. Yüzyıl Osmanlı Devletinde Cülûs ve Cenaze Törenleri.* Ankara: Kültür Bakanlığı, 1999.

Ervynck, Anton. "Sedentism or Urbanism? On the Origin of the Commensal Black Rat (*Rattus rattus*)." In *Bones and the Man: Studies in Honour of Don Brothwell*, edited by Keith Dobney and Terry Patrick O'Connor, 95–109. Oxford: Oxbow, 2002.

Etker, Şeref. "Paul-Louis Simond ve Bakteriyolojihane-i Osmani'nin Çemberlitaş'ta açılışı (21 Eylül 1911)." *Osmanlı Bilimi Araştırmaları* 10, no. 2 (2009): 13–33.

Evered, Emine Ö., and Kyle T. Evered. "Sex and the Capital City: The Political Framing of Syphilis and Prostitution in Early Republican Ankara." *JHMAS* 68, no. 2 (2013): 266–99.

Evered, Kyle T., and Emine Ö. Evered. "Governing Population, Public Health, and Malaria in the Early Turkish Republic." *Journal of Historical Geography* 37, no. 4 (2011): 470–82.

———. "State, Peasant, Mosquito: The Biopolitics of Public Health Education and Malaria in Early Republican Turkey." *Political Geography* 31, no. 5 (2012): 311–23.

———. "Syphilis and Prostitution in the Socio-Medical Geographies of Turkey's Early Republican Provinces." *Health and Place* 18, no. 3 (2012): 528–35.

Fahmy, Khaled. "An Olfactory Tale of Two Cities: Cairo in the Nineteenth Century." In *Historians in Cairo: Essays in Honor of George Scanlon*, edited by J. Edwards, 155–87. Cairo: American University in Cairo Press, 2002.

Fahmy, Ziad. "Coming to Our Senses: Historicizing Sound and Noise in the Middle East." *History Compass* 11, no. 4 (2013): 305–15.

Faroqhi, Suraiya. *Animals and People in the Ottoman Empire*. Istanbul: Eren, 2010.

———. *Pilgrims and Sultans: The Hajj under the Ottomans, 1517–1683*. London: Tauris, 1994.

———. "Sixteenth-Century Periodic Markets in Various Anatolian *Sancaks*, İçel, Hamid, Karahisar-ı Sahib, Kütahya, Aydın, and Menteşe." *JESHO* 22, no. 1 (1979): 32–80.

———. "Textile Production in Rumeli and the Arab Provinces: Geographical Distribution and the Internal Trade (1560–1650)." *Osmanlı Araştırmaları* 1 (1980): 61–83.

———. *Towns and Townsmen of Ottoman Anatolia: Trade, Crafts and Food Production in an Urban Setting, 1520–1650*. Cambridge: Cambridge University Press, 1984.

Fazlıoğlu, İhsan. "İlk dönem Osmanlı ilim ve kültür hayatında İhvânu's-safâ ve Abdurrahmân Bistâmî." *Dîvân: İlmî Araştırmalar* 2 (1996): 229–40.

Fedorov, V. N. "Plague in Camels and Its Prevention in the USSR." *Bulletin of the WHO* 23, nos. 2–3 (1960): 275–81.

Finkel, Caroline. *Osman's Dream: the History of the Ottoman Empire, 1300–1923*. New York: Basic Books, 2006.

Fleet, Kate. *European and Islamic Trade in the Early Ottoman State: The Merchants of Genoa and Turkey.* Cambridge: Cambridge University Press, 1999.

———. "Ottoman Grain Exports from Western Anatolia at the End of the Fourteenth Century." *JESHO* 40, no. 3 (1997): 283–93.

———. "The Turkish Economy, 1071–1453." In *The Cambridge History of Turkey: Vol. 1. Byzantium to Turkey, 1071–1453*, edited by Kate Fleet, 227–65. Cambridge: Cambridge University Press, 2009.

Fleischer, Cornell H. *Bureaucrat and Intellectual in the Ottoman Empire: The Historian Mustafa Âli (1541–1600)*. Princeton, NJ: Princeton University Press, 1986.
———. "The Lawgiver as Messiah: The Making of the Imperial Image in the Reign of Süleymân." In *Soliman le magnifique et son temps*, edited by Gilles Veinstein, 159–77. Paris: La Documentation française, 1992.
———. "Preliminaries to the Study of the Ottoman Bureaucracy." *Journal of Turkish Studies* 10 (1986): 135–41.
Foucault, Michel. *The Birth of Biopolitics: Lectures at the Collège de France, 1978–79*. New York: Palgrave Macmillan, 2008.
———. *The History of Sexuality*. London: Penguin, 1998.
Frandsen, Karl-Erik. *The Last Plague in the Baltic Region, 1709–1713*. Copenhagen: Museum Tusculanum Press, 2010.
Gage, Kenneth L., and Michael Y. Kosoy. "Natural History of Plague: Perspectives from More Than a Century of Research." *Annual Review of Entomology* 50, no. 1 (2005): 505–28.
Galanté, Abraham. *Histoire des juifs de Turquie*. Istanbul: Isis, 1985.
———. *Histoire des juifs d'Istanbul*. Istanbul: Imprimerie Hüsnütabiat, 1941.
Gallagher, Nancy. *Egypt's Other Wars: Epidemics and the Politics of Public Health*. Syracuse, NY: Syracuse University Press, 1990.
———. *Medicine and Power in Tunisia, 1780–1900*. Cambridge: Cambridge University Press, 1983.
Geltner, Guy. "Healthscaping a Medieval City: Lucca's Curia Viarum and the Future of Public Health History." *Urban History* 40, no. 3 (2013): 395–415.
———. "Public Health and the Pre-Modern City: A Research Agenda." *History Compass* 10, no. 3 (2012): 231–45.
Gibbons, Herbert Adams. *The Foundation of the Ottoman Empire: A History of the Osmanlis up to the Death of Bayezid I, 1300–1403*. New York: Century, 1916.
Ginio, Eyal. "Neither Muslims nor Zimmis: The Gypsies (Roma) in the Ottoman State." *Romani Studies* 14, no. 2 (2004): 117–44.
Gökbilgin, Tayyip. "Edirne." *EI²*.
Golem, Bilal, and Kemal Özsan. "Türk Veba Suşlarında Biyoşimik Karakter Farkları." *Türk İjiyen ve Tecrübi Biyoloji Dergisi* 12, no. 1 (1952): 29–51.
Goodwin, Godfrey. "Gardens of the Dead in Ottoman Times." *Muqarnas* 5 (January 1, 1988): 61–69.
Gordon, Daniel. "Confrontations with the Plague in Eighteenth-Century France." In *Dreadful Visitations: Confronting Natural Catastrophe in the Age of Enlightenment*, edited by Alessa Johns, 3–29. New York: Routledge, 1999.
Goubert, Jean-Pierre, ed. *La Médicalisation de la société française, 1770–1830*. Waterloo, ON: Historical Reflections Press, 1982.
Green, Monica H. "Editor's Introduction to *Pandemic Disease in the Medieval World: Rethinking the Black Death*." *The Medieval Globe* 1 (2014): 9–26.
Griffin, J. P. "Venetian Treacle and the Foundation of Medicines Regulation." *British Journal of Clinical Pharmacology* 58, no. 3 (2004): 317–25.
Grosrichard, Alain. *The Sultan's Court: European Fantasies of the East*. London: Verso, 1998.
Günalan, Rıfat. "XVI. Yüzyılda Bab-ı Defteri Teşkilatı ve Maliye Ahkam Defterleri." PhD diss., Marmara University, Istanbul, 2005.

Haensch, Stephanie, Raffaella Bianucci, Michel Signoli, Minoarisoa Rajerison, Michael Schultz, Sacha Kacki, Marco Vermunt et al. "Distinct Clones of *Yersinia pestis* Caused the Black Death." *PLoS Pathogens* 6, no. 10 (2010): e1001134.

Halevi, Leor. *Muhammad's Grave: Death Rites and the Making of Islamic Society*. New York: Columbia University Press, 2007.

Harbeck, Michaela, Lisa Seifert, Stephanie Hänsch, David M. Wagner, Dawn Birdsell, Katy L. Parise, Ingrid Wiechmann et al. "*Yersinia pestis* DNA from Skeletal Remains from the 6th Century AD Reveals Insights into Justinianic Plague." *PLoS Pathogens* 9, no. 5 (2013): e1003349.

Hasluck, F. W. *Christianity and Islam under the Sultans*. 2 vols. Oxford: Clarendon Press, 1929.

Hatt, Robert T. *The Mammals of Iraq*. Ann Arbor: University of Michigan, 1959.

Hecker, J. F. C. *The Epidemics of the Middle Ages*. Translated by B. G. Babington. London: Trübner, 1859.

Heier, Lise, Geir O. Storvik, Stephen A. Davis, Hildegunn Viljugrein, Vladimir S. Ageyev, Evgeniya Klassovskaya, and Nils Chr. Stenseth. "Emergence, Spread, Persistence and Fade-out of Sylvatic Plague in Kazakhstan." *Proceedings of the Royal Society, Series B*: 278, no. 1720 (2011): 2915–23.

H-Environment Discussion Network. *Roundtable Reviews* 3, no. 8 (2013): 1–26. http://www.h-net.org/~environ/roundtables/env-roundtable-3-8.pdf.

Hess, Andrew C. "The Ottoman Conquest of Egypt (1517) and the Beginning of the Sixteenth-Century World War." *IJMES* 4, no. 1 (1973): 55–76.

Heyd, Uriel. "The Jewish Community of Istanbul in the Seventeenth Century." *Oriens* 6 (1953): 311–13.

Heyd, W. *Histoire du commerce du Levant au moyen-âge*. Amsterdam: Hakkert, 1983.

Heywood, Colin. "Filling the Black Hole: The Emergence of the Bithynian Atamanates." In *The Great Ottoman Turkish Civilisation*, edited by Kemal Çiçek, Ercüment Kuran, Nejat Göyünç, and İlber Ortaylı, 4 vols, 1: 107–15. Ankara: Yeni Türkiye Yayınevi, 2000.

———. "Sickness and Death in an Ill Climate: The Detention of the Blackham Galley at Izmir 1697–8." In *Ottoman Izmir: Studies in Honour of Alexander H. de Groot*, edited by Maurits H. van den Boogert, 53–74. Leiden: Nederlands Instituut voor het Nabije Oosten, 2007.

Hinnebusch, B. J. "The Evolution of Flea-Borne Transmission in *Yersinia pestis*." *Current Issues in Molecular Biology* 7 (2005): 197–212.

Houhamdi, Linda, Hubert Lepidi, Michel Drancourt, and Didier Raoult. "Experimental Model to Evaluate the Human Body Louse as a Vector of Plague." *Journal of Infectious Diseases* 194, no. 11 (2006): 1589–96.

Hrabak, Bogumil. "Kuga u balkanskim zemljama pod Turcima od 1450 do 1600 godine." *Istoriski glasnik* 1–2 (Belgrade, 1957): 19–37.

Hubálek, Zdenek. "An Annotated Checklist of Pathogenic Microorganisms Associated with Migratory Birds." *Journal of Wildlife Diseases* 40, no. 4 (2004): 639–59.

Hymes, Robert. "Epilogue: A Hypothesis on the East Asian Beginnings of the *Yersinia pestis* Polytomy." *The Medieval Globe* 1 (2014): 285–308.

İhsanoğlu, Ekmeleddin. "Endülüs Menşeli Bazı Bilim Adamlarının Osmanlı Bilimine Katkıları." *Belleten* 58 (1994): 565–605.

_____, ed. *Osmanlı Tıbbi Bilimler Literatürü Tarihi* [History of the literature of medical sciences during the Ottoman period]. 4 vols. Istanbul: IRCICA, 2008.

Imber, Colin. "The Legend of Osman Gazi." In *The Ottoman Emirate (1300–1389): Halcyon Days in Crete 1: A Symposium Held in Rethymnon 11–13 January 1991*, edited by Elizabeth A. Zachariadou, 67–73. Rethymnon: Crete University Press, 1993.

_____. *The Ottoman Empire, 1300–1650: The Structure of Power*. Houndmills, UK: Palgrave, 2002.

İnal, Onur. "Environmental History as an Emerging Field in Ottoman Studies: An Historiographical Overview." *Osmanlı Araştırmaları* 38 (2011): 1–25.

İnalcık, Halil. *An Economic and Social History of the Ottoman Empire. Vol. I: 1300–1600*. Cambridge: Cambridge University Press, 1994.

_____. "Bursa." *EI²*.

_____. "Bursa and the Commerce of the Levant." *JESHO* 3, no. 2 (1960): 131–47.

_____. "Edirne'nin Fethi (1361)." In *Edirne: Edirne'nin 600. Fetih Yıldönümü Armağan Kitabı*, 137–59. Ankara: TTK, 1993.

_____. "Istanbul." *EI²*.

_____. "Mehemmed II." *EI²*.

_____. "Ottoman Galata, 1453–1553." In *Essays in Ottoman History*, edited by Halil İnalcık, 275–376. Istanbul: Eren, 1998.

_____. "Ottoman Methods of Conquest." *Studia Islamica* 2 (January 1, 1954): 103–29.

_____. "Selim I." *EI²*.

_____. *The Ottoman Empire: The Classical Age 1300–1600*. Translated by Norman Itzkowitz and Colin Imber. London: Weidenfeld and Nicolson, 1973.

Jennings, Ronald C. *Christians and Muslims in Ottoman Cyprus and the Mediterranean World, 1571–1640*. New York: New York University Press, 1993.

_____. "Plague in Trabzon and Reactions to It According to Local Judicial Registers." In *Humanist and Scholar: Essays in Honor of Andreas Tietze*, edited by Heath W. Lowry and Donald Quataert, 27–36. Istanbul: Isis Press, 1993.

_____. "Urban Population in Anatolia in the Sixteenth Century: A Study of Kayseri, Karaman, Amasya, Trabzon, and Erzurum." *IJMES* 7, no. 1 (1976): 21–57.

Johns, Alessa, ed. *Dreadful Visitations: Confronting Natural Catastrophe in the Age of Enlightenment*. New York: Routledge, 1999.

Jones, Colin. "Montpellier Medical Students and the Medicalisation of 18th-Century France." In *Problems and Methods in the History of Medicine*, edited by R. Porter and A. Wear, 57–80. London: Croom, Helm, 1987.

_____. "Plague and Its Metaphors in Early Modern France." *Representations* 53 (1996): 97–127.

Jones, Colin, and Roy Porter, eds. *Reassessing Foucault: Power, Medicine, and the Body*. London: Routledge, 1994.

Kacki, Sacha, and Dominique Castex. "Réflexions sur la variété des modalités funéraires en temps d'épidémie. L'exemple de la peste noire en contextes urbain et rural." *Archéologie Médiévale* 42 (2012): 1–21.

Kafadar, Cemal. *Between Two Worlds: The Construction of the Ottoman State*. Berkeley: University of California Press, 1995.

Kafesçioğlu, Çiğdem. *Constantinopolis/Istanbul: Cultural Encounter, Imperial Vision, and the Construction of the Ottoman Capital.* University Park: Penn State University Press, 2009.

Karlsson, Gunnar. "Plague without Rats: The Case of Fifteenth-Century Iceland." *Journal of Medieval History* 22, no. 3 (1996): 263–84.

Kasaba, Reşat. *A Moveable Empire: Ottoman Nomads, Migrants, and Refugees.* Seattle: University of Washington Press, 2009.

Kastritsis, Dimitris J. *The Sons of Bayezid: Empire Building and Representation in the Ottoman Civil War of 1402–1413.* Leiden: Brill, 2007.

Keeling, M. J., and C. A. Gilligan. "Bubonic Plague: A Metapopulation Model of a Zoonosis." *Proceedings of the Royal Society of London, Series B* 267, no. 1458 (2000): 2219–30.

———. "Metapopulation Dynamics of Bubonic Plague." *Nature* 407, no. 6806 (2000): 903–6.

Kermeli, Eugenia, and Oktay Özel, eds. *The Ottoman Empire: Myths, Realities and "Black Holes": Contributions in Honour of Colin Imber.* Istanbul: Isis Press, 2006.

Kiel, Machiel. "Ottoman Building Activity along the Via Egnatia, the Cases of Pazargah, Kavalla and Ferecik." In *The Via Egnatia under Ottoman Rule (1380–1699)*, edited by Elizabeth A. Zachariadou, 145–58 (Rethymnon: Crete University Press, 1996).

Kılıç, Orhan. *Eskiçağdan Yakınçağa Genel Hatlarıyla Dünyada ve Osmanlı Devletinde Salgın Hastalıklar.* Elazığ: Fırat Üniversitesi Rektörlüğü, 2004.

Kinzelbach, Annemarie. "Infection, Contagion, and Public Health in Late Medieval and Early Modern German Imperial Towns." *JHMAS* 61, no. 3 (2006): 369–89.

Konkola, Kari. "More Than a Coincidence? The Arrival of Arsenic and the Disappearance of Plague in Early Modern Europe." *JHMAS* 47, no. 2 (1992): 186–209.

Konyalı, İbrahim Hakkı. *Konya tarihi.* Konya: Enes Kitap Sarayı, 1997.

Kōstēs, Kōstas. *Ston kairo tēs panōlēs: eikones apo tis koinōnies tēs Hellēnikēs chersonēsou, 14os-19os aiōnas.* Hērakleio: Panepistēmiakes Ekdoseis Krētēs, 1995.

Krekic, B. "Europe centrale et balkanique." *Annales: Économies, Sociétés, Civilisations* 18, no. 3 (1963): 594–95.

Kuhnke, LaVerne. *Lives at Risk: Public Health in Nineteenth-Century Egypt.* Berkeley: University of California Press, 1990.

Kumrular, Özlem. *The Ottoman World, Europe and the Mediterranean.* Istanbul: Isis Press, 2012.

Kunt, Metin I. "State and Sultan up to the Age of Süleyman: Frontier Principality to World Empire." In *Süleyman the Magnificent and His Age: The Ottoman Empire in the Early Modern World*, edited by Metin Kunt and Christine Woodhead, 3–29. London: Longman, 1995.

———. *The Sultan's Servants: The Transformation of Ottoman Provincial Government, 1550–1650.* New York: Columbia University Press, 1983.

Kuran, Abdullah. "A Spatial Study of Three Ottoman Capitals: Bursa, Edirne, and Istanbul." *Muqarnas* 13 (1996): 114–31.

Laayouni, Hafid, Marije Oosting, Pierre Luisi, Mihai Ioana, Santos Alonso, Isis Ricaño-Ponce, Gosia Trynka et al., "Convergent Evolution in European and

Rroma Populations Reveals Pressure Exerted by Plague on Toll-like Receptors," *PNAS* 111, no. 7 (2014): 2668–73.

Langer, Lawrence N. "The Black Death in Russia: Its Effects upon Urban Labor." *Russian History* 2, no. 1 (1975): 53–67.

Laqueur, Hans-Peter. *Hüve'l-Baki: İstanbul'da Osmanlı Mezarlıkları ve Mezar Taşları.* Translated by Selahattin Dilidüzgün. Istanbul: Tarih Vakfı Yurt Yayınları, 1997.

Lefort, Jacques. "Population and Landscape in Eastern Macedonia during the Middle Ages: The Example of Radolibos." In *Continuity and Change in Late Byzantine and Early Ottoman Society*, edited by Anthony Bryer and Heath W. Lowry, 11–21. Birmingham: The University of Birmingham, Centre for Byzantine Studies, 1986.

———. "Rural Economy and Social Relations in the Countryside." *Dumbarton Oaks Papers* 47 (1993): 101–13.

Le Roy Ladurie, Emmanuel. "Un concept: l'unification microbienne du monde (XIVe-XVIIe siècles)." *Revue Suisse d'Histoire* 23, no. 4 (1973): 627–96.

Li, Yanjun, Yujun Cui, Yolande Hauck, Mikhail E. Platonov, Erhei Dai, Yajun Song, Zhaobiao Guo et al. "Genotyping and Phylogenetic Analysis of *Yersinia pestis* by MLVA: Insights into the Worldwide Expansion of Central Asia Plague Foci." *PLoS ONE* 4, no. 6 (2009): e6000.

Lien-Teh, Wu. "The Original Home of Plague." In *Far Eastern Association of Tropical Medicine, Transactions of the Fifth Biennial Congress Held at Singapore, 1923*, edited by A. L. Hoops and J. W. Scharff, 286–304. London: John Bale/Danielsson, 1924.

Lindner, Rudi Paul. *Nomads and Ottomans in Medieval Anatolia*. Bloomington: Research for Inner Asian Studies, Indiana University, 1983.

Little, Lester K. "Plague Historians in Lab Coats." *Past and Present* 213, no. 1 (2011): 267–90.

Lopez, Pasquale. *Napoli e la peste 1464–1530: politica, istituzioni, problemi sanitari*. Naples: Jovene, 1989.

Low, Michael Christopher. "Empire and the Hajj: Pilgrims, Plagues, and Pan-Islam under British Surveillance, 1865–1908." *IJMES* 40, no. 2 (2008): 269–90.

Lowry, Heath W. *Fifteenth Century Ottoman Realities: Christian Peasant Life on the Aegean Island of Limnos*. Istanbul: Eren, 2002.

———. *Ottoman Bursa in Travel Accounts*. Bloomington: Indiana University Ottoman and Modern Turkish Studies Publications, 2003.

———. "Pushing the Stone Uphill: The Impact of Bubonic Plague on Ottoman Urban Society in the Fifteenth and Sixteenth Centuries." *Osmanlı Araştırmaları* 23 (2003): 93–132.

Lybyer, A. H. "The Ottoman Turks and the Routes of Oriental Trade." *The English Historical Review* 30, no. 120 (1915): 577–88.

Mackenzie, Mordach. "Extracts of Several Letters of Mordach Mackenzie, M.D. Concerning the Plague at Constantinople." *Philosophical Transactions (1683–1775)* 47 (1751–52): 384–95.

MacLean, Gerald M. *The Rise of Oriental Travel: English Visitors to the Ottoman Empire, 1580–1720*. New York: Palgrave Macmillan, 2004.

Magdalino, Paul. "The History of the Future and Its Uses: Prophecy, Policy and Propaganda." In *The Making of Byzantine History: Studies Dedicated to Donald*

M. Nicol on His Seventieth Birthday, edited by Roderick Beaton and Charlotte Rouché, 3–34. Aldershot, UK: Variorum, 1993.

———. "The Maritime Neighborhoods of Constantinople: Commercial and Residential Functions, Sixth to Twelfth Centuries." *Dumbarton Oaks Papers* 54 (2000): 209–26.

Malkinson, Mertyn, Caroline Banet, Yoram Weisman, Shimon Pokamunski, Roni King, Marie-Thérèse Drouet, and Vincent Deubel. "Introduction of West Nile Virus in the Middle East by Migrating White Storks." *Emerging Infectious Diseases* 8, no. 4 (2002): 392–97.

Malkinson, Mertyn, C. Banet, Y. Weisman, S. Pokamonski, R. King, and V. Deubel. "Intercontinental Transmission of West Nile Virus by Migrating White Storks." *Emerging Infectious Diseases* 7, no. 3(Suppl.) (2001): 540.

Manolova-Nikolova, Nadja I. *Čumavite vremena: (1700–1850)*. Sofia: IF-94, 2004.

Mantran, Robert. *Istanbul au siècle de Soliman le Magnifique*. Paris: Hachette, 1994.

Marien, Gisele. "The Black Death in Early Ottoman Territories: 1347–1550." MA thesis, Bilkent University, 2009.

Marshall, John. *John Locke, Toleration and Early Enlightenment Culture*. Cambridge: Cambridge University Press, 2006.

Marushiakova, Elena, and Vesselin Popov. *Gypsies in the Ottoman Empire: A Contribution to the History of the Balkans*. Hatfield: University of Hertfordshire Press, 2001.

Masters, Bruce. "Hajj." In Ágoston and Masters, ed., *Encyclopedia of the Ottoman Empire*, 246–48.

Matar, Nabil. *Turks, Moors, and Englishmen in the Age of Discovery*. New York: Columbia University Press, 1999.

Matschke, Klaus-Peter. "Research Problems Concerning the Transition to Tourkokratia: The Byzantinist Standpoint." In *The Ottomans and the Balkans: A Discussion of Historiography*, edited by Fikret Adanır and Suraiya Faroqhi, 79–113. Leiden: Brill, 2002.

May, Jacques M. "Map of the World Distribution of Plague." *Geographical Review* 42, no. 4 (1952): 628–30.

Mazak, Mehmet. *Orijinal Belge ve Fotoğraflar Işığında Osmanlı'da Sokak ve Çevre Temizliği*. Istanbul: İSTAÇ, 2001.

McCormick, Michael. "Rats, Communications, and Plague: Toward an Ecological History." *The Journal of Interdisciplinary History* 34, no. 1 (2003): 1–25.

McNeill, J. R. "The Eccentricity of the Middle East and North Africa's Environmental History." In *Water on Sand: Environmental Histories of the Middle East and North Africa*, edited by Alan Mikhail, 27–50. Oxford: Oxford University Press, 2012.

McNeill, William. *Plagues and Peoples*. Garden City, NY: Anchor Press, 1976.

Mehmed Yazıcıoğlu. *Muhammediye*. Edited by Amil Çelebioğlu. Istanbul: Milli Eğitim Bakanlığı, 1996.

Mengel, David C. "A Plague on Bohemia? Mapping the Black Death." *Past and Present* 211, no. 1 (2011): 3–34.

Meriç, Rıfkı Melûl. "Şeyyad Hamza'nın Kızına Ait Mezartaşı." *Taşpınar Mecmuası* 28 (1935): 60–63.

Meserve, Ruth I. "Striped Hyenas and 'Were-Hyenas' in Central Eurasia." In *Archivum Eurasiae Medii Aevi*, edited by T. T. Allsen, P. B. Golden, R. K. Kovalev, and A. P. Martinez, 199–220. Wiesbaden: Harrassowitz, 2012.

Mikhail, Alan. "An Irrigated Empire: The View from Ottoman Fayyum." *IJMES* 42, no. 4 (2010): 569–90.

———. *Nature and Empire in Ottoman Egypt: An Environmental History*. Cambridge: Cambridge University Press, 2011.

———. "The Nature of Plague in Late Eighteenth-Century Egypt." *Bulletin of the History of Medicine* 82, no. 2 (2008): 249–75.

———, ed. *Water on Sand: Environmental Histories of the Middle East and North Africa*. New York: Oxford University Press, 2012.

Miller, T. S. "The Plague in John VI Cantacuzenus and Thucydides." *Greek, Roman and Byzantine Studies* 17, no. 4 (1976): 385–95.

Miller, William. "The Historians Doukas and Phrantzes." *The Journal of Hellenic Studies* 46, no. 1 (1926): 63–71.

———. *Trebizond, the Last Greek Empire*. Amsterdam: Hakkert, 1968.

Millingen, Alexander van, Ramsay Traquair, Walter S. George, and Arthur E. Henderson. *Byzantine Churches in Constantinople: Their History and Architecture*. London: Macmillan, 1912.

Milwright, Marcus. "The Balsam of Matariyya: An Exploration of a Medieval Panacea." *Bulletin of the School of Oriental and African Studies* 66, no. 2 (2003): 193–209.

Misonne, Xavier. "Mammifères de la Turquie sud-orientale et du nord de la Syrie." *Mammalia* 21, no. 1 (1957): 53–68.

Mitler, Louis. "The Genoese in Galata: 1453–1682." *IJMES* 10, no. 1 (1979): 71–91.

Mordtmann, J. H. "Isfendiyār Oghlu." *EI²*.

Morelli, Giovanna, Yajun Song, Camila J Mazzoni, Mark Eppinger, Philippe Roumagnac, David M. Wagner, Mirjam Feldkamp et al. "*Yersinia pestis* Genome Sequencing Identifies Patterns of Global Phylogenetic Diversity." *Nature Genetics* 42, no. 12 (2010): 1140–43.

Morris, Christopher. "The Plague in Britain." *The Historical Journal* 14, no. 1 (1971): 205–15.

Necipoglu, Gülru. *Architecture, Ceremonial, and Power: The Topkapi Palace in the Fifteenth and Sixteenth Centuries*. New York: Architectural History Foundation, 1991.

———. "A Kânûn for the State, a Canon for the Arts: Conceptualizing the Classical Synthesis of Ottoman Art and Architecture." In *Soliman le magnifique et son temps*, edited by Gilles Veinstein, 195–216. Paris: La Documentation française, 1992.

———. "Süleyman the Magnificent and the Representation of Power in the Context of Ottoman-Hapsburg-Papal Rivalry." *The Art Bulletin* 71, no. 3 (1989): 401–27.

Necipoğlu, Nevra. *Byzantium between the Ottomans and the Latins: Politics and Society in the Late Empire*. Cambridge: Cambridge University Press, 2009.

———. "Circulation of People between the Byzantine and Ottoman Courts." In *The Byzantine Court: Source of Power and Culture; Papers from the Second International Sevgi Gönül Byzantine Studies Symposium, Istanbul 21–23 June 2010*, edited by Ayla Ödekan, Engin Akyürek, and Nevra Necipoğlu, 105–108. Istanbul: Koç University Press, 2013.

Nehama, Joseph. *Histoire des Israélites de Salonique*. Thessaloniki: Librairie Molho, 1935.

_____. *Salonique: La ville convoitée*. Tarascon, France: Cousins de Salonique, 2004.

Neuhäuser, Gabriele. *Die Muriden von Kleinasien*. Lucka (Bez. Leipzig): Druck von Reinhold Berger, 1936.

Neustadt [Ayalon], David. "The Plague and Its Effects upon the Mamluk Army." *Journal of the Royal Asiatic Society* 66 (1946): 67–73.

Nguyen-Hieu, Tung, Gérard Aboudharam, Michel Signoli, Catherine Rigeade, Michel Drancourt, and Didier Raoult. "Evidence of a Louse-Borne Outbreak Involving Typhus in Douai, 1710–1712 during the War of Spanish Succession." *PLoS ONE* 5, no. 10 (2010): e15405.

Norris, J. "East or West? The Geographic Origin of the Black Death." *Bulletin of the History of Medicine* 51, no. 1 (1977): 1–24.

_____. "Response." *Bulletin of the History of Medicine* 52, no. 1 (1978): 114–20.

Nutku, Özdemir. "Nahil," *TDVİA*.

Nutton, Vivian, ed. *Pestilential Complexities: Understanding Medieval Plague*. Medical History 27. London: Wellcome Trust Centre for the History of Medicine at UCL, 2008.

_____. "The Reception of Fracastoro's Theory of Contagion: The Seed That Fell among Thorns?" *Osiris* 6 (1990): 196–234.

_____. "The Seeds of Disease: An Explanation of Contagion and Infection from the Greeks to the Renaissance." *Medical History* 27, no. 1 (1983): 1–34.

Ocak, Ahmet Yaşar. *Kültür Tarihi Kaynağı Olarak Menâkıbnâmeler: Metodolojik Bir Yaklaşım*. Ankara: TTK Basımevi, 1992.

Oral, Zeki M. "Durağan ve Bafra'da İki Türbe." *Belleten* 20, no. 79 (1956): 385–410.

Orhonlu, Cengiz. *Osmanlı İmparatorluğu'nda Aşiretlerin İskânı*. Istanbul: Eren, 1987.

Özaydın, Zuhal, and H. Hüsrev Hâtemî. *Türk Tıp Tarihi Araştırmalarının Son 30 Yılda (1970–2002) Yönelişleri ve Bir Bibliografya Denemesi*. Istanbul: Cerrahpaşa Tıp Fakültesi Vakfı, 2002.

Öztürk, Said, ed. *Afetlerin Gölgesinde İstanbul: Tarih Boyunca İstanbul ve Çevresini Etkileyen Afetler*. Istanbul: İstanbul Büyükşehir Belediyesi, 2009.

Panagiotakopulu, Eva. "Pharaonic Egypt and the Origins of Plague." *Journal of Biogeography* 31, no. 2 (2004): 269–75.

Panzac, Daniel. "Alexandrie: peste et croissance urbaine (XVIIe-XIXe siècles)." *Revue de l'Occident musulman et de la Méditerranée* 46, no. 1 (1987): 81–90.

_____. *La peste dans l'empire ottoman, 1700–1850*. Leuven: Éditions Peeters, 1985.

_____. "La peste à Smyrne au XVIIIe siècle." *Annales: Économies, Sociétés, Civilisations* 28, no. 4 (1973): 1071–93.

_____. "La population de l'empire ottoman et de ses marges du XVe au XIXe siècle: Bibliographie (1941–1980) et bilan provisoire." *Revue de l'Occident musulman et de la Méditerranée* 31, no. 1 (1981): 119–37.

_____. "Mourir à Alep au XVIIIe siècle." *Revue du monde musulman et de la Méditerranée* 62, no. 1 (1991): 111–22.

_____. *Osmanlı İmparatorluğu'nda Veba: 1700–1850*. Translated by Serap Yılmaz. Istanbul: Türkiye Ekonomik Toplumsal Tarih Vakfı, 1997.

———. "Plague." In Ágoston and Masters, ed., *Encyclopedia of the Ottoman Empire*, 462–63.

———. "Population." In Ágoston and Masters, ed., *Encyclopedia of the Ottoman Empire*, 467–69.

———. *Quarantaines et lazarets: l'Europe et la peste d'Orient, XVIIe – XXe siècles.* Aix-en-Provence: Édisud, 1986.

———. "Wabā'." *EI²*.

Parkhill, J., B. W. Wren, N. R. Thomson, R. W. Titball, M. T. G. Holden, M. B. Prentice, M. Sebaihia et al. "Genome Sequence of *Yersinia pestis*, the Causative Agent of Plague." *Nature* 413, no. 6855 (2001): 523–27.

Parmenter, R. R., E. P. Yadav, C. A. Parmenter, P. Ettestad, and K. L. Gage. "Incidence of Plague Associated with Increased Winter-Spring Precipitation in New Mexico." *The American Journal of Tropical Medicine and Hygiene* 61, no. 5 (1999): 814–21.

Pawlowski, David R., Daniel J. Metzger, Amy Raslawsky, Amy Howlett, Gretchen Siebert, Richard J. Karalus, Stephanie Garrett, and Chris A. Whitehouse. "Entry of *Yersinia pestis* into the Viable but Nonculturable State in a Low-Temperature Tap Water Microcosm." *PLoS ONE* 6, no. 3 (2011): e17585.

Perho, Irmeli. *The Prophet's Medicine: A Creation of the Muslim Traditionalist Scholars.* Helsinki: Finnish Oriental Society, 1995.

Piarroux, Renaud, Aaron Aruna Abedi, Jean-Christophe Shako, Benoit Kebela, Stomy Karhemere, Georges Diatta, Bernard Davoust, Didier Raoult, and Michel Drancourt. "Plague Epidemics and Lice, Democratic Republic of the Congo." *Emerging Infectious Diseases* 19, no. 3 (2013): 505–6.

Pitcher, Donald Edgar. *Osmanlı İmparatorluğu'nun Tarihsel Coğrafyası.* Translated by Bahar Tırnakcı. Istanbul: Yapı Kredi Yayınları, 2001.

de Planhol, Xavier. "Le boeuf porteur dans le Proche-Orient et l'Afrique du Nord." *JESHO* 12, no. 3 (1969): 298–321.

Pobst, Phyllis. "Should We Teach That the Cause of the Black Death Was Bubonic Plague?" *History Compass* 11, no. 10 (2013): 808–20.

Porter, Roy. *The Greatest Benefit to Mankind: A Medical History of Humanity from Antiquity to the Present.* London: HarperCollins, 1997.

Pratt, Mary Louise. *Imperial Eyes: Travel Writing and Transculturation.* London: Routledge, 1992.

Prinzing, Friedrich. *Epidemics Resulting from Wars.* Oxford: Clarendon Press, 1916.

Rahimi, Babak. "Nahils, Circumcision Rituals and the Theatre State." In *Ottoman Tulips, Ottoman Coffee: Leisure and Lifestyle in the Eighteenth Century*, edited by Dana Sajdi, 90–116. London: Tauris Academic Studies, 2007.

Raoult, Didier, Olivier Dutour, Linda Houhamdi, Rimantas Jankauskas, Pierre-Edouard Fournier, Yann Ardagna, Michel Drancourt et al. "Evidence for Louse-Transmitted Diseases in Soldiers of Napoleon's Grand Army in Vilnius." *Journal of Infectious Diseases* 193, no. 1 (2006): 112–20.

Raoult, Didier, Nadjet Mouffok, Idir Bitam, Renaud Piarroux, and Michel Drancourt. "Plague: History and Contemporary Analysis." *Journal of Infection* 66, no. 1 (2013): 18–26.

Redhouse, Sir James W. *A Turkish and English Lexicon.* Beirut: Librarie du Liban, 1880.

Robarts, Andrew. "A Plague on Both Houses? Population Movements and the Spread of Disease across the Ottoman-Russian Black Sea Frontier, 1768–1830s." PhD diss., Georgetown University, 2010.

Rosen, William. *Justinian's Flea: Plague, Empire, and the Birth of Europe.* New York: Viking, 2007.

Royer, Katherine. "The Blind Men and the Elephant: Imperial Medicine, Medieval Historians, and the Role of Rats in the Historiography of Plague." In *Medicine and Colonialism: Historical Perspectives in India and South Africa*, edited by Poonam Bala, 99–110. London: Pickering and Chatto, 2014.

Rozen, Minna. *A History of the Jewish Community in Istanbul: The Formative Years, 1453–1566.* Leiden: Brill, 2002.

Ruffino, Lise, and Eric Vidal. "Early Colonization of Mediterranean Islands by *Rattus rattus*: A Review of Zooarcheological Data." *Biological Invasions* 12, no. 8 (2010): 2389–94.

Saeed, Abdulaziz A. Bin, Nasser A. Al-Hamdan, and Robert E. Fontaine. "Plague from Eating Raw Camel Liver." *Emerging Infectious Diseases* 11, no. 9 (2005): 1456–57.

Şahin, Kaya. "Constantinople and the End Time: The Ottoman Conquest as a Portent of the Last Hour." *Journal of Early Modern History* 14, no. 4 (2010): 317–54.

———. *Empire and Power in the Reign of Süleyman: Narrating the Sixteenth-Century Ottoman World.* Cambridge: Cambridge University Press, 2013.

Sajdi, Dana. "Decline, Its Discontents and Ottoman Cultural History: By Way of Introduction." In *Ottoman Tulips, Ottoman Coffee: Leisure and Lifestyle in the Eighteenth Century*, edited by Dana Sajdi, 1–40. London: Tauris Academic Studies, 2007.

Sakaoğlu, Necdet. "Osmanlı'da Salgınlar." *Toplumsal Tarih* 22 (1995): 23–25.

Sallares, Robert. "Ecology, Evolution, and Epidemiology of Plague." In *Plague and the End of Antiquity: The Pandemic of 541–750*, edited by Lester K. Little, 231–89. Cambridge: Cambridge University Press, 2007.

Sarı, Nil. "Osmanlı Hekimliğinde Tıp Ahlâkı." In *Osmanlılarda Sağlık*, edited by Coşkun Yılmaz and Necdet Yılmaz, 207–35. Istanbul: Biofarma, 2006.

——— (Akdeniz). *Osmanlılarda Hekimlik ve Hekimlik Ahlakı.* Istanbul, 1977.

Sarıyıldız, Gülden. *Hicaz Karantina Teşkilatı (1865–1914).* Ankara: TTK, 1996.

———. "Karantina Meclisi'nin Kuruluşu ve Faaliyetleri." *Belleten* 58, no. 222 (1994): 329–76.

———. "Karantina Teşkilatının Kuruluşu ve Faaliyetleri (1838–1876)." MA thesis, Istanbul University, 1986.

Savinetsky, A. B., and O. A. Krylovich. "On the History of the Spread of the Black Rat (*Rattus rattus* L., 1758) in Northwestern Russia." *Biology Bulletin* 38, no. 2 (2011): 203–7.

Schamiloglu, Uli. "Preliminary Remarks on the Role of Disease in the History of the Golden Horde." *Central Asian Survey* 12, no. 4 (1993): 447–57.

———. "The Rise of the Ottoman Empire: The Black Death in Medieval Anatolia and Its Impact on Turkish Civilization." In *Views from the Edge: Essays in Honor of Richard W. Bulliet*, edited by Neguin Yavari, Lawrence G. Potter, and Jean-Marc Ran Oppenheim, 255–79. New York: Columbia University Press, 2004.

Schmidt, Jan. *Pure Water for Thirsty Muslims: A Study of Mustafā Âli of Gallipoli's Künhü'l-ahbar*. Leiden: Het Oosters Instituut, 1991.

Schreiber, Werner. *Infectio: Infectious Diseases in the History of Medicine*. Basel: Roche, 1987.

Scott, James C. *Seeing Like a State: How Certain Schemes to Improve the Human Condition Have Failed*. New Haven, CT: Yale University Press, 1998.

Scott, Susan, and Christopher J. Duncan. *Biology of Plagues: Evidence from Historical Populations*. Cambridge: Cambridge University Press, 2001.

_____. *Return of the Black Death: The World's Greatest Serial Killer*. Chichester, UK: John Wiley, 2004.

Sebbane, Florent, Clayton O. Jarrett, Donald Gardner, Daniel Long, and B. Joseph Hinnebusch. "Role of the *Yersinia pestis* Plasminogen Activator in the Incidence of Distinct Septicemic and Bubonic Forms of Flea-Borne Plague." *PNAS* 103, no. 14 (2006): 5526–30.

Şehsuvaroğlu, Bedi. "Karantina Tarihi." PhD diss., Istanbul University, 1956.

Seng, Yvonne J. "The Üsküdar Estates (Tereke) as Records of Everyday Life in an Ottoman Town, 1521–1524." PhD diss., University of Chicago, 1991.

Shakow, Aaron. "Marks of Contagion: The Plague, the Bourse, the Word and the Law in the Early Modern Mediterranean, 1720–1762." PhD diss., Harvard University, 2009.

_____. "'Oriental Plague' in the Middle Eastern Landscape: A Cautionary Tale." *IJMES* 42, no. 4 (2010): 660–62.

Shay, M. L. *The Ottoman Empire from 1720 to 1734 as Revealed in Despatches of the Venetian Baili*. Urbana: University of Illinois Press, 1944.

Shefer-Mossensohn, Miri. "Communicable Disease in Ottoman Palestine: Local Thoughts and Actions." *Korot* 21 (2012): 19–49.

_____. "Health as a Social Agent in Ottoman Patronage and Authority." *New Perspectives on Turkey* 37 (2007): 147–75.

_____. *Ottoman Medicine: Healing and Medical Institutions, 1500–1700*. Albany: State Univeristy of New York Press, 2009.

_____. "A Tale of Two Discourses: The Historiography of Ottoman-Muslim Medicine." *Social History of Medicine* 21, no. 1 (2008): 1–12.

Shrewsbury, John Findlay Drew. *A History of Bubonic Plague in the British Isles*. Cambridge: Cambridge University Press, 1970.

Simond, Paul-Louis. "La propagation de la peste." *Annales de l'Institut Pasteur* 12, no. 10 (1898): 625–87.

Simond, M., M. L. Godley, and P. D. Mouriquand. "Paul-Louis Simond and His Discovery of Plague Transmission by Rat Fleas: A Centenary." *Journal of the Royal Society of Medicine* 91, no. 2 (1998): 101–4.

Singer, Amy. "Ottoman Palestine (1516–1800): Health, Disease, and Historical Sources." In *Health and Disease in the Holy Land: Studies in the History and Sociology of Medicine from Ancient Times to the Present*, edited by Manfred J. Waserman and Samuel S Kottek, 189–206. Lewiston, NY: Edwin Mellen Press, 1996.

Skinner, Bruce. "Plague and the Geographical Distribution of Rats." *The British Medical Journal* 1, no. 2314 (May 6, 1905): 994–95.

Slack, Paul. *The Impact of Plague in Tudor and Stuart England*. London: Routledge and Kegan Paul, 1985.

———. Introduction to *Epidemics and Ideas: Essays on the Historical Perception of Pestilence*, edited by Paul Slack and Terence Ranger, 1–20. Cambridge: Cambridge University Press, 1992.

———. *Plague: A Very Short Introduction*. New York: Oxford University Press, 2012.

Solak, İbrabim. "Anadolu'da Nüfus Hareketleri ve Osmanlı Devleti'nin İskan Politikası." *Türk Dünyası Araştırmaları* 127 (2000): 157–92.

Soliman, S., A. J. Main, A. S. Marzouk, and A. A. Montasser. "Seasonal Studies on Commensal Rats and Their Ectoparasites in a Rural Area of Egypt: The Relationship of Ectoparasites to the Species, Locality, and Relative Abundance of the Host." *Journal of Parasitology* 87, no. 3 (2001): 545–53.

Soucek, Svat. "Rodos." *EI²*.

Stathakopoulos, Dionysios C. "Crime and Punishment: The Plague in the Byzantine Empire, 541–749." In *Plague and the End of Antiquity: The Pandemic of 541–750*, edited by Lester K. Little, 99–118. Cambridge: Cambridge University Press, 2007.

———. *Famine and Pestilence in the Late Roman and Early Byzantine Empire: A Systematic Survey of Subsistence Crises and Epidemics*. Aldershot, UK: Ashgate, 2004.

Stearns, Justin K. *Infectious Ideas: Contagion in Premodern Islamic and Christian Thought in the Western Mediterranean*. Baltimore: Johns Hopkins University Press, 2011.

———. "New Directions in the Study of Religious Responses to the Black Death." *History Compass* 7, no. 5 (2009): 1363–75.

Stenseth, Nils Chr, Bakyt B. Atshabar, Mike Begon, Steven R. Belmain, Eric Bertherat, Elisabeth Carniel, Kenneth L. Gage, Herwig Leirs, and Lila Rahalison. "Plague: Past, Present, and Future." *PLoS Medicine* 5, no. 1 (2008): e3.

Sticker, Georg. *Abhandlungen aus der Seuchengeschichte und Seuchenlehre*. 2 vols. Giessen: Töpelmann, 1908–12.

Stoianovich, Traian. "Pour un modèle du commerce du Levant: economie concurrentielle et economie de bazar 1500–1800." In *Istanbul à la jonction des cultures balkaniques, méditerranéennes, slaves et orientales, aux XVIe-XIXe siècles*. Bucharest: Association internationale d'études du Sud-Est européen, 1977.

Sublet, Jacqueline. "La peste prise aux rêts de la jurisprudence: le traité d'Ibn Ḥaǧar al-ʿAsqalānī sur la peste." *Studia Islamica*, no. 33 (1971): 141–49.

"Su," *Dünden Bugüne İstanbul Ansiklopedisi*, 7:47–49.

Sussman, George D. "Was the Black Death in India and China?" *Bulletin of the History of Medicine* 85, no. 3 (2011): 319–55.

Tabak, Faruk. *The Waning of the Mediterranean, 1550–1870: A Geohistorical Approach*. Baltimore: Johns Hopkins University Press, 2008.

Tavukçu, Orhan. "Şeyyâd Hamza'nın Bilinmeyen Bir Şiiri Münasebetiyle." *International Journal of Central Asian Studies* 10, no. 1 (2005): 181–95.

Tenenti, Alberto. *Piracy and the Decline of Venice, 1580–1615*. Translated by Janet and Brian Pullan. Berkeley: University of California Press, 1967.

Theilmann, John, and Frances Cate. "A Plague of Plagues: The Problem of Plague Diagnosis in Medieval England." *Journal of Interdisciplinary History* 37, no. 3 (2007): 371–93.

Thorndike, Lynn. "The Blight of Pestilence on Early Modern Civilization." *The American Historical Review* 32, no. 3 (1927): 455–74.

Tran, Thi-Nguyen-Ny, Cyrille Le Forestier, Michel Drancourt, Didier Raoult, and Gérard Aboudharam. "Brief Communication: Co-Detection of *Bartonella quintana* and *Yersinia pestis* in an 11th–15th Burial Site in Bondy, France." *American Journal of Physical Anthropology* 145, no. 3 (2011): 489–94.

Traub, Robert. "The Fleas of Egypt: Two New Fleas of the Genus *Nosopsyllus* Jordan, 1933." *Proceedings of the Entomological Society of Washington* 65, no. 2 (1963): 81–97.

Traweger, Doris, Rita Travnitzky, Cornelia Moser, Christian Walzer, and Guenther Bernatzky. "Habitat Preferences and Distribution of the Brown Rat (*Rattus norvegicus* Berk.) in the City of Salzburg (Austria): Implications for an Urban Rat Management." *Journal of Pest Science* 79, no. 3 (2006): 113–25.

Tsiamis, Costas, Effie Poulakou-Rebelakou, and Spyros Marketos. "Earthquakes and Plague during Byzantine Times: Can Lessons from the Past Improve Epidemic Preparedness?" *Acta Medico-Historica Adriatica* 11, no. 1 (2013): 55–64.

Tsiamis, Costas, Effie Poulakou-Rebelakou, Athanassios Tsakris, and Eleni Petridou. "Epidemic Waves of the Black Death in the Byzantine Empire (1347–1453 AD)." *Le Infezioni in Medicina: Rivista Periodica Di Eziologia, Epidemiologia, Diagnostica, Clinica E Terapia Delle Patologie Infettive* 19, no. 3 (2011): 194–201.

Turan, Ebru. "The Marriage of İbrahim Pasha (ca. 1495–1536)." *Turcica* 41 (2009): 3–36.

Turna, Nalan. "İstanbul'un Veba ile İmtihanı: 1811–1812 Veba Salgını Bağlamında Toplum ve Ekonomi." *Studies of the Ottoman Domain* 1, no. 1 (2011): 23–58.

Twigg, Graham. *The Black Death: A Biological Reappraisal*. London: Batsford Academic and Educational, 1984.

Üçel-Aybet, Gülgün. *Avrupalı Seyyahların Gözünden: Osmanlı Dünyası ve İnsanları 1530–1699*. Istanbul: İletişim, 2003.

Uluçay, Çağatay. "Yavuz Sultan Selim Nasıl Padişah Oldu?" *Tarih Dergisi* 7, no. 10 (1954): 117–42.

Ünver, Süheyl. "Buğdan Voyvodası Oğlunun Vebadan Ölümü." *Türk Tıp Tarihi Arkivi* 12 (1939): 147–50.

———. "İstanbul Halkının Ölüm Karşısındaki Duyguları." *Yeni Türk* 68 (1938): 312–21.

———. "Les épidemies de choléra dans les terres balkaniques aux XVIIIe et XIXe siècles." *Études Balkaniques (Sofia)* 4 (1973): 89–97.

———. "Mezar Taşlarında Veba ve Tauna Ait Kayıtlar." *Dirim* 11–12 (1965): 268–72.

———. "Romanya Tıb Tarihine Ait Bir Vesika." *Türk Tıp Tarihi Arkivi* 9 (1938): 25–27.

———. "Taun Nedir? Veba Nedir?" *Dirim* 3–4 (1978): 363–66.

———. "Türkiyede Veba (Taun) Tarihçesi Üzerine." *Tedavi Kliniği ve Laboratuvarı Mecmuası* 5 (1935): 70–88.

———. "Türk Tıb Tarihinde Veba Hastalığına Karşı Kına Tatbiki." *Türk Tıp Tarihi Arkivi* 7 (1938): 82–85.

Uzunçarşılı, İsmail Hakkı. *Osmanlı Devletinin Saray Teşkilâtı*. Ankara: TTK, 1988.

van den Bossche, Willem, Peter Berthold, Michael Kaatz, Eugeniusz Nowak, and Ulrich Querner. *Eastern European White Stork Populations: Migration Studies and Elaboration of Conservation Measures.* Bonn: Bundesamt für Naturschutz (BfN)/German Federal Agency for Nature Conservation, 2002.

van Ess, Josef *Der Fehltritt des Gelehrten: Die "Pest von Emmaus" und ihre theologischen Nachspiele.* Heidelberg: Universitätsverlag C. Winter, 2001.

Varlık, Nükhet. "Attitudes toward Plague Epidemics in Ottoman Society of the Nineteenth Century." *Proceedings of the 37th International Congress on the History of Medicine,* edited by Chester R. Burns et al., 359–64. Galveston: University of Texas Medical Branch, Institute for the Medical Humanities, 2002.

———. "Conquest, Urbanization, and Plague Networks in the Ottoman Empire, 1453–1600." In *The Ottoman World,* edited by Christine Woodhead, 251–63. London: Routledge, 2012.

———. "Disease and Empire: A History of Plague Epidemics in the Early Modern Ottoman Empire (1453–1600)." PhD diss., University of Chicago, 2008.

———. "From '*Bête Noire*' to '*le Mal de* Constantinople': Plagues, Medicine, and the Early Modern Ottoman State." *Journal of World History* 24, no. 4 (2013): 741–70.

———. "New Science and Old Sources: Why the Ottoman Experience of Plague Matters." *The Medieval Globe* 1 (2014): 193–227.

———. "Plague, Conflict, and Negotiation: The Jewish Broadcloth Weavers of Salonica and the Ottoman Central Administration in the Late Sixteenth Century." *Jewish History* 28, nos. 3–4 (2014): 261–88.

———. "The Study of a Plague Treatise: Tevfikatü'l-Hamidiyye fi Def'i'l-Emrazi'l-Veba'iyye." MA thesis, Boğaziçi University, 2000.

———. "Tâun." In *TDVİA.*

Vatin, Nicolas. "La conquête de Rhodes." In *Soliman le magnifique et son temps,* edited by Gilles Veinstein, 435–54. Paris: La Documentation française, 1992.

Vatin, Nicolas, and Stefanos Yerasimos. *Les cimetières dans la ville: statut, choix et organisation des lieux d'inhumation dans Istanbul intra muros.* Istanbul: Institut français d'études anatoliennes Georges Dumézil, 2001.

Veinstein, Gilles. "Süleyman." *EI².*

Vernin, Colette Establet. "Daniel Panzac (1933–2012)." *Revue des mondes musulmans et de la Méditerranée,* no. 134 (2013): 307–14.

Villard, Pierre. "Constantinople et la peste (1467). (Critoboulos, V, 17)." In *Histoire et société/La mémoire, l'écriture et l'histoire,* edited by Georges Duby, 143–50. Aix-en-Provence: Université de Provence, 1992.

von Hammer-Purgstall, Joseph. *Histoire de l'empire ottoman depuis son origine jusqu'à nos jours.* Paris: Bellizard, Barthès, Dufour, et Lowell, 1835–43.

Vogler, Amy J., Fabien Chan, David M. Wagner, Philippe Roumagnac, Judy Lee, Roxanne Nera, Mark Eppinger et al. "Phylogeography and Molecular Epidemiology of *Yersinia pestis* in Madagascar." *PLoS Neglected Tropical Diseases* 5, no. 9 (2011): e1319.

Watts, Sheldon J. *Epidemics and History: Disease, Power, and Imperialism.* New Haven, CT: Yale University Press, 1997.

Webb, Nigel, and Caroline Webb. *The Earl and His Butler in Constantinople: The Secret Diary of an English Servant among the Ottomans.* London: I. B. Tauris, 2009.

White, Hayden. "The Value of Narrativity in the Representation of Reality." *Critical Inquiry* 7, no. 1 (1980): 5–27.

White, Sam. *The Climate of Rebellion in the Early Modern Ottoman Empire*. Cambridge: Cambridge University Press, 2011.

———. "The Little Ice Age Crisis of the Ottoman Empire: A Conjuncture in Middle East Environmental History." In *Water on Sand*, ed. Alan Mikhail, 71–90.

———. "Rethinking Disease in Ottoman History." *IJMES* 42, no. 4 (2010): 549–67.

Wing, Patrick. "The Jalayirids and Dynastic State Formation in the Mongol Ilkhanate." PhD diss., University of Chicago, 2007.

———. "'Rich in Goods and Abounding in Wealth:' The Ilkhanid and post-Ilkhanid Ruling Elite and the Politics of Commercial Life at Tabriz, 1250–1400." In *Politics, Patronage and the Transmission of Knowledge in 13th–15th Century Tabriz*, edited by Judith Pfeiffer, 301–20. Leiden: Brill, 2014.

World Health Organization (WHO). *Plague Manual: Epidemiology, Distribution, Surveillance and Control*. WHO/CDS/CSR/EDC/99.2. Geneva: WHO, 1999.

Wunder, Amanda. "Western Travelers, Eastern Atiquities, and the Image of the Turk in Early Modern Europe." *Journal of Early Modern History* 7, nos. 1–2 (2003): 89–119.

Xoplaki, Eleni, Panagiotis Maheras, and Juerg Luterbacher. "Variability of Climate in Meridional Balkans during the Periods 1675–1715 and 1780–1830 and Its Impact on Human Life." *Climatic Change* 48, no. 4 (2001): 581–615.

Yerasimos, Stefanos. "Alberti, Tommaso." *Dünden Bugüne İstanbul Ansiklopedisi*, 1:181.

———. *Kostantiniye ve Ayasofya Efsaneleri*. Translated by Şirin Tekeli. Istanbul: İletişim, 1993.

———. "La Communauté juive d'Istanbul à la fin du XVIe siècle." *Turcica* 27 (1995): 327–28.

———. *La fondation de Constantinople et de Sainte-Sophie dans les traditions turques: légendes d'empire*. Istanbul: Institut français d'études anatoliennes; Librairie d'Amérique et d'Orient J. Maisonneuve, 1990.

———. *Les voyageurs dans l'empire ottoman, XIVe–XVIe siècles: bibliographie, itinéraires et inventaire des lieux habités*. Ankara: TTK, 1991.

Yersin, Alexandre. "La peste bubonique à Hong-Kong." *Annales de l'Institut Pasteur* 8 (1894): 662–67.

Yi, Eunjeong. *Guild Dynamics in Seventeenth-Century Istanbul: Fluidity and Leverage*. Leiden: Brill, 2004.

Yiğit, N., and E. Çolak. "Contribution to the Geographic Distribution of Rodent Species and Ecological Analyses of Their Habitats in Asiatic Turkey." *Turkish Journal of Biology* 22 (1998): 435–46.

Yiğit, N., E. Çolak, M. Sözen, and Ş. Özkurt. "A Study on the Geographic Distribution along with Habitat Aspects of Rodent Species in Turkey." *Bonner Zoologische Beiträge* 50, no. 4 (2003): 355–68.

Yıldırım, Nuran. *A History of Healthcare in Istanbul: Health Organizations, Epidemics, Infections and Disease Control, Preventive Health Institutions, Hospitals, Medical Education*. Istanbul: Istanbul University, 2010.

———. "Salgınlar." *Dünden Bugüne İstanbul Ansiklopedisi*, 6:423–25.

Yıldız, Netice. "Ottoman Decorative Arts in Cyprus." In *Proceedings of the 11th International Congress of Turkish Art, Utrecht, the Netherlands, August 23–28, 1999*, edited by Machiel Kiel, Nico Landman, and Hans Theunissen, 1–25. Utrecht: Universiteit Utrect, 2001.

Yılmaz, Coşkun, and Necdet Yılmaz, eds. *Osmanlılarda Sağlık*. 2 vols. Istanbul: Biofarma, 2006.

Yücel, Yaşar. *Çoban-oğulları Candar-oğulları Beylikleri: XIII–XV. Yüzyıllar Kuzey-Batı Anadolu Tarihi*. Ankara: TTK, 1980.

Yüksel, Emrullah. "Birgivî." *TDVİA*.

Zachariadou, Elizabeth A. "The Emirate of Karasi and That of the Ottomans: Two Rival States." In *The Ottoman Emirate (1300–1389): Halcyon Days in Crete 1: A Symposium Held in Rethymnon 11–13 January 1991*, edited by Elizabeth A. Zachariadou, 225–36. Rethymnon: Crete University Press, 1993.

———. "Manuel II Palaeologos on the Strife between Bāyezīd I and Ḳāḍī Burhān Al-Dīn Aḥmad." *Bulletin of the School of Oriental and African Studies* 43, no. 3 (1980): 471–81.

———. "Notes sur la population de l'Asie mineure turque au XIVe siècle." *Byzantinische Forschungen: Internationale Zeitschrift für Byzantinistik* 12 (1987): 221–31.

———, ed. *The Via Egnatia under Ottoman Rule (1380–1699)*. Rethymnon: Crete University Press, 1996.

Zarinebaf, Fariba. *Crime and Punishment in Istanbul: 1700–1800*. Berkeley: University of California Press, 2010.

Ze'evi, Dror. *Producing Desire: Changing Sexual Discourse in the Ottoman Middle East, 1500–1900*. Berkeley: University of California Press, 2006.

Zinsser, Hans. *Rats, Lice, and History*. Boston: Little, Brown, 1935.

Zlatar, Zdenko. *Dubrovnik's Merchants and Capital in the Ottoman Empire (1520–1620): A Quantitative Study*. Istanbul: Isis Press, 2011.

Index